POWER YOGA

the total strength and flexibility workout

BERYL BENDER BIRCH

PHOTOGRAPHS BY NICHOLAS DeSCIOSE

A FIRESIDE BOOK

PUBLISHED BY SIMON & SCHUSTER

NEW YORK   LONDON   TORONTO   SYDNEY   TOKYO   SINGAPORE

FIRESIDE
Rockefeller Center
1230 Avenue of the Americas
New York, New York 10020

FIRESIDE and colophon are registered trademarks
of Simon & Schuster Inc.

Designed by Jennifer Dossin
Manufactured in the United States of America
10   9   8   7   6   5   4

Library of Congress Cataloging-in-Publication Data
Birch, Beryl Bender.
Power yoga: the total strength and flexibility workout /
by Beryl Bender Birch; photographs by Nicholas DeSciose.
p.   cm.
"A Fireside book."
Includes bibliographical references and index.
1. Astanga yoga.   I. Title
RC781.68.B57   1995
613.7'046—dc20   93–48099
CIP
ISBN 0-02-058351-6

CONTENTS

ACKNOWLEDGMENTS

Ever since 1981, when I first began work on this book, I thought about whom I would thank if and when it was ever finished. Although at that time I didn't have a clue as to what the finished form would be like (or even have the tools to complete the task), I did know that I would probably feel a lot of gratitude to those faces and forces, both seen and unseen, that had helped me to get it done.

Now, as the project reaches completion, the gratitude I feel most strongly is for the eight-limbed path of *astanga yoga* and the practice itself. Without the practice, I would never have developed the focus and concentration needed to complete this project—especially in the midst of New York City, while running a full-time yoga business. Consequently, I find myself feeling an enormous sense of appreciation running backward through time to all the yogis who took the time and effort to practice *astanga yoga,* especially this particular form, and keep it alive over the millennia.

First, I would obviously like to thank my teacher, Norman Allen, and his teacher, Sri K. Pattabhi Jois, for their dedication to *astanga yoga.* I would like to thank Norman for beginning the process of teaching me to be regular and consistent and earnest in all aspects of my yoga practice. He gave me my first copy of the Yoga Sutras and the Hatha Yoga Pradapika. He will always be the person I remember as my "teacher."

It is interesting, as you write an acknowledgment, how you begin to see what the Buddhists refer to as the interconnectedness of all things. If I hadn't moved to California in 1971, I might never have taken that first yoga class at UCLA. And if I hadn't gotten into yoga, I probably wouldn't have gone to India. And if I hadn't gone to India, I wouldn't have had the opportunity to travel with the Jain nuns, study meditation, practice silence, learn about nonviolence, and continue my spiritual search—which eventually led me to New York City and *astanga yoga.*

If any little thing had been different, I wouldn't be sitting here typing out these acknowledgments today. Who then to thank? Everyone and every experience of life leading up to now. And not only every one of my experiences but every one of everyone else's experiences that put them where they were when they connected with me and my path.

More than anything, I would like to thank my soul mate and husband, Thom Birch, for his faith, devotion, love, and support. Through his example as a world-class long-distance runner, he taught me the meaning of discipline and dedication, and the importance of staying in one place and digging your well, long after everyone else has bounced around from spot to spot and given up on ever finding water. Without his encouragement and coaching, I might never have found the method, the mental strength, or the endurance to successfully complete this work.

I would like to thank Fred Lebow for his courage in supporting the Power Yoga program in the early eighties, when very few other people did, and offering me the opportunity to teach it to all fitness-minded people through the prestigious New York Road

Runners Club. I would also like to thank Elizabeth Phillips for her early faith and support, without which I could never have approached Fred Lebow.

I would like to thank Syracuse University and all my teachers there in the early sixties, for awakening me to Western physics and Eastern mysticism, both of which have captivated me ever since. I will always be grateful for their general efforts to educate me, despite my dyslexia and the death of my mother, neither of which were much acknowledged in those days.

I would like to especially thank Edward Ruscha, who first encouraged me as a writer and photographer back in 1971 and taught me to trust my own creativity and imagination. I am grateful to Virginia Miller Cornell, who took my yoga classes in Winter Park, Colorado, in the midseventies and told me I should forget everything else and concentrate on teaching yoga because that's what I did the best.

I am also most grateful to Vine Deloria, who in 1975 encouraged me to believe that I could actually be a writer and tackle a major project—and then taught me that the way to get through any ambitious undertaking is to just chip away at it one day at a time. I thank all my formal and informal teachers over the years, those who have become friends and those whom I've only known through their workshops or writings. For helping me to find, and begin travel on my path in the early seventies, special thanks to Paramahansa Yogananda's *Autobiography of a Yogi,* John Lilly's *Center of the Cyclone,* Alice Bailey's *The Reappearance of the Christ,* Carlos Casteneda's *A Separate Reality,* Baba Ram Dass's *Be Here Now,* Robert DeRopp's *Drugs and the Mind* and *The Master Game,* Fritjof Capra's *The Tao of Physics* Krishnamurti's *The Flight of the Eagle* and *The Impossible Question,* Joseph Campbell's *The Mythic Image,* Al Huang's *Embrace Tiger, Return to Mountain,* Suzuki Roshi's *Zen Mind, Beginner's Mind,* Chogyam Trungpa's *Meditation in Action,* and Allan Watts's *Psychotherapy East and West.* I am greatly indebted

to many other teachers as well who have continued to inspire me through their writings or our meetings over the years. Especially thanks to David Rappaport for patient support and encouragement.

I would like to thank Dr. Dean Ornish for his total dedication to his belief in the prevention and reversibility of heart disease through lifestyle changes, which include diet, meditation, and yoga practice. As a result of his persistent effort to follow through and confirm this as fact to the medical community, he has helped to establish the credibility of yoga as a serious healing modality. Thanks to Thich Nhat Hahn, whom I first met in 1981 at the Reverence for Life Conference in New York City, for *The Miracle of Mindfulness,* and his dedication to the dharma. Thank you to everyone who is awake and working to make this planet and its inhabitants mindful and at peace.

I would like to thank our friend and fellow *astanga* practitioner, Clifford Sweatte, not only for his loyalty, and mindful effort to truly practice yoga, but also for his long hours of pouring through early drafts of this manuscript, checking for errors and inconsistencies. I would like to thank our friend Bob Allen, for his unfailing ability to provide true western hospitality and respond to any cry for help at any time of the day or night, but especially for his help in preparation of the initial book proposal for Macmillan.

I would like to thank my many thousands of students and clients who help me to stay in shape mentally and physically by faithfully showing up for class, which continually inspires me to be at my best at all times for each of them. And I would like to thank the many special friends and students who hung in there with me while I did the major work on this manuscript. Especially thanks to David Rappaport for patient support and encouragement.

I would especially like to thank my friend and student, Sharon Dynak, of Macmillan Publishing Company, who first thought to ask after class one day if I had ever considered writing a book. She is the person responsible for introducing this project to Macmillan.

I would like to thank the universe for my editor, Mark Chimsky, and one of the most balanced, joyful, and rewarding people to work with on the planet earth. Thanks to Mark for his faith in this project from the start, his accessibility, his genuine participation, and his positive feedback every step of the way. I would also like to thank Mark's assistant, Rob Henderson, for all the long hours of work he put into making this book possible. Thanks also to my editor at Simon & Schuster, Bill Rosen, and his assistant, Gillian Sowell, and all the talented production people at Simon & Schuster who had the extremely difficult and challenging job of actually putting this book together so beautifully.

And I would like to thank my superb photographer, Nicholas DeSciose, for his hard work and dedication to his art and for his enthusiasm for this project. His appreciation throughout the shoot encouraged me to relax, have fun, and be myself! And also thanks to Body Design by Gilda for all the great workout clothes that I wear in the photographs.

I would like to thank my guru, Timber, the wolf I ran with from 1972 until 1984, for teaching me mindful meditation through example, for saving my life, and for sharing endless hours of joy in the mountains, deserts, fields, and forests. And to Grandfather and Jesse, the wolves I have run with since, thanks for teaching me to follow a trail, find my way home, smell the wind, howl at the moon, and sense whom I can trust.

Lastly, I thank my parents for my life and genes: my mother especially for teaching me about *karma yoga,* the path of service, and my father especially for teaching me about *jnana yoga,* the path of knowledge. I wish they could be around to see the completion of this long-dreamed-of work.

POWER YOGA

1

the hard & the soft

The Nature of Mind

Confined in the dark, narrow cage of our own making which we take for the whole universe, very few of us can even begin to imagine another dimension of reality. Patrul Rinpoche tells the story of an old frog who had lived all his life in a dank well. One day a frog from the sea paid him a visit.

"Where do you come from?" asked the frog from in the well.

"From the great ocean," he replied.

"How big is your ocean?"

"It's gigantic."

"You mean about a quarter the size of my well here?"

"Bigger."

"Bigger? You mean half as big?"

"No, even bigger."

"Is it . . . as big as this well?"

"There's no comparison."

"That's impossible! I've got to see this for myself."

They set off together. When the frog from the well saw the ocean, it was such a shock that his head just exploded into pieces.

SOGYAL RINPOCHE, *The Tibetan Book of Living and Dying*

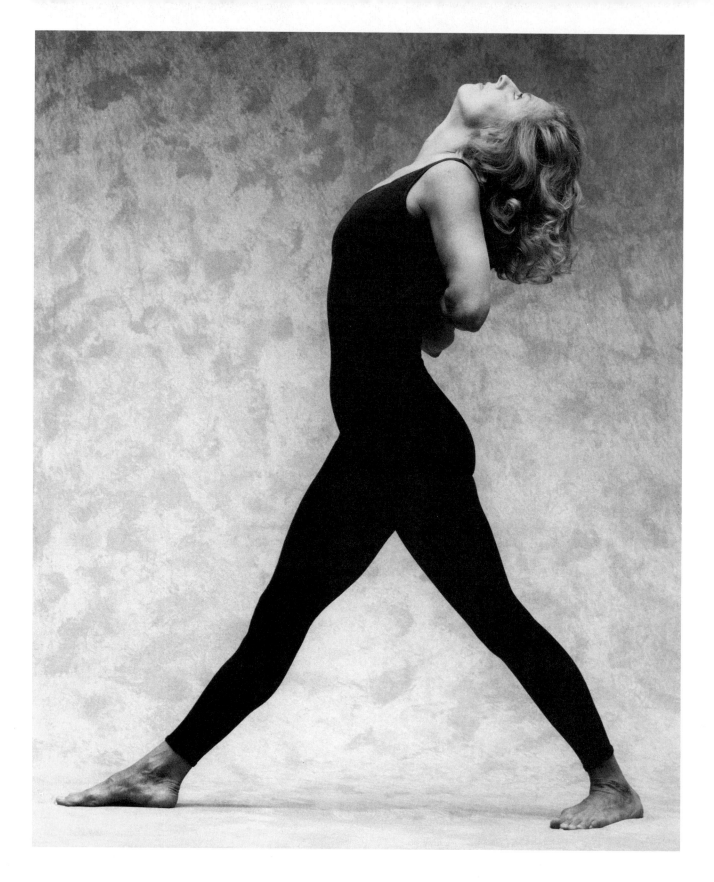

THE QUEST

Everywhere I went the search continued. Four years in California. I looked in the sea. Seven in Colorado. I looked in the mountains. In 1974 I even traveled to India for six months and looked there in the cities and the mountains. The pretext for the trip was to cover—as a photojournalist for *East West Journal*—Kumbha Mela, a huge spiritual festival held only once every twelve years on the banks of the Ganges River. Hundreds of thousands of Hindus from all over India make a pilgrimage to Hardwar, a small town north of Delhi, and all try to bathe in the Ganges at the same auspicious moment. I was in India to search. Photographing and writing about monks, mystics, and myriads of spiritual sojourners was just a way to validate my own ethereal wandering.

One evening in the swarming marketplace of Bombay, weeks before I was due in Hardwar for Kumbha Mela, I was hard at work on my search. In Bombay at night, small fires of burning dried buffalo dung are omnipresent, and a hazy yellow-orange curtain hangs over the churning sea of night life. The smell is intoxicating. And the dark, turbulent mystery of a Far Eastern city at night was irresistible to a young photojournalist.

I was so curious to find what I was looking for. I was so innocent. When those two polite gentlemen in the open-collared white shirts and loose jackets, with armloads of books on their hips, wanted to talk politics, I thought it might lead me to the answer. I was compliant. They said all Americans only wanted to stay in the Taj Mahal Hilton and have toilet paper and sheets and didn't have a clue about Indian life.

That's not me! Let me show you some of us care, some of us are down-to-earth, I thought. "Let's sit in this brightly lit tea stall," they said. I'm thinking, *Gee, yes, let's sit in this quaint little shop with the pictures of Lord Ganesha, the elephant god, on the walls and discuss the socioeconomic implications of Third World countries visited by First World tourists! Yes! Almost as good as Paris cafés in the thirties with Chopin and Liszt.*

When the picture of Ganesha and the clock next to him started to melt visually down the wall, I realized instantly I was in trouble. As a voice audibly said, "Get out of here now!" I jumped up, knocked over my chair, and lurched out the door. I did get out, barely. Even as I escaped into the taxi, which miraculously appeared out of nowhere in front of the tea stall, a hand reached out unsuccessfully toward the cab door to follow me into the covering darkness of the backseat. The cab pitched forward and we bumped off toward my destination. Where was this search to end?

I sat all night on a veranda overlooking the Sea of Bombay, in shock. Searching the string of pearl lights along the harbor, encircling the city, I wondered what in the hell I was looking for. I watched the lights melt and drain into the sea and then rebirth themselves as fireworks. What was in that lime drink those men insisted I drink instead of *chai,* the ubiquitous tea served in India? And the voice I heard? *What* was that, and where did it come from? Perhaps it was Lord Ganesha the Elephant, patron of travelers, and favorably regarded in Hindu mythology as the remover of obstacles. Alone, out at night, in Bombay? Are you serious? What was I thinking? I wasn't thinking. I was looking for God.

God had very nearly let me get offed that night. It never fully dawned on me until I returned to New York City five months later that I had been drugged, almost kidnapped, and very nearly ended up a casualty of the white slave trade. I came within microseconds of disappearing off the face of the known earth. Things never seem real till you live them. You can cry and sympathize and shake your head, but whether it's a movie or TV news about a hijacking, a bombing, or an earthquake in San Francisco, it isn't real. It isn't real till you feel it, smell it, taste it, live it.

What was I looking for that night in Bombay? The same thing I had been looking for as long as I can remember. The same thing all of us seek in one way or another. The "answer" to life, whatever that might mean. The "truth." The reason for living, dying, or being "here" at all. What is the point to it all? I guess I expected to turn a dark corner and stumble upon a soul—preferably a good-looking male, someone like Christ or Buddha—who would materialize a couple of bananas and show me the secret to life.

Well, it didn't take long to realize that if what you are looking for is someone to pull out a couple of wrist watches from his sleeve, then that is what you will find, and that being impressed with magic tricks is a serious deterrent to the genuine search for truth. Finding the truth takes hard work. I finally found what I was looking for in February of 1981 in New York City.

From California to Colorado

As a philosophy and comparative religion major at Syracuse University in the early sixties, it seemed only fitting for me to move to the West Coast for the early seventies. It was the early days of the human potential and New Age movements, and California was the epicenter. I was taking pictures and working as a biofeedback researcher in Los Angeles, studying the brain-wave patterns of meditation. One day while walking across the UCLA campus, where I was taking an anatomy and physiology course, I literally stumbled up some steps. I sat down for a few moments to compose myself and noticed a flyer advertising a yoga course on Tuesday and Thursday evenings. I took the course.

It was okay—it wasn't what I was looking for, but it was okay. Other people in the course got all fired up about the guru who taught the course and the wild breathing we did, and they joined on—changing their names, their dress, their eating habits—to become enlightened. I thought this guy was reasonable, but no enlightened master. I finished the course, said thank you, and went back to my search. It was 1971 in California. If you were an introspective type, except for the smog it was heaven on earth. Over the years, I continued to study yoga and everything else California had to offer, taking a variety of courses and workshops.

After I returned from India in 1974, I moved to Winter Park, Colorado, to continue my quest in a more environmentally friendly milieu, and began to teach yoga. Naturally, I taught skiers. I worked with the ski patrol, the ski school, and the handicapped-skiers program. By routine yoga standards, my class was pretty conventional. Oh, perhaps it was a bit more energetic than the average yoga class because we were all skiers. Most of us skied every day from nine to five, and we were used to being in motion, training. We didn't rest between postures, the way you do in many yoga classes. But basically, from a physical standpoint this was a (shudder!) "stretch" class.

I was able, however, to utilize many of the techniques I had learned while working in the field of biofeedback. So we did lots of visualization and progressive relaxation in class. We did autonomic training, which consisted of repeating phrases like "I am relaxed, I am calm, I am at my center." Most of the students in my class were also competitive skiers, so during racing season we would practice a technique called Visual Motor Behavior Rehearsal, or VMBR, as it was called. This was a visualization technique where you would simply rehearse an event, such as a ski race, in your mind step-by-step before you actually did it.

The classes were fun and popular, and pretty soon just about everyone in this mountain valley was onto my yoga program. When the U.S. Nordic Ski Team came to town for a few months to train at Devil's Thumb Ranch (an international cross-country facility in nearby Fraser), it was only a matter of hours before Marty Hall, the coach of the team, ran into a local skier who told him about the yoga classes. Marty called me up to see if I could do a session for the team.

Well, I guess I was a little overenthusiastic, or these kids were tighter than average, because the day after their first class, Marty called me again to say that everybody on the team was so sore they couldn't walk, much less ski. That night while reading a book of Zen stories, I came across a proverb that said "Only when you can be extremely soft and pliable can you be extremely hard and strong." It didn't sink in right away, as Zen *koans,* or teaching puzzles, tend not to. But a few weeks later, one morning on waking I saw the letters THE HARD & THE SOFT laid out on the side of a mountain in my mind, like the HOLLYWOOD sign in L.A.

The Hard & The Soft became the name of my yoga program and the underlying philosophy for everything I either entertained or actually experienced from that moment on. Every challenge in life seemed to me to be a question of finding the balance between hard and soft in any given situation. The men and women on the ski team came back to class. We did a little stretching, but mostly I did visualization and VMBR with them. They loved it. But thinking back to that first experience, wasn't it odd that here were world-class athletes, yet they couldn't move outside the range of their specificity of training without being incapacitated? What had caused them to get so sore?

Well, for one thing, although they were very fit, they were also very tight. Tight in the back, the shoulders, the thighs especially, and the ankles. They were all hard and no soft. No wonder they all got injured so easily and frequently, I thought. When they fall, there is no "give," no malleability. They tumble through an unaccustomed range of motion, and something tears as a result of being so tight. I tried to visualize what the stretching had done to them. The muscles didn't want to stretch, and had resisted. The muscles were used to contraction, not surrender.

For another thing, all they did was ski. They took the same biomechanical path through the woods, day after day. I had asked them to take a different route. They had used new muscles in new ways, and were feeling the effects. Third, I had given them too much too soon. And last, it seemed to me that if the muscles had been warmed up a bit, they might have been willing to stretch a little more easily.

These were some of my first musings about the role of heat in yoga, the importance of what twenty years later would be called "cross-training," and the significance of balance between hard and soft, or strength and flexibility. I realized that no matter how fit a person might be at his or her particular sport, he or she had to *ease* into activities that were not muscularly familiar to avoid strain, soreness, or even injury.

In my classes, I began to introduce beginners to the work a bit more gently. Instead of drop-in classes, I started to offer yoga "semesters," where the intensity of the class increased progressively as the course went along. I encouraged students to start at the beginning and slowly accustom themselves to the practice. I began to be more sensitive to the temperature of the room. I always tried to turn the heat on before class so that the room was at least 70°F for practice—which in Winter Park, Colorado, in the winter, was always welcome. The Hard & The Soft yoga system was evolving, but still not where I felt it should or could be.

By 1980 I had pretty much taught yoga to everyone in Winter Park. After seven years in the mountains I was restless and hungry for cultural stimulation. I was hosting a talk show on public television in Denver on Friday nights and thinking about moving to Denver. I thought, "Well, if I'm going to move to Denver, I might as well move back to New York."

THE SEARCH ENDS

Just about the time I started giving energy to thoughts of returning east, I received a call from the Jain Meditation International Center in New York City. They invited me to conduct a yoga teacher-training program at their center in Manhattan. I had returned frequently to New York over the years to study Jain meditation and was somewhat familiar with their organization. So in the autumn of 1980, I traveled back to the East Coast, planning to spend a few months and see what evolved.

It was here, in February of 1981, that I walked into a Saturday morning yoga workshop and experienced a totally unique form of yoga unlike anything I had ever seen in my ten years of prior training. The workshop was given by a dark-haired, bearded American just recently returned from India. His name was Norman Allen, and from the first moment I saw him, I had the feeling I had met him before.

The first half of the program was a demonstration. Allen and his student, a woman in her early fifties, began to practice. They started with warm-ups, or Sun Salutations, as they are called. I was familiar with Sun Salutations, but these were different from the ones I had been practicing and teaching. They then began to flow though a series of yoga postures—or *asanas,* as they are called in the yoga language of Sanskrit—going from one to the next without stopping.

I was completely riveted by this youthful man in his forties, doing yoga in front of me. I could hardly believe this was yoga. This was stronger than any other yoga practice I had ever seen, and it looked like what I always felt yoga was supposed to be: a balance between strength and flexibility. Hard and soft. I knew immediately it was something I had to learn. It motivated me in a way no other yoga training had.

I had never seen such strength, grace, and fluidity in a yoga practice before. Every posture was connected to every other posture with movement. The whole practice flowed along like a dance. The minute I saw this form, I knew that I had found what I had been searching for all these years. It looked familiar to me, like something I had lost and then found again after a long time. And in the second half of the program, when we began to do the practice itself, it felt as though I had come home.

THE EIGHTFOLD PATH

The particular yoga practice I watched that Saturday morning was called *astanga yoga,* named by an Indian Brahman and Sanskrit scholar whose teacher purportedly recovered the lost form from an ancient manuscript he found while traveling through India. In Sanskrit, the word *astanga* means "eight limbs," from the two root words *ashta,* meaning "eight," and *anga,* meaning "limb" or "part." It refers to the classical eight-limbed yogic path as described in the famous *Yoga Sutras of Patanjali,* the primary text of the science of classical yoga, written (according to most estimates) between 400 and 200 B.C. by the great Indian philosopher and spiritual leader Patanjali. Patanjali did not "invent" yoga, but rather collated and systematized existing techniques and knowledge, giving Yoga credibility as one of the six orthodox schools of Indian philosophical thought.

I was familiar with most of the postures Norman Allen was doing and teaching. It wasn't the postures that were new, different, and captivated my attention. What was it, then? I slowly realized that there were a number of aspects to this practice that made it distinctive. One was the *vinyasa,* or connecting movement between the postures. Another was the sequential linking of the postures—or as it is called in *astanga yoga,* the "series."

Then there was the strength of the postures, the powerful breathing technique that accompanied the practice, and the resultant "heat," all combining to make this form unique. Also, the emphasis wasn't on how flexible or weird you could look. The emphasis was on strength and constancy, on concentration and flow. Watching Norman do his practice was like watching an Olympic gymnast work out. As he moved effortlessly through an awesome and challenging nonstop series of postures, his body began to glisten with sweat, which poured off him throughout the entire routine. I had never seen anybody continuously sweat while doing yoga before.

FINDING THE FORM

Norman Allen had gone to India in 1971 on his own quest. One day on the beach in Goa, he happened to see a young Indian man doing a totally awesome yoga practice, unlike anything he had ever seen before. After watching respectfully for several hours, Norman approached the yogi and asked him where he had learned yoga.

"From my father, Pattabhi Jois," was the response.

"Where is he?" asked Norman.

"In Mysore," came the answer, "but don't bother going to see him, because he wouldn't teach you."

"Why not?" Norman had asked.

"Because you aren't Indian and you aren't Brahman," was the answer. Of course, Norman went immediately to Mysore, sat on the senior Jois's doorstep for weeks, and steadfastly asked to be taught this incredible yoga form, only to be ignored.

According to doctrine in the Hindu caste system, Brahmans, or the priest class, are the highest station and associate socially and professionally only with other male Brahmans. Jois was raised as a traditional

Brahman and had never even taught this system to lower-class Indians, much less any foreigners. Jois spoke no English and could only have looked at this crazy American on his doorstep with bewilderment.

Apparently, Norman was not willing to be chased off, because he continued to sit there. Eventually, Jois relented, perhaps disregarding old dogma, or perhaps concluding that this persistent spirit, being American, must be Brahman, and agreed to teach him. Perhaps Jois even thought nostalgically back to the way his teacher, Krishnamacharya, had met his teacher before him—going off to the mountains in the north to find this yogi of whom he had heard, and then sitting on his doorstep and refusing to eat until the sage agreed to take him on as a student.

Norman Allen was the first foreigner and American to learn *astanga yoga* from Jois. He went on to become a serious and uncompromising yogi, mastering all four series of the *astanga* form, spending a number of years in India learning the native Kannada language that Jois spoke so they could communicate, and taking a master's degree in Indian studies from a local university.

THE *YOGA KORUNTA*

Sri K. Pattabhi Jois (Pa-TAH-bi Joyce) is a renowned Sanskrit scholar and yogi in India who came from a prosperous Brahman family in the southern city of Mysore. As a young man, Jois was surrounded by the lingering aroma of the still-plentiful sandalwood trees of southern India, and he was schooled, as are all good Brahman boys, in the ancient texts and scriptures of Indian philosophy. As a college student in the 1930s, his mentor was the renowned Sanskrit scholar and elder yoga teacher Krishnamacharya. Jois was an eager and dedicated yoga student. He spent years studying the rigorous path of a young Brahman priest, and became one of Krishnamacharya's leading students and disciples.

Krishnamacharya spent much time traveling

throughout India as an invited guest, giving lectures and demonstrations on yoga. During one such tour, Krishnamacharya supposedly traveled to Calcutta, and while doing research in the archives of the National Library, came across an old manuscript, the *Yoga Korunta.* The manuscript was bound together, written on some kind of leaves, and as he started going through the crumbling pages, he discovered a lengthy and intricate description of a system of *hatha yoga,* written in Sanskrit by an ancient seer named Vamana Rishi. You can easily imagine the excitement of this Sanskrit scholar, finding an ancient Sanskrit manuscript with much of the work intact. It would be like a team of archaeologists uncovering a dinosaur with all the bones in place!

Sanskrit is generally regarded in both Eastern and Western thought as the most ancient of any human language and the oldest continuously used language on the planet today (at least as far as it can be determined). Even though Sanskrit is commonly associated with India and its ancient history, there is a common bond between our modern European languages and Sanskrit.

Sanskrit was the precursor of Greek and Latin, and many, many Greek and Latin words have roots in Sanskrit. It is still uncertain, though, as to whether the European languages were actually derived from Sanskrit or whether they go back still further to a common source. For many years European scholars attributed the presence of Sanskrit in India to an 1800 B.C. invasion by seminomadic Aryan tribes from the steppes of southern Russia. These groups were believed to have spoken an archaic form of Sanskrit. However, that theory has recently been challenged by some Eastern scholars and the American Sanskrit scholar David Frawley, who believe that Sanskrit actually originated in ancient India and was in use before 6000 B.C.

The form of Sanskrit that has been used for the past 2,500 years is called classical Sanskrit. According to another American scholar, Vyaas Houston, in his *Sanskrit and the Technological Age,* the standards and style of classical Sanskrit grammar were set down by ancient grammarians who had the difficult task of organizing and codifying a scientific approach to language. All classical Hindu writings and much of Buddhist and Jain literature are written in Sanskrit, and it has long been a primary language of religious scholars in these traditions.

Thus Krishnamacharya, as a renowned Sanskrit scholar, could easily look over the *Yoga Korunta* manuscript and estimate the age of the work from the grammatical style. According to his evaluation, the manuscript itself was about 1,500 years old, but the style of the language used derived from an oral tradition predating classical Sanskrit, and possibly going back as far as 5,000 years.

The *Yoga Korunta* manuscript reportedly consisted of hundreds of stanzas of rhymed, metered *sutras,* or phrases, much like the *Yoga Sutras.* A separate stanza dealt with each movement, or individual posture, and explained how to get into the posture, how to get out of it, how many breaths to take in the posture, and the total number of movements required for completion. In addition, there was specific information on the breathing and so-called secret techniques for enhancing performance, concentration, strength, and so forth.

The *asanas,* (postures) had been known over the years and handed down from teacher to student through a variety of traditions. Each yoga school had its own way of doing the postures, and a recommended grouping. But this was the first time that a manuscript had ever been found explaining in detail not only the postures, but all the connecting movements and the correct order of the postures as well.

According to Pattabhi Jois, Krishnamacharya recited these *slokas,* or verses, from the *Yoga Korunta* to him, and he faithfully recorded them. Jois subsequently became the primary proponent of this system from the *Yoga Korunta,* naming it *astanga yoga,* as he believed it to be the authentic and original *asana* practice as intended and known by Patanjali.

The word *yoga* comes from the Sanskrit root *yug,* which means "to yoke or harness." Since 500 B.C., yoga has traditionally referred to the art of "yoking," or hooking up, the lower (or individual) consciousness with the higher (or universal) consciousness. Over the centuries the word *yoga* has also been used to mean "union," and often refers not only to the union between lower and higher levels of consciousness, but union between mind and body.

Practice of the physical exercises—the yoga *asanas*—is generally referred to as *hatha yoga. Hatha* commonly means "force" or "forceful," but the word also has a deeper esoteric significance. The two component roots of the word, *ha* and *tha,* are often defined as standing for "sun" and "moon." I like to think of yoga as also referring to the union between these two basic energies of the universe—the solar or contracting energy, and the lunar or expanding energy.

These two forces can also be understood in terms of direction. One moves toward you and one moves away from you. They are the same energies that hold the planets in place and your organs in place. They are also called the male and female energies, the yang and the yin, or the *pingala* and the *ida,* as they are named in yoga. You could go on forever citing the two polarities in the universe and their expressions. I call them hard and soft. Simple. One makes you solid, strong, focused, grounded, powerful, effective, and unyielding. The other makes you fluid, gentle, expansive, compassionate, sensitive, spacious, and yielding. We all need them both in varying amounts from moment to moment. It depends on what is appropriate at any given point.

▼

BEGINNING PRACTICE

All I know is that the minute I saw this form, it reached out and grabbed my attention. And whether it came from an ancient manuscript as sacred as the Dead Sea Scrolls, from an ancient culture like Atlantis, from outer space, or from somebody's imagination, didn't matter in the least to me. I didn't know

it at the time, but here was a 5,000-year-old tradition come to life in front of me in twentieth-century New York City. There was something very exciting about that day and that discovery. I had been wanting something stronger in my teaching. I had always taught a somewhat vigorous yoga class, especially when I had been working with skiers. But still, something had been missing. That missing "something" was here in front of me.

I began to study the *astanga* form with Norman Allen at 6:00 A.M. the day after I first saw the practice, and every day after that for nearly two years. I practiced in earnest with this man, and then one day he moved 6,000 miles away from New York and I never saw him again. I eventually tracked down his teacher, Sri K. Pattabhi Jois, and over the years I spent many months studying with Jois directly, and slowly learned of the origins of this unique yoga form.

More than anything physical, what I learned is that you start slowly, do what you can, go one day at a time, and appreciate the moment. You build strength and discipline the way you build a sand castle: a couple of grains at a time. I guess, now that I think back on it, what really captured my heart about *astanga* was the discipline, or more correctly, the way in which this system enabled me to learn focus and discipline. It forced me to be constantly vigilant in practice, and over the years this began to carry over into all aspects of my life.

The way most yoga was taught in the 1970s and early eighties, a posture would be performed, followed by rest. Then another posture and more rest. It always felt to me as if the class would start and stop. You are at it for a few minutes and then the mind has its own free time. This is changing in the nineties—in part because of the influence of *astanga* and in part because of the needs of the times—but much *hatha yoga* is still taught in a fragmented way. You do some work and then you discuss it. This method is okay, even necessary, for beginners. But you don't ever really have the yoga experience (which is the sustained quieting of the mind, the literal cessation of mind activity or chatter) through these forms of yoga practice. Or at least I never did.

In this practice, however, you don't concentrate for a minute or two, then rest or space out. In *astanga* you are training yourself in mental endurance. You are training the body to build physical endurance in order to flow through the form without stopping. But more important, you are training the mind through continuous practice to stay focused for the duration and not break concentration. This was extraordinary to me! And many years later, after many thousands of hours of practice and much study of the ancient yoga literature, especially the *Yoga Sutras,* I would come to my own understanding of the authentic and original nature of this form of *hatha yoga.*

"Focus"

In 1971 my friend Edward Ruscha, the famous American artist from Los Angeles, gave me a painting of his called *Focus,* which still hangs over my desk. At the time, although my life wasn't in total disarray, I hadn't a clue as to the meaning of the word. It would be ten years before I realized the significance of that word in my life. Here I was attempting to learn something that, when I first saw it, seemed overwhelming, awesome. I wanted to be "there." But I really didn't know how to find the discipline to get there.

So I just started. I didn't start with handstands and headstands and back walkovers. I started with the warm-ups, which is the way you will start in chapter 3. Then I went on to the standing postures, which are the beginning of the Primary Series and the foundation of the Power Yoga workout. They follow in chapter 4. Like me and everyone else who studies this form, you will find that there are some postures that are easier than others and some that are more difficult. In the beginning you may struggle,

but after time, as you learn the sequence and correct alignment, you will start to notice greater strength and fluidity, and better concentration.

The Early Days

A year after I had begun to study the routine of *astanga* yoga, I began to teach the form as I was learning it. This was the "real stuff," as Norman Allen had called it, or the "correct yoga method," according to Pattabhi Jois, and practicing or teaching anything else for me would have been a waste of time and unthinkable. The first place I taught the Power Yoga workout, as I eventually came to call it, was the New York Road Runners Club (NYRRC). At first I was afraid to call it yoga, for fear the word was too loaded with preconceived notions of pretzel positions and foreign-sounding words, and no one, at least not any runners, would come to the class. So I continued to call it The Hard & The Soft.

The NYRRC had just bought a townhouse on East Eighty-Ninth Street, near Central Park, and the first couple of years we held classes in the front room on the second floor of the club. The room was big enough to handle about twelve to fifteen people maximum, which was fine because when we started, there was plenty of extra space in the room. But slowly, people started to tell their friends and other runners about the classes, and by 1983 we had begun to spill out into the hall. As the classes continued to grow and we began to see more and more runners, I began to realize how desperately runners, and everyone else for that matter, needed this program. They were so tight! They were constantly injured not only from their training, but from tension, imbalance, and life in general. Many were actually disabled by their tightness!

In the early eighties, practically no one came to class unless they were injured. So in those days the

Power Yoga workout was basically a rehab class for injured runners. Over the years I watched as people with joint pain, back problems, muscle pulls, tendinitis, strains, and sprains would come to class and begin to practice. Slowly their pain and injuries would disappear. I watched them increase range of motion, agility, flexibility, strength, lung capacity, endurance, and general body awareness. If there was ever any secret or miracle to the practice, that was it! From a physical standpoint, the bottom line was this: People did this and got better—better in terms of healing and rehabilitation, better in terms of practice, better in terms of strength and flexibility, and better in terms of the elimination of pain. I thought back to my experience with the U.S. Nordic Ski Team and realized how great this practice would have been for them!

Order, Flow, and Heat

As the NYRRC wellness director to 30,000 international members, I've seen literally hundreds of so-called stretching programs, exercise devices, gimmicks, and the like come across my desk for sampling or evaluation over the years. Many include slick promises to increase speed, range of motion, strength, flexibility, and solve a vast array of ailments and injuries for all sports. For a number of reasons, no workout, no machine, no device—*nothing*—has ever come close to being as complete, effective, thorough, or well rounded as the form of *astanga yoga.*

First of all, the sequence of postures in the system is brilliant and extremely well balanced. Successive postures within the series are uniquely complementary, developing strength and flexibility both concurrently and alternatively. *Astanga* is the most sophisticated form of physical therapy I have ever been exposed to. I have analyzed in detail every posture in the Primary Series, or first grouping of postures, and have looked at each of them not only as a single unit but as a piece of a synergistic system. Af-

ter many years of practicing and teaching this form, I am still amazed at the contemporary relevance of the practice.

Second, the idea of connecting postures together with movement and a unique breathing technique to keep the whole practice flowing and alive is completely original. This concept of uninterrupted flow, or *vinyasa* in Sanskrit, tied to an empowering breath, sets the practice apart from every other form of yoga. This is what starts and maintains the heat, which is what enables the healing and therapy to take place. *Vinyasa,* along with the particular breathing technique explained in chapter 2, and other "mindfulness" techniques explained in later chapters, is what makes this authentically yoga.

As early as the sixth century B.C. the word *yoga* referred to the spiritual endeavor of controlling or harnessing the mind. By all accounts, this requires dedicated practice and presence. Patanjali in the *Yoga Sutras* says that yoga is the suspension of the mind's waves or vacillations (*vrttis*), and that to learn to control these waves requires constant practice (*abhaysa*) and nonattachment (*vairagya*). Yoga isn't about fluctuation; it is about constancy and focus and being present in the moment. As long as you are practicing the postures, for example, and the breathing, you pretty much have to be focused on the moment and cannot be attached to a thought about the past or future. Once you stop and start in your practice, though, you lose concentration and tend to think more, which invariably takes you into the past or the future. So because of the uninterrupted, flowing nature of this practice, it is possible to actually experience the *state* of yoga through the *practice* of yoga. Constancy and focus are standard equipment. They are built into the training, which is the thing that is so ideal about this form. The practice itself compels continuity and attention, as you will see.

Third, whoever figured out that without heat, any attempt to stretch or realign the body was a complete waste of time, had the jump on current thought in the sports medical community by 5,000 years. As recently as 1980, I was practically the only one saying,

"You have to be hot to stretch" (Axiom No. 1 of the Power Yoga workout). At that time, most people still thought that you did stretching to "warm up" for sports, not vice versa. The next step, which I propose in this book, is that not only do you have to warm up to stretch, you have to be warm *while* stretching—and not only warm, but hot and sweating. This is accomplished by doing strength work concurrently and continuously along with the stretch.

I often tell people in my classes that for an active sports or fitness-minded person, the traditional "stretching" routines are the biggest waste of time imaginable, and that they might as well stay home and eat paper towels expecting to become more flexible. What?! People don't expect me to say this. Wait a minute, they think. Isn't this about stretching?

No. This is not about stretching. There is no study in the body of sports medical literature (that I have ever seen) that shows "stretching" does any good whatsoever. Why not? Because all the studies have obviously been done on some funky type of passive stretching, often done cold or on muscles mildly warmed by some previous activity. It just doesn't work, especially for athletic-type people.

Many professional athletes, for example—both men and women—have *tried* various "stretching" programs of one sort or another, only to end up injured or with a feeling of wasting valuable training time. Additionally, since stretching by itself sort of represents the "soft" aspect of training, it is often regarded as too "feminine" by the male coaches or athletes themselves, and not something that should be practiced by "real" men. This is probably good, because it keeps more tight male athletes from getting injured by trying to push themselves into doing something that they think is "good" for them.

It's funny. Most of us are way too tight, and we do seem to think we need to be more flexible. Ask practically anyone you know who is athletically active, "Do you stretch?" A few people will look proud and say, "Yes, I stretch religiously," and look all proud. But most will look guilty and say something like, "I know I should, but . . ."

We *are* on the right track with this. We *are* too tight and our intuition that we need to be more flexible is correct. It *will* help us to prevent injury. It *will* improve performance. But the stretching programs that have been available up until now are for the most part a complete waste of time and totally ineffective. To undo all the negative effects of our fitness quest—shortened muscles, limited range of motion, and imbalanced or misaligned musculature—it takes something more *intense* than just leaning up against a tree after we run or bouncing a little before we strap on our Rollerblades.

The major question then is, How in the world do you stretch intensely without injuring yourself? You do Power Yoga! Power Yoga is about strength. Flexibility comes as a result of the strength work. Axiom No. 2 of Power Yoga states, "Strength, not gravity, develops flexibility." And without the strength work, the heat is not there and, consequently, the stretch work is not effective, safe, or even possible.

ALL SPORTS INJURY IS CAUSED BY IMBALANCE

Obviously, the idea of a yoga workout specifically designed to build and maintain complete strength, flexibility, fitness, and health is unique in the world of sports and fitness today. But it is catching on like wildfire and is filling a tremendous gap. The answer to fitness and balance certainly isn't found in sports. Yes, sports are fun. They give us exercise. Most get us out of doors. Some are even good for us. But if you are considering taking up a sport to get in shape or lose some weight, or if you are already fitness-minded and working out regularly, you should know that, according to Axiom No. 3 of Power Yoga, "Sports do not get us in shape. In fact, sports get us out of shape."

Sports develop tight muscles and create imbalance because of repetitive training and uneven use of muscle groups, or the uneven use of one side of the body.

Running, for instance, is great for the cardiovascular system. But it dramatically tightens the muscles at the back of the legs and does virtually nothing for the rest of the body. This intense shortening or disproportionate strengthening results in mind-boggling muscular and structural imbalance.

The harder you train, the tighter your body will become, and this is true of nearly any sport. One aspect of this tightening will be positive, especially if you are new to fitness or exercise. You'll probably lose a few pounds, burn a little fat, get a little fitter, and feel terrific about yourself. Another aspect, however, will be disastrous, almost guaranteeing that if you continue training without Power Yoga work, you will become injured and have to stop exercising for a period of time, or until you take up a "new" sport.

Invariably, a lack of awareness about either an existing imbalance or the need for total fitness training and what that entails is what ultimately leads to injury in sports. Axiom No. 4 of the Power Yoga system says, "All injury in sports is caused by structural and muscular imbalance," with the obvious exceptions of falling off your bike or getting hit over the head with a hockey stick. If you come into a training program with a structural imbalance that may have developed over the years from poor posture, an old injury, genetic bad luck, or whatever, this imbalance will definitely make its presence known sooner or later through your training. The same thing is true of developing muscular and structural imbalance as a result of training.

Because the old-fashioned stretching isn't something most people like, have time for, or find effective, many athletes watch—at first perhaps with pride and then with remorse—as their bodies get tighter and tighter. They enviously recall their pretraining days when they could still touch their toes. In the mornings they crawl from bed to a hot shower to their training clothes, perhaps downing an aspirin or two on the way. They prowl the streets in search of chiropractors, physical therapists, and orthopedists. They will only stop training when threatened with paralysis, permanent disability, divorce, or murder. And sometimes not even then!

And although chronic injury in most cases (see the Appendix) comes on slowly as the body goes further and further out of alignment, the day eventually comes when the imbalance breaks through as debilitating pain. And this is the point where we absolutely have to do something about the imbalance or face stopping our training. If we were paying closer attention, we might have been able to notice the slow, incremental decrease in our range of motion and agility that has come about from training. But generally we aren't paying attention, or if we are, we're looking the other way. We're focused on our training. We like being fit. We want to stay fit. Being fit makes us feel good. It's worth the little inconveniences, like getting tight! But all of a sudden, there it is: a very noticeable pain and (gasp!) an injury! Ah yes. Injury is a very effective means used by the body to get your attention.

CROSS-TRAINING IS NOT THE TOTAL SOLUTION

So how do you correct imbalances? Some try other sports. In hopes of reducing the injuries, they may begin to follow various types of cross-training regimens where they depend on other sports or activities to keep them in shape while the muscles needed for the primary sport rest or heal. "Well, if I can't run, maybe I can bike or skate or swim."

Training for other sports helps, but it is not the end solution. Even though it may help to counter the effects of sport specificity (training at only one sport), or allow you to continue one or another aspect of your exercise during injury, it is not the complete answer to injury prevention, injury rehabilitation, and balanced training. There are two fundamental reasons why it is not.

First of all—and this is extremely important to remember—discontinuing a specific sport or exercise does not fix an imbalance that has resulted from or been aggravated by that same sport! Rest may give torn connective tissue or muscle tissue a chance to heal, but it doesn't eliminate the source of the problem. Once you start training again, the same imbalance will cause the same injury over and over again. The tightness never goes away. Muscles don't get longer by themselves. For example, if you ran track in high school or college, and are now forty-five and haven't run a day since then, your muscles are as tight as they were the day you stopped running. You will have lost your strength or your running fitness, of course, but the muscles, unless you have done something about it, are exactly the same length as they were twenty-five years ago. And there is a good chance that if you developed an injury as a result of that tightness, when you start running again the same injury will return like a ghost to haunt you.

A good analogy for this might be to imagine you have driven your car over a major pothole and this has knocked the front end out of alignment. You continue to drive the car, not realizing that it's a little out of balance. Without your awareness, one of the tires begins to wear unevenly, getting thinner and thinner in one spot until, eventually, the tire wears through and one day goes flat! Uh-oh, you think. Flat tire! You are forced to stop driving, yes? So you sit for a while (you rest the injury). You put on a new tire (new tissue forms, the pain and inflammation are gone). If you start to drive again without getting the car aligned and correcting the imbalance, the new tire will begin to wear in the same place and eventually go flat, too.

I generally use this analogy in the first class of every Power Yoga session I teach at the New York Road Runners Club. Then I ask if anyone in the class has had the experience of developing an injury, resting, then resuming training and developing the same injury again. It's amazing. There are tons of people in every class who answer yes.

So what do you do? You straighten the frame! "Muscular imbalance and structural irregularities don't fix themselves" (Axiom No. 5 of the Power Yoga program). You have to do something about it.

And that is what you use the Power Yoga workout for, among other things. If you carried a baby on one hip for two years, and now you are running and have a knee problem, it may take having another baby and carrying that baby on the other hip for two years to solve the problem. It might also mean doing Power Yoga for two years.

Second, no one sport perfectly balances and complements any other in strict biomechanical terms. Some sports complement one another well, like cross-country skiing and distance running; others not so well, like basketball and distance running. Some sports have a good direct muscular crossover effect, like Rollerblading and cycling, or climbing and kayaking. Others have very little muscular crossover effect, like cycling and running. Besides, most of us hate to shift our exercising priorities to the point where we would be backing off from the level of achievement that we worked so hard to reach. Only a program designed to specifically open, realign, and build power and flexibility will work effectively as an antidote to the negative effects of exercise and keep us on the road.

EVEN IRON WILL BEND

If the fender of our car gets banged up, what do we do? We take the car to a body shop where the "body workers" will heat up the frame and then remold it to take out the dent. "Even iron will bend if you heat it up" (Axiom No. 6 of Power Yoga). In many of us who've been active exercisers for years, our muscle and connective tissue are starting to feel like the iron in our cars. The only way to get rid of a dent (unless you just want to hammer it out cold—and some of you actually try that method!) is to heat up our frame and remold it.

Let's say we have a serious injury and need surgery. The surgery might repair a bone or reconnect a severed ligament or muscle, but it does not restore the tissue to the preinjured elastic, supple state.

The "memory" of the injury will stay there forever until we do some body work.

More often our injuries are less traumatic. Yet we feel pain. So for relief many of us seek out a sports medical specialist or an orthopedist and expect some miracle. We might get some information about what specifically is wrong with us. Frequently, as is the procedure in allopathic medicine, the doctor will give us drugs, generally painkillers, muscle relaxants, or anti-inflammatories. Then what? We may get rid of pain, spasm, or inflammation. But *something* caused the pain, spasm, or inflammation. Did we get rid of the cause of the problem? Probably not. Surgery might correct a structural imbalance, but drugs rarely do!

Perhaps we stop all activity and rest. But Axiom No. 7 of the Power Yoga system states: "Stopping training doesn't correct an imbalance." It may give the injury time to heal, but as soon as we begin to train again, as I mentioned previously, the injury will come back. Why is that? Imagine misaligned moving parts rubbing against one another, causing friction, or what we feel as pain. If we stop exercising, the friction stops, so the pain diminishes and the inflammation subsides. But when we start things up again, the moving parts are still in the same biomechanical relationship to one another. And the moment we start using them in the same way, the rubbing starts and the pain returns.

You have to take out the "dent" to stop the rubbing! How do you do that? You have to get in there and knead it around like bread dough and work out the trauma. You have to take the tissue in every direction, both in a stretch and in a contraction. And in order to remold and reshape the tissue while you are doing this pushing and pulling, you have to heat it up. Without the heat, the realignment is not safely possible.

THE ALCHEMICAL PROCESS

The primary ingredient of the Power Yoga practice—and what makes it so particularly effective as physical therapy—is heat. Think of what a glassblower can do with a piece of glass tubing when it is heated. The glass can be shaped into swans, baskets, and unicorns. But imagine trying to reshape the glass without the heat? What would happen? You would end up with a pile of shattered glass.

The heat does more, though, than allow us to realign our frame without breaking. As the connective tissue becomes heated by our practice, it becomes less "solid" and more "liquid." We become pliable for reshaping. In this pliable state, we apply the form of the practice that begins the remolding process. Tight, "dead" spaces that may have been shut down and in shock for years begin to open up and allow increased circulation. Thus, old clumps of gnarly scar tissue, debris, and other by-products of the healing process get moved out, not to mention environmental toxins that accumulate in the body.

The practice can then undo the rigidity and create more space for intercellular fluids to circulate and bring in nutrients while carrying off toxins. So not only does the practice work on restoring function to an injured area and facilitating realignment, but it also works to detoxify the organs and tissue and revitalize the entire system.

When gold is mined it comes in the form of ore. It looks kind of dirty and not much like the gold we think of in coins or jewelry. In order to persuade the gold to come loose from its setting in the ore, we must heat it. Gold can only be purified in the presence of heat. In the same way, to develop the "gold" in ourselves, we must apply heat and cleanse ourselves of the unwanted "ore."

Every injury, whether old or recent, is embedded in "ore." The Power Yoga practice works to restore the gold luster of the tissue, joint, or bone by applying heat and helping the bodily systems of circulation and elimination carry off the unwanted elements.

It's funny how when something goes wrong with

us, most of us expect medicine to make it right. Sometimes it can. But what we will learn with our yoga practice is that much of our healing potential is in our own hands, and our active participation is frequently the essential element in effective medical therapy and long-lasting health.

MACHINES CAN'T REPLACE YOGA

The primary series of *astanga yoga* in Sanskrit is called *yoga chikitsa,* which means "yoga therapy." The series is specifically designed to therapeutically align the body and protect and rehabilitate it from injury. Nothing else seems to work as well or in quite the same way.

For example, riding a bike for a while instead of running may allow a running injury to heal and enable you to keep up your aerobic fitness level. And although cycling is a great form of exercise, the act of the bike-riding itself isn't healing the injury. Or let's suppose you have shin splints. A sports doctor might suggest that you sit on the edge of a table, hang a bucket over your toes, and then do toe lifts with the bucket hanging on your feet. This will strengthen (tighten) the muscles at the front of your legs in the hope that you will subsequently get rid of the shin splints. But doing bucket lifts with your toes isn't healing the injury! In fact, now instead of just having tight calf muscles (which is almost always the primary cause of shin splints), you have tight muscles on *both* sides of the bone. Since muscles tend to work in pairs, and these two are now competing for power, neither of them can let go (or be flexible enough) to accommodate the strength of the other. So you are trying to solve the cause of the shin splints—tight calf muscles—by overpowering them with the muscles in the front of the legs. Oooooh!

Individual muscle strengthening can be effective in the context of an all-around fitness program. But according to yoga therapy, it is much better to do something that will stretch the calf muscles and strengthen the anterior tibialis muscles (the front of

the shin) at the *same time!* The incredibly effective and unique thing about this system is that it works on the whole person, from the inside out, which is essentially different from the fragmented solutions offered by a wide range of products and services. The marvel of the Power Yoga program is its completeness, its simplicity, and its accessibility to anyone, anywhere, at any age. There is always a place for you to start.

A PLACE TO START
AND A WAY TO CONTINUE

Doing Power Yoga is an ideal way to start a fitness program and an ideal aid to continue a sport or fitness program for life. It can be done on its own or as a companion to sport. It will slowly teach you discipline and self-awareness—not rigid, unyielding discipline, but doable discipline. It will teach you to be hard with yourself as well as soft—to work hard and sweat and to rest and recover. It will work on your body, your mind, your whole self.

However, you should know that it won't happen overnight. If you are in a hurry, you are in the wrong place. For one thing, and this is one of my favorite Power Yoga axioms (No. 8): "No matter how fit you are at what you do, when you start something new you have to ease into it." You are using new muscles in new ways, and you can't expect to perform at the same level as you do in your own sport. If you do expect the same level of performance, you'll either be surprised or sore.

Second, no matter how unfit you may be, you have to ease into a new training program. You can't try to make up for years of inactivity by rushing out and cramming all the lost time into one workout or trying to pick up where you left off years back. This applies in the case of illness or injury, too. Whenever you lay off training, whether for a week or a year, you have to ease back into it, not pick up where you left off.

So let it be clear that this program does not promise or even remotely hint that we can get you fit overnight, or from one-sided to balanced, injured to healed, unconscious to conscious, out of control to in control, sloppy to disciplined, or fat to fit in twenty-one days or less. This practice encourages you to begin slowly, practice regularly, breathe deeply, pay attention, and build on the small, gradual changes you observe as you progress.

THERE IS ALWAYS A FASTER BOAT

There is a wonderful story in the yogic literature about an eager student who comes to the shore of a river and is most anxious to get to the other side, where he believes the answer to life can be found. He sees a little rowboat go by, and eagerly flags it down for a ride. The people in the rowboat kindly stop and pick him up, and he begins to make his way across the river in the rowboat. A sleek and beautiful sailboat passes by. Captivated by the smooth efficiency of the sailboat and its progress across the river, and tired of the hard work of rowing, our friend gestures wildly to the sailboat to pick him up, and as it comes by, he jumps from the rowboat into the sailboat.

But shortly thereafter, the wind dies and the sailboat comes to an abrupt halt; now it is being carried downstream by the current, not across. Impatient with the turn of events, the student jumps to a motorized boat passing by that is obviously the best transportation to the other shore. But shortly after jumping onto the motorboat, he becomes irritated with the noise and fumes from the motor, and then doubly annoyed when the boat runs out of fuel. Now he looks around and sees that the rowboat, with its hardworking rowers, is steadfastly making its way to the other shore. Ahhhh. If only he had stayed in the rowboat.

POWER YOGA WORKOUT

One day in early autumn of '92, we received a call at our yoga center (The Hard & The Soft Astanga Yoga Institute) in New York from an enthusiastic triathlete in his mid thirties. He had just moved to New York from California and was referred to us by friends in L.A. I figured he was in a bit of culture shock and needed all the help he could get. He was mostly interested in the physical aspects of what this yoga program could do for him.

"A yoga system that builds strength?" he asked.

"Yes, strength and endurance," I replied. I try to keep it simple, especially when I'm attempting to tell an endurance athlete that yoga builds strength.

"Well, how does it build strength?"

Uh-oh! This could get complicated. "Through static muscular contractions and weight work," I explained.

"You use weights in yoga?!!"

Oh boy, now I've done it! "No, but you do lift the weight of the body and its parts, in various ways and combinations, which is similar to using the arms and legs to lift anywhere from ten pounds to your body weight." He was quiet for a minute.

"Is it aerobic?"

"No. Though the heart rate for a beginner at yoga might occasionally go up close to aerobic levels, it's not aerobic. I'm guessing that yours won't go up as high as someone who is not aerobically fit. The idea of yoga is to slow the heart rate and the respiration, as well as the activity of the mind. It's not supposed to be aerobic. Through conscious effort and concentration, you slowly learn control of the functions of the autonomic nervous system, like heart rate, muscle contractions, brain-wave patterns, etc. You then use that control to build heat and power."

"Wow! Sounds heavy!"

I guess I did go a little overboard for a first phone call. But I figured he was from California and could handle it!

He continued, "Didn't you say it builds endurance, too?"

"Yes."

"Well, how does it build endurance if it isn't aerobic?"

Good question. These people from California are hot! Okay, I think to myself. I'm gonna lay it on him.

"With this practice you are training the lungs to increase their volume and uptake while training the heart to increase its efficiency. Studies on advanced practitioners of this yoga system show that the resultant effects on the heart and lungs are very similar to the effects of aerobic sports—the resting heart rate slows, the capacity of the heart and lungs to deliver oxygen to the muscles increases, and the anaerobic threshold moves farther away."

"R-r-really?"

Yes, really.

DEVELOPING MINDFULNESS

Needless to say, it is incredibly difficult to try and explain this program to people over the phone. My favorite question to grapple with is the one that goes something like this: "Power Yoga? Isn't that a contradiction in terms?" Most people know that yoga is soft and relaxing. What most of them don't know is that it is equally hard and energizing. Yoga, when properly taught, should be a discipline that gives you the mental and physical strength to cope with and fight back the onslaught of a current environmental condition. Thus, yoga is very much about power—personal power.

Although yoga has become a bit more mainstream in recent years, to many people the word *yoga* still tends to elicit rolling eyes and conjure up thoughts of hocus-pocus and impressions of strange sounds and incantations. In large part, this is because yoga has been proffered to the American public under such a wide variety of banners and causes. Many people do not realize that yoga is simply about learning to pay attention. And since it is through this practice of paying attention, as all spiritual traditions tell us, that life

is lived most fully, more and more people are becoming able to see the relevance of such a practice in their own lives, and its compatibility with their own religious beliefs.

Once we actually begin this yoga practice and start to pay attention a little more closely, we begin to notice how much of the time we *aren't* paying attention and how much of our life passes us by in unawareness. We see for ourselves how the mind goes off and is pulled away from the present moment by a sight or sound. We begin to become aware of how much time is actually spent not here in the present moment, but off somewhere in the past or future. As a friend of mine used to say, "The lights are on, but nobody's home." We fret about how we could have done or said something differently. Or how we should do something in the future. This busyness of the mind in the past and future is a major contributing element to worry, stress, anxiety, and consequently, to tightness, tension, injury, and dis-ease. Later in this chapter I talk about the techniques we use in this practice to control this tendency of the mind to drift off.

Astanga yoga and the Power Yoga workout is a method for developing mindfulness, and thus a tool for dealing with the stress and conflict of existence. It clears out the confusion and congestion of the mind and body. As you gain proficiency in the practice, it makes you feel in control, empowered—as if there is something you can do to direct your life, rather than feeling adrift at sea, subject to the whimsical storms of life. It gives you a feeling of power. We're not talking political power here, or socioeconomic power, but power to liberate oneself from the grasp of stress, disease, inner enemies, and inappropriate behavior, and to see clearly. It enables us to slowly develop the personal power to take control of our own physical and mental wellness. But trying to explain what this practice will be like for you in two months or two years is like trying to explain to people over the phone what they will do in class. You cannot possibly "know" what the practice will be like until you start. I'm not sure I can tell you exactly why that is except by analogy. You can't put the top of the sand castle on until you build the foundation.

In this practice the focus, or discipline, happens mentally a beat before it happens physically. As a result of the breathing or the strength work or the heat or the eventual stillness in a posture, some small confusion or craving will clear. But not overnight or all at once. Only a grain of sand, a breath at a time. For one instant, the clouds part, and bang, the Grand Canyon comes into full, spectacular view, and *whoosh,* something releases in your body, some tangled old neuromusculature untangles, and life flows through anew. You feel it. But you can't possibly understand it *until you feel it.*

THE PATH TO MASTERY

Learning how to master something, whether it's the computer or the guitar, mathematics, dance, art, or any other endeavor in life, requires spending long periods of time on plateaus. You go along for weeks or months thinking you'll never get any better, but you plod along doing regular practice and paying attention (that's the key, I think). Then one day, when you least expect it, something changes and the gears grind forward a few notches, and lo and behold, you are suddenly on the next plateau! But plateaus can be boring for the mind that wants constant stimulation and entertainment. If we haven't been on the path to mastery, we don't realize what it takes to get good at something—whether it's yoga, running a marathon, or playing the piano. The path of yoga is the path of mastery. I often describe this practice as an analogy for mastering anything in life, because it teaches you the discipline of working at something every day, without expecting immediate gratification.

Let's say we watch the New York City Marathon on television and see all those different types of people running twenty-six-plus miles. We're feeling a little lethargic and chubby and think, "Well, gee, if they can do it, I can do it." We go out and buy some shoes the next day, get some sleek-looking running tights, and off we go. But soon we realize that in order to get any good at this, or have it be effective for weight loss or fitness or mental de-stressing, or whatever, we need to practice at least four or five times a week. In the heat, in the cold, in the sun, in the rain, in the snow. Ugh! Maybe this running isn't so great after all. Maybe this isn't the right sport. Maybe we should try something else. A few weeks of enthusiasm go by and then the enthusiasm begins to wane. This is the first plateau. It's not so much fun. It's lonely sometimes. It's cold. It's (uh-oh, here it comes) boring! Pretty soon the running shoes are gathering dust in the closet.

By being in constant touch with your breathing, which is what you will be doing in this practice (see chapter 2), you are training yourself to be in touch with the process of life and growth—to be aware, day to day, of the subtle tensions, toxins, tightness, and limitations of the body and mind. And to be mindful of how all of these change and move and evaporate. This gets you used to being on the plateau, which is a constant companion on the path of learning just about anything.

BE YOURSELF

Some people come to my classes to learn to relax or be more flexible. They have been working at some job or training at some sport for twenty-five years. They are incredibly tight. Not just physically, but mentally as well. Their brains are tight. Perhaps some doctor has told them they need to relax or be more flexible. So here they are in class telling me, "My doctor says I need to relax." This always amazes me! My experience has shown me that it doesn't do any good to tell these people they are tight or that they need to be more flexible. They *know* they are tight! They know they need to relax! But they don't know *how* to be more flexible, either physically or mentally. They need to learn how. Jon Kabat-Zinn, the director of the University of Massachusetts Stress Clinic, tells a similar story in his book *Full Catastrophe Living,* "One man who came to the stress clinic ten years ago with back pain . . . was very stiff and his legs were as hard as rocks as a result of stepping on a land mine in Vietnam . . . his doctor told him he had to relax . . . it didn't do this man any good to be told to relax. He knew he needed to relax more. But he had to learn *how* to relax . . . Once he started [yoga], he was able to learn to relax, and his leg muscles eventually regained a healthy tone." Until these people begin to feel the process of letting go and opening up in their own minds and bodies, anything anyone says is useless. So they come to yoga class to learn.

I see the tightness causing them anxiety and the anxiety causing impatience and the impatience causing more tension. So I tell them to be patient, that they aren't going to regain their flexibility overnight. But often they don't really hear that. They are too busy mentally, looking around and comparing themselves to someone else in class. "Wow," they might think, while I am trying to explain the virtue of patience and practice. "Look at that guy! He is so flexible!" The following week these people haven't made any progress. They never heard me talk about patience, because they weren't "home" when I was talking to them. All they can see is that they still aren't as flexible or relaxed as this other person in class, and they get irritated. They then go off to the chiropractor or physical therapist or doctor to find out why they are chronically stressed, injured, or ill.

The worst thing you can possibly do is to look around and compare yourself to somebody else, whether it is in yoga or any other field of endeavor. It wastes energy, it saps your self-esteem, and it has nothing to do with your own path. As Kabat-Zinn says in *Full Catastrophe Living,* "It is impossible to become like somebody else. Your only hope is to become more fully yourself. That is the reason for practicing [yoga] in the first place."

Diana Vreeland, the longtime editor of *Vogue* magazine, was once asked if she ever worried about what the other fashion magazines were doing, and

she remarked that she was too busy. She didn't have time to look left and right to see what everybody else was doing. She knew that nobody else saw what she saw. She just kept her eyes focused straight ahead on where she was going and what she wanted.

If you have a desire to be a master of yourself and anything else, you can put this book to very good use. Go through it one step and one page at a time, just as you are going through medical school or writing your thesis or running a marathon or building a business or painting a picture or photographing wildlife or dancing *Swan Lake* or composing a symphony. And slowly you will find yourself enjoyably learning how to build discipline and work on yourself every day. For those of you who have already realized this lesson in life, this will be a familiar process and a welcome tool to fine-tune all aspects of mindfulness, concentration, and practice.

THE REAL STUFF

The word *yoga* derives from the Sanskrit word *yug,* as I explained earlier, which means "to yoke, bind, join, or direct one's attention." It can also mean "union" or "fusion." Around the third or fourth century B.C., at the time of the composition of the *Bhagavad Gita* (probably the most famous of all yoga scriptures and an important text on Yoga philosophy), *yoga* generally referred to the Hindu tradition of spiritual discipline comprising different approaches to "enlightenment" or "self-realization."

In Patanjali's *Yoga Sutras,* the complete definition of yoga in the second *sutra* of Book One is given as *Yogas-citta-vrtti-nirodhah,* or "the cessation of the fluctuations of the mind." Another translation might be "the selective elimination of mental activity in the field of consciousness." The word *nirodhah* means "cessation" and *vrtti* literally means "waves," or fluctuations of thought.

So what Patanjali is saying is that if you can learn to control the rising of the mind into ripples and waves, you will experience yoga! When the mind is free from *vrttis,* you will experience your true nature, which is joyous equipoise. You will then be free of the mind's perilous highs and lows and the commotion and pain of going from one extreme to the other. In the twelfth *sutra* of Book One, Patanjali goes on to say that there are two ways to get a grip on these *vrttis:* through practice (*abhyasa*) and nonattachment (*vairagya*). In the next two *sutras,* he defines practice as "effort or vigilance toward steadiness of mind," and says that the practice becomes effective when it is "well attended to for a long time (*durga kala*), without a break (*nairantarya*) and in all earnestness (*satkara*)."

In Book Two, Patanjali goes on to explain the means (*sadhana*) of the yoga practice. In *Sutra* 29 he details the eight limbs of the yoga path: (1) *yama,* which literally means "restraint" or "abstinence"; (2) *niyama,* or "observance" (There are five *yamas* and five *niyamas,* which I will list later in chapter 3); (3) *asana,* or "posture," which is what we will primarily be working with in this book; (4) *pranayama,* which, again, quite literally means "restraint (or control) of the life force," generally through awareness of the breathing; (5) *pratyahara,* or "withdrawal of the senses"; (6) *dharana,* or "concentration"; (7) *dhyana,* or "meditation"; and (8) *samadhi,* or "bliss, superconsciousness."

One of the things I found to be fairly unique about the *astanga* practice was the way in which each of the limbs is actually incorporated in some small way into the practice of the postures. For example, with the focus on breathing during the practice, you are actually able to *experience* the beginning levels of *pranayama,* or control of *prana* (life force) through the breath. You have to pay attention to what you are doing, so the senses begin to be drawn in or curbed, as Patanjali describes the process of *pratyahara.* The whole practice trains you in concentration, or *dharana,* which leads to meditation, or *dhyana.* Thus, this practice, certainly like none I had ever done be-fore, actually gives you a tangible way to engage the eight limbs and develop the "practice," and "nonattachment," that Patanjali says is necessary to learn control of our mental activity and find peace of mind and equipoise.

As I have pursued my practice over the years, I have come to realize that this form, from the *Yoga Korunta,* or wherever it came from, has to be an original and very ancient form of *asana* practice well known to Patanjali and the rishis (wise men) who preceded him. This yoga practice is "practice." The *vinyasa,* or connecting movement, feels to me like threads, or *sutras,* hooking up the main verses, or postures. The practice does exactly what Patanjali says must be done to attain the yogic state of consciousness. There must be constant effort toward steadiness of mind, as you will see, or you don't get it! And one way of learning to control the mind's waves (*vrttis*) is through practice—the constant, uninterrupted, vigilant practice of watching the mind and its activities (mindfulness). And that is exactly what this Power Yoga practice trains you to do.

The other way to control the *vrttis,* says Patanjali, is through *vairagya,* which means nonattachment or freedom from desire. Now, this covers a whole host of stuff, but one practical application of how this might get in the way of being in control of one's own mind is to think of *vairagya* as nonattachment to previous experience. In my classes people will often say to me, "I can't do that!" I will say to them, "Forget that you think you can't do this! Breathe!" They will cling to some past notion that they are clumsy, uncoordinated, or slow, and as long as the *vrtti* from the past is there, the resistance is there, and the experience of yoga is not there. So I am saying to them, Forget that previous experience. Pay attention to your breath now. Be mindful. See what is happening here. Be willing to let that go. Be willing to take a risk here.

The mind generally gets attached through the senses, most frequently by seeing or hearing something. The *vrttis* are generally stirred up by the eyes and the ears as the mind goes out to satisfy its desires.

We see or hear something we either want or don't want, like or don't like. We either crave it or run from it. Either way it is an attachment to a past experience. According to yoga philosophy, this limits our ability to appreciate the moment, realize the Self, and live life fully.

The *astanga* practice right away has a method to deal with these tendencies of the mind to avoid discipline and seek stimulation through the ears and eyes. The eyes are trained to focus in on a *drishti,* or "gazing point," and the ears are trained to listen to an audible breathing technique. Then, in addition, the nonstop organic flow of postures helps to keep the attention on the practice. The postures and the connecting movement between them are actual *sutras,* or "threads" woven into a magnificent tapestry. The practice feels to me like a Sanskrit manuscript following an "organic and logical development."

In an essay entitled "The Yoga of Learning Sanskrit," Vyaas Houston wrote that "Sanskrit is a perfect language. Its construction, from the placement of each letter of the alphabet to the building of words and their relationships, follows an *organic and logical development.* Anything that is missed is like losing supports for the floors of a building." It had long become clear to me, after many years of study of other schools of yoga, and many years of practice at *astanga,* that in the *astanga* sequence the placement of each posture followed an "organic and logical development." When I was teaching, I came to notice that if any student's attention lapsed so that they missed a critical piece of information, sooner or later I had to fill them in on the missing piece before they could be up to speed with everyone else.

Some people come to yoga for psychological or spiritual reasons—to learn to relax or meditate. Some people come to yoga for physical reasons—to exercise or fix an injury, to heal an illness, or to be more balanced, strong, and flexible. The few who come looking to learn to levitate or be psychic or see auras or whatever, I tend not to encourage. Instead I ask them if they can touch their toes. They don't generally like that.

Whatever a person's reason for beginning the study of yoga, *everyone* must begin with the physical work. I am a great believer in reality. I think you have to be able to find your toes before you can find your aura or your astral body! So it makes sense to me that *asana,* for example, the third "limb," which works on healing and balancing the physical body through the postures, precedes *dhyana,* or meditation (the seventh limb), which is an extremely difficult discipline for the mind. Organic and logical development! Sometimes members of the yoga community, used to softer practices than the Power Yoga workout, will look at this practice and say, "Oh, it's so physical," implying that it therefore must be less "spiritual" than practices that cater more to esoteric pursuits.

This always makes me shake my head. The body and mind are inextricably linked—whether we like it or not. We can't just hope to control our mind and ignore the body. If the body is out of control (or out of shape or alignment), the mind cannot possibly be in control. I have found through many years of teaching and practicing yoga that it is generally easier for most people to learn to control a particular muscle first before some remote, intangible portion of the brain or psyche.

Since many of my students are initially interested in the physical yoga therapy and the strength and flexibility aspects of the practice, as I imagine you are, a primary concern of this book is the early therapeutic stages of yoga that work on aligning, healing, and purifying the body. But essential to the body work is the attention of the mind. Without mindfulness, this isn't yoga.

So in the next chapter we start with bringing our toes together. This is not necessarily easy for many people. I have to bang up against their consciousness like a biofeedback device: "Hey, bring your feet together." Yoo-hoo, wake up. Feet together. Feet together. Is anybody home? Are you here? Being here is truly the first step to levitation.

2

breathing for life

*Our breath is the bridge from our body to our mind, the element which reconciles
our body and mind and which makes possible oneness of body and mind.
Breath is aligned to both body and mind and it alone is the tool
which can bring them both together, illuminating
both and bringing both peace and calm.*

THICH NHAT HANH, *The Miracle of Mindfulness*

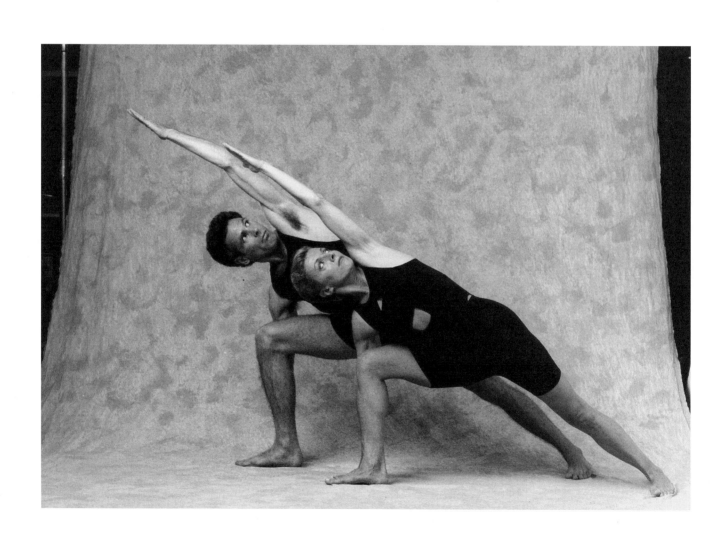

BREATHING BACKWARD

If you take a room full of people and tell them to stand up with their arms at their sides, then take a deep breath and hold it, at least half of them will breathe only from the middle of the chest up, and this includes athletes and fitness-minded individuals. They suck in the belly and puff out the upper chest, with the shoulders hunching up around the ears. After years of beginning my classes with that simple directive, and watching people breathe, I realize that many people are unaware of their breathing and are not utilizing full lung capacity.

We all know how to breathe when we are infants. Somewhere along the way about half of us get turned around and start to breathe upside down. For one reason or another we get "shut down," either emotionally or physically, in the area of the solar plexus and refuse, perhaps unconsciously, to allow full expression of our breath, full lung capacity—or, taking it further, fullness of life and fullness of emotional expression.

A plexus is a main energy storehouse of the nervous system and an aggregation of nerves and ganglia. The solar or epigastric plexus supplies all the organs in the abdomen with "nerve" energy. According to yogic tradition, this center is a great storehouse of *prana,* or "life force," and the word *solar* is most appropriate, since this abdominal "brain" radiates strength and energy. Whether you look at Eastern or Western traditions, most agree that the solar plexus, located in front of the spine and behind the stomach,

is traditionally thought of as the area of emotional storage.

Often when we shut off our emotions, what can result is incomplete and shallow upper-chest breathing. However, constant worry and stress can also result in shallow breathing. So whether the "gut" is closed down to emotional response, or so knotted up with anxiety that it blocks the breath, either way our solar center is deprived of full, radiant energy, and the subsequent distribution of this energy to the abdominal viscera is withheld.

CHECK YOUR OWN BREATHING

Here is a simple test you can do to see how your own breathing pattern stacks up: Stand up. Hook your thumbs over the waist of your skirt or pants so the thumbs are about even with your belly button. Then let your hands lay across your lower belly. Now take a deep breath. Which way does your belly move?

If your belly sucks in and flattens on the in breath, and all the air seems to go to your shoulders, you are breathing backward. If, however, your belly relaxes and even expands slightly on the inhale, you are breathing naturally, as babies do, and correctly.

Let's assume now that many of you have made the discovery that your breathing is upside down and not nearly as effective as it could be. What now? Well, let's give you a preliminary exercise to do. Everyone should learn and practice this beginning breathing technique to prepare for learning the more advanced breathing that is done with the practice of Power Yoga.

But first you may be wondering, What happened? How come I'm doing it wrong? Why me? You may be saying, "I knew it, I knew my breathing was shallow."

First of all, *you* are not backward, only your breathing—and that can be adjusted. There are lots of reasons people begin "breathing backward," as the great operatic tenor Luciano Pavarotti is fond of saying. It may be simply that as a child, a parent told you constantly to hold in your stomach. Or a gym teacher or drill instructor told you to suck it in. Maybe you had the wind knocked out of you emotionally somewhere along the line (most of us did), and consequently it felt safer to shut down the gut a little bit, as we described above. Your environmental stress levels, whether on the job or at home, may be quite high. Why else? You may come up with your own reason why your breath is restricted and insubstantial.

As we discussed, *prana* is the Sanskrit word for "life force" or "life current" in Yoga philosophy. It refers to the energy that circulates through the body and sustains life, and that is also drawn in when we inhale. It is the link between matter and energy, and body and mind. Obviously it is difficult to define. *Prana* is carried by the breath, but is a great deal more than simply air or oxygen.

Many students of yoga and, indeed, many books on yoga erroneously define *prana* as only breath. *Prana* is a vital universal force that keeps up the activities of the mind and body in the same way it keeps up the activities of the planets and stars. It is not just some mysterious power that exists within the body and cosmos, maintaining equilibrium and guarding against imbalance or disorder. It is a real current, with a tangible basis, yet it is different from other definable mechanisms. Only very recently has the state of our technology even begun to be capable of actually measuring a force as subtle as *prana.* Ultimately, the control and management of *prana* is what this practice is all about.

The vehicle for this *prana* is not the dense physical body that we wash, dress, train, feed, and rest, among other things, but a subtler vehicle interpenetrating the physical body and working in conjunction with it. This ethereal or magnetic body is a counterpart to the physical body. Currents of *prana* run through it in well-marked channels, or *nadis,* as they are called in yoga. They supply energy to every organ and cell of the body, vitalizing them in unique ways. Although there is a difference between breath and *prana,* there is also a close connection between them.

The first step of increasing *prana* in the body is the practice of deep, mindful breathing. Not only does deep breathing promote mental and physical health in many ways through the increased intake of oxygen and energy, but being conscious of—we will call it "mindful" of—the breath brings the attention to the present moment. This attentiveness to the now helps us to be more fully appreciative of what our life actually is at any given moment. Once you begin to rehearse mindfulness, as you will do with this practice, and to watch the nature of your mind, you will be amazed how much of the present you actually miss because the mind is busy with the past or future. This regret or worry wastes huge amounts of energy and leaves you exhausted, enervated, and vulnerable to imbalance and illness. When we practice mindfulness, or attentiveness to "now," through awareness of the breath, it calms this frenetic activity of the "monkey mind," as the yogis describe it, and brings peacefulness and increased energy. The short quote at the beginning of this chapter heading actually comes from a longer quote from Thich Nhat Hanh's *The Miracle of Mindfulness.* It is a simple little illustration that helps us to see just how we can begin to use the breath as a powerful tool in our lives: "Suppose there is a towering wall from the top of which one can see vast distances—but there is no apparent means to climb it, only a thin piece of thread hanging over the top and coming down both sides. A clever person will tie a thicker string onto one end of the thread, walk over to the other side of the wall, then pull on the thread bringing the string to the other side. Then he will tie the end of the string to a strong rope and pull the rope over. When the rope has reached the bottom of one side and is secured on the other side, the wall can be easily scaled.

"Our breath is a such fragile piece of thread. But once we know how to use it, it can become a wondrous tool to help us surmount situations which would otherwise seem hopeless. Our breath is the bridge from our body to our mind, the element which reconciles our body and mind and which makes possible one-ness of body and mind. Breath is aligned to both body and mind and it alone is the tool which can bring them both together, illuminating both and bringing both peace and calm."

THE OPENING-UP PROCESS: *ACTIVE EXHALATION*

The first lesson in letting go, opening up, and allowing some *prana* into all the tight, closed-down, or injured areas of your body is learning a technique I call *active exhalation.* It involves putting all your attention on the exhale and forgetting about the inhale. And although this is the opposite of what happens naturally when we breathe—namely active inspiration and passive expiration—it is an excellent technique to put you in touch with the motion of the diaphragm, and reawaken, if necessary, the area around the solar plexus.

Sit or stand up straight. Close your mouth. Put your palms on your lower belly. First, focus on the outbreath. Exhale, with the mouth closed, and press the lower rib cage down and back while simultaneously contracting the belly back toward the spine and lifting it up into the thoracic cavity. This will push all the air out of your lungs. Hold for a second. Then let go. Do this a few times. What happens?

Ideally, what will happen is that when you "let go" and relax the belly and ribs, the in-breath will get sucked in all by itself. Let's use the analogy of an accordion. If you take an accordion and push the two ends in, squeezing out all the air, then set it down in the middle of the room all by itself, what will happen? It will slowly expand on its own, drawing in air and returning to its original shape.

It is the same with your lungs. If you use the abdominals and intercostal (between ribs) muscles like an accordion and push them in toward the spine to press out all the air, when you let go or relax them, the air will get sucked back in practically by itself.

Try it again a few times. Just focus on the exhale: Push the exhale. Hold. Let the belly and rib cage go. Push the exhale. Hold. Let go. Make sure you keep your mouth closed for both exhale and inhale. This breathing exercise is done through the nose only.

If it's not working too well, simply think about "allowing" the inhale to happen as you relax. Don't try to inhale. Let yourself inhale. Push the exhale. Relax. Push the exhale. Relax. Eventually, what will happen is that you will feel the diaphragm, the major muscle of respiration, lifting up into the chest on your exhale, then automatically contracting and descending into the belly on the inhale.

As you practice this you will become more comfortable with what eventually will be correct breathing, and the whole process of paying attention to your breath will get easier and more natural. Then you can start to play around a bit—drawing the breath out, and even starting to actively draw the breath in. Longer and longer. Eventually, you will replace active exhalation with the more advanced technique used in Power Yoga called *ujjayi* breathing, which we will begin to learn in the following pages. But for now, active exhalation is an excellent technique for improving the breath and developing mindfulness.

THE SEVEN *CHAKRAS*

In yoga tradition there are seven major *chakras,* or energy centers, in the body. *Chakra* means "nerve center" and is also a Hindu word meaning "circle of light." These nerve centers are aggregates of *prana* in the magnetic body that we discussed earlier. They correspond to zones within the spinal column where the *nadis* (the channels that carry *prana*) cross one another. These nerve crossings create energy fields, or "circles of light," according to yogic thought. Interestingly, they roughly correspond with the major plexuses, or aggregations of nerves and ganglia, of the central nervous system. Let's look for a moment at what the yogis say about these different centers.

The first center, located at the base of the spine just above the anus, coincides with the sacral plexus and is called *muladhara chakra* in Sanskrit. *Mula* means "root" or "source." *Adhara* means "support" or "vital part." This first *chakra* is the root or foundation that supports our structure. According to yogic theory it corresponds to the element earth. This center is our seat of security and supplies us with our most basic and instinctual survival skills. However, here in our earth center also resides our very earthly desire to possess, to acquire, to hoard, to compete. Thus, all of our most basic fears and insecurities stem from this *chakra*. When this center is balanced and filled with *prana*, we will feel secure, calm, and connected to the earth. We will be grounded within ourselves, without depending on external objects for our sense of security.

The second *chakra*, located just above the genitals, corresponds with the lumbar or hypogastric (lower, middle region of the abdomen) plexus and is called *svadhisthana* in Sanskrit, which means "the place of our origin." *Sva* means "your own" and *adhisthana* means "dwelling," "residence," or "origin." As the element of the first center is earth, representing our foundation, so the element of the second is water, symbolizing our creative energy. This *chakra* is the source of our physical, sexual, and creative energy. It is the place of our physical origin and the animation behind our urge to reproduce. When this center is truly flowing, there is unlimited creativity and love. We are in touch with our intuitive voice, and indecision gives way to certainty. However, this center also

gives rise to such things as jealousy, anger, promiscuity, sexual codependency, and preoccupation with sex as the basis for all relationships.

The third *chakra,* or *manipura chakra* is located at the navel and coincides with the solar plexus. *Mani* in Sanskrit means "jewel" and *puram* means "city" or "dwelling place." Thus, *manipura* is that city or place where the bright jewel of inner power is felt. This is the center of power, expression, and expansion and is associated with the element fire, the nature of which is always to move upward, radiating light and heat. Tuning into this center, the yogis say, you begin to break the constricting nature of ego and experience a deepening communion with your true nature. Since this *chakra* is the focus for much of our breathing—and the development of heat, a critical aspect to the practice—I will talk more about this center later in the book, especially in chapter 4.

The fourth *chakra* is called *anahata* in Sanskrit, and means "that which is ever new, that which is constantly resounding without being struck, or that which is self-sustaining." This *chakra* is situated at the heart and coincides with the cardiac and pulmonary plexus. This is the center of compassion and unconditional love. Love for everyone and everything regardless of color, background, species, or form. This center is associated with the element air. When the yogis meditate on this fourth *chakra*, they will take time to be aware of the element air, moving in and around them, sustaining life within and without. According to the yogis, when you connect with life around you through the heart center, your love will flow like air, both in reverence toward those who have realized their perfection more fully than you have, and in benevolent service to your fellow beings who are in need on the path of life.

The fifth *chakra* is the *vishuddha chakra*, which is located at the throat and aligns with the brachial or pharyngeal plexus. *Vishuddha* means "pure amidst all purity." It is the center of abundance and is also known as *jalandhara-pitha,* or "the great doorway to liberation." It is allied with the element space. As we let go of all impure elements—all resentments, anger, bitterness—we are set free to enjoy the boundless reaches of space. Our speech is pure and we become masterful speakers and teachers, according to yogic thought.

The *ajna,* or the sixth *chakra,* corresponds to the choroid plexus. *Ajna* is the third eye, the eye of inner awareness. It is located at the center of the eyebrows, and is said to control both incoming and outgoing thought. According to Yoga philosophy the third eye is the vertical eye of wisdom and that which takes us out of physical or horizontal reality and connects us to the vertical plane of divinity. The element of this center is the mind and thought.

The Sanskrit name for the seventh center is *sahas-rara,* which means "a thousand petals." It is the highest *chakra* in terms of location and consciousness, and is located at the crown of the head. It coincides with the choroid plexus, or the upper cerebral center, and is represented by a thousand-petaled lotus flower. Symbolically, there are a thousand rays of light emanating from the center of this *chakra,* like a thousand spokes radiating from the hub of a wheel. Meditating on this center, one experiences duality merging into oneness with universal life force. There is no longer separation between "me" and "everything else," or between "I" and "Thou." There is only oneness.

THE SECRET TECHNIQUES

While it is fascinating to look at the more flowery and philosophical aspects of the yogic energy centers, it is important to remind ourselves that this book focuses primarily on the very tangible aspects of the *astanga* practice, which are to align the physical body, purify the nervous system, and develop concentration and mindfulness—all of which combine to prevent and reduce injury, stress, pain, suffering, and dis-ease.

However, while it is also interesting to note the similar pattern between the layout of the seven *chakras* in the magnetic body and the plexuses in the physical body, for example, it is equally important to realize that the *chakras* are not simply the physical plexuses. They are not tangibly situated in the body. We cannot see them with X rays, and a doctor cannot physically locate them while performing surgery. However, even though they are intangible, they do affect the physical and mental body to a great degree.

The purpose of experimenting with active exhalation is certainly to develop our awareness of our breath and increase lung capacity. But couldn't we also say that its purpose is to stimulate our awareness of the third *chakra*? With improper or shallow breathing, the nerve cells (neurons) in the solar plexus are not fully nourished. A nerve cell's job is to generate and conduct electrochemical energy forms called nerve impulses. Without sufficient *prana,* the cells become inefficient conveyors of nerve force. In a physical sense all the abdominal viscera, fed by the solar plexus, suffer. In a psychological sense the emotional "center" is deprived of full "feeling" as well, as I mentioned earlier. Thus, whether the third *chakra* is blocked, asleep, or just simply not as "conscious" as it could be, it begins to benefit from active exhalation. The practice puts you more fully in touch with this physical and emotional "center" of yourself, so to speak. And once we go on to learn the actual yogic breathing practice of *ujjayi,* the benefits are even greater.

In yoga, the third *chakra,* symbolized by a flame, has always been the center thought to control the development of psychic power. Correspondingly, in both Chinese and Japanese martial art traditions, this area irradiating out from the navel is also thought to be the center of psychic power, the source of the *chi* (Chinese) or the *ki* (Japanese), like *prana* or "life force" in yoga. One of the so called secret techniques in esoteric yogic literature for enhancing lung capacity and maximizing performance, for example, has been to stoke the "fire" in the lower part of the thoracic cavity through breathing and meditation techniques.

Couldn't we apply this to our own practice, if only metaphorically? Couldn't we, through relaxation and "opening" of the abdominal "center," learn to utilize this fire to purify a particular toxin or simply to send heat and energy, out into our bodies, minds, and lives? So even though we are just trying to develop our breathing at the moment, it's kind of fun to look at some of the philosophical aspects of the practice, and ponder our untapped potential as humans.

SCIENCE STUDIES *PRANA*

Although there may be a scarcity of scientific studies that measure the actual effect of this directed *prana*, or energy, on improved performance or increased strength, there are some. And there is certainly no scarcity of references in Eastern as well as Western literature to extraordinary feats accomplished by yogis, Zen masters, martial artists, athletes, and even ordinary individuals who refer to "bringing up" this power.

Recently, I was interviewed for a magazine article on breathing. The writer was telling me that a number of exercise physiologists and sports medical people she had spoken with said that there were no studies to show that any breathing exercises could improve performance or increase strength or lung capacity. "What do you think of that?" she wanted to know, expecting me to disagree.

"They are right," I responded. "Unless they just misread their data, the experimenters obviously looked at breathing techniques that didn't affect lung capacity or performance. That doesn't mean anything except that the particular breathing exercises they tested didn't affect performance! That certainly doesn't mean that there are not *any* breathing techniques that affect performance."

Actually, there was an extensive study done at the University of Toledo in 1986. A group of cyclists and triathletes were tested before and after using active exhalation and simple yogic breathing techniques,

and in virtually every instance researchers observed improved physiological function as related to performance. According to the August 1986 issue of *Ultra Sport* magazine, "test subjects were able to reduce blood pressure and pulse rate by 10 to 15 percent while performing at the same work rate, and their V02 max [the maximum amount of oxygen the body can utilize with each breath] indicated a similar increase. The athletes were also able to burn fats at a slower rate, postponing the point of total fatigue."

What we are talking about here are truly some of the ancient secret techniques known formerly to only an elite few. Many of these methods were handed down orally from teacher to student over thousands of years. Other sophisticated performance-enhancing techniques such as those described in the *Yoga Korunta,* the ancient manuscript on which Power Yoga is based, were just not available to the general public. For example, the specific order of postures of *astanga yoga* and the concept of *vinyasa,* or the connecting movement between the postures, was only brought to light some fifty years ago and is just now beginning to be taught in the United States. This is the first time the ancient teaching of the *astanga* order and method of postures have been available in English in book form.

The world is changing incredibly rapidly, so some information that may truly have been esoteric and secret a few years back is public domain in this age. Think of all the places that once seemed remote and mysterious and inaccessible, with names like Tibet, Tierra del Fuego, the Galápagos, the Seychelles, and the Himalayas. Nowadays you can pick up any travel magazine and find chic ecotours going to them all.

TRAINING THE DIAPHRAGM

The diaphragm is a muscle, and can be trained and strengthened like any other muscle. I find that most fitness-minded folks don't know any more about the diaphragm than they do about the pancreas. But with practice and concentration it can be brought under conscious control. And along with other muscles of respiration, it can be trained to measurably increase lung capacity and improve performance.

It was always difficult for me to visualize what the diaphragm must look like. Was it a big rubber balloon stretched across the middle of the chest? What was above it? What was below it?

After considerable research on the anatomy of the diaphragm, I had a much better idea of how it looked. I'm spending some time trying to describe it here because I think it will give you a better idea, as it has done for me, of how breathing works—and what happens when you add the yogic *bandhas,* or locks, which we will learn later in the practice (see chapter 4).

So let's try to visualize a wide, fan-shaped muscle that separates the chest cavity (thorax) and its contents from the abdominal cavity and its contents. This is the main muscle of inhalation. Its outer edge is made up of fibrous tissue that originates from the inner wall of the entire chest cavity. These muscle fibers pass upward and inward and converge in a central tendon. When viewed from below, the diaphragm would look like the sky as seen from the earth—the underside of an arched dome. When viewed from above, it would look like a protruding rounded surface, like a hill.

Inhalation begins as the muscular fibers of the diaphragm contract and are drawn downward. The hill becomes less arched or nearly flat, and this pulls down on the central tendon, lowering the "floor" of the chest cavity. As a result of this, the vertical diameter of the chest is increased, creating more space in the lungs. At the same time the intercostal muscles, the little muscles between the ribs, begin their work. The external intercostals contract and the internal intercostals relax (on exhalation it is the opposite). This creates expansion of the rib cage and, along with the action of the diaphragm, reduces air pressure in the thorax to the point where it is lower than atmospheric pressure. Thus, air from the outside surges in to fill the vacuum.

When descending, the diaphragm presses on the abdominal organs. The right portion forms a complete arch molding over and pushing gently against the convex surface of the liver. Resting on top of the right side of the diaphragm is the concave base of the right lung. So the base of the right lung and the top of the liver fit together like two spoons, with the diaphragm in between.

The left portion is arched in a similar way but is narrower because of the intrusion of the pericardium, the membranous sac that contains the heart. The left part of the diaphragm covers the large end of the stomach, the spleen, and the left kidney, and supports the base of the left lung.

As the diaphragm descends and presses on the liver, stomach, and other organs, it gently massages them, stimulates their actions, and encourages normal functioning. Internal organs need exercise much the way external muscles do. The diaphragm is nature's principal instrument for this internal exercise. Its motion vibrates the important organs of digestion and elimination, massaging and kneading them at each inhale and exhale, forcing blood into the organs and then squeezing it out.

Naturally, exhalation takes place passively and is effortless movement. The walls of the thorax simply return to a condition of rest because of their own natural elasticity and that of the lungs. But what happens in forced, or active, exhalation? This action is performed mainly by the flat muscles of the abdomen (oblique and transverse) and the internal intercostal muscles, the little muscles between the ribs on the inner side. When the internal intercostals contract, they pull the rib cage in and help to force residual air, the air that remains in the lungs after exhalation, out of the lungs.

In order to allow the in-breath to penetrate to the depths of the lungs, there can't be any blocks of any type. Any hindrance will cause the breath to be shallow. When you practice active exhalation, and you "push" the exhalation out with your abdominals and intercostals, then relax or "let go," you are actually experimenting with a simple technique that begins to open up and dislodge any obstacles in the power *chakra.*

How is this different from "belly" breathing? you might ask. Belly breathing is a practice taught in many stress management courses and in some yoga classes. It was adapted, as nearly all Western breathing exercises have been, from ancient Eastern techniques. Is it the same as what we are doing here?

Well, yes and no. Yes, in that both methods encourage the practitioner to take the in-breath down into the abdominal area. But no in every other aspect. Belly breathing focuses on inhalation instead of exhalation, and teaches you to actively stick out the belly on the in-breath in order to take the breath down past the chest. It takes a lot more energy than active exhalation. And if someone is used to backward breathing, it is more difficult to learn.

The preliminary Power Yoga practice of "allowing" the passive in-breath to enter instead of desperately sucking in the energy teaches you, in yoga fashion, to learn greater control of your breath. It teaches you to empty before you fill up. To get rid of the toxins and clean out the lungs before you try to fill them. A similar practice that can help illustrate the advantage of emptying before filling is the yogic health recommendation to empty the bowels in the morning before putting any more food in the body. You don't eat until you get rid of what came into your system from the previous meal.

THE REAL STUFF—*UJJAYI* BREATHING

The next step after learning active exhalation and getting comfortable with that is learning *ujjayi* breathing technique itself. It is important to realize that in the Power Yoga practice, the breath changes and evolves with the practice. You cannot master the advanced levels of breathing in the first couple of weeks or months, any more than you can master the advanced postures. In chapter 4, for example, we will take the breath another step by adding internal locks,

called *bandhas,* to the practice. This process further helps to train and strengthen the intercostal and diaphragm muscles, thus increasing lung capacity, and strengthen the mind, thus increasing concentration. But for most of us, we can't possibly understand *bandhas* without learning the basics first.

People often ask actors how in the world they remember all those lines. As any actor knows, learning lines is only step one, the most basic of the basic. It's like learning steps in dance or scales in music. Only when you can do the lines or steps or scales forward, backward, and upside down can you begin to explore the true essence of your performing art.

In Sanskrit the prefix *uj* means "to expand," and the word *jayi* means "success: or "victory." Learning *ujjayi* breathing is the first step in learning the language of Power Yoga. Like an actor or dancer practices their lines or steps, we practice the conscious breathing of the *ujjayi* method in order to "expand" into our own "fullness" or "success." The yoga tradition tells us that if we can learn to control the breath, then we can one day control the mind.

If we wish to control the flow of something, for example people, traffic, water, or our breath, generally what we do is narrow the passageway through which these things move. Think of how when three lanes of traffic merge into one lane the flow of traffic is drawn out for what can seem like hours. It is the same with our breath. By consciously narrowing the passageway of the throat through which the air is moving, we are able to draw out and control the flow of our breath. *Ujjayi* breathing creates a unique hissing sound that is caused by this slight conscious constriction of the throat as the breath travels through the larynx and over the vocal cords. When we whisper, the same action that softens the speech, creates the sound in *ujjayi.* As the throat passageway is narrowed, the velocity of the air traveling through it is increased. This is what generates the sound. Although *ujjayi* is done with the mouth closed, the easiest way to learn it at first is with the mouth open.

Begin by whispering an "ahhh" or "urrr" sound with the mouth open on an exhalation. Completely empty the lungs with the sound. Then inhale by whispering the "ahhh" or "urrr" sound. Completely fill the lungs with the inhale. Then do it with the mouth closed. You will notice a soft aspirant sound on the inhale and a throaty sibilant sound on the exhale—much like a closed-mouth whisper. This is *ujjayi* breathing, or at least the beginnings of it.

If you will watch your breath while you are exercising or just going about your daily activities, you will notice tremendous fluctuation. Sometimes it is slow, sometimes fast, sometimes deep, sometimes shallow. This invariably relates to the level of stress present, whether physical or psychological. If you are running or climbing stairs or lifting weights, obviously the breath is faster. If you are scared or anxious, the breath is more shallow.

But more than the level of stress, the breath relates to the activities of the mind. When the mind is level, the breath is level. When the mind is excited and jumping around, the breath is irregular. When the mind is heavy and lethargic, the breath is often labored and laden.

In Yoga philosophy, *prana,* or life force, is said to be the master of the mind. And the master of *prana* is sound. The sound created in *ujjayi* breathing is an important aspect of the practice. The sound of the breath gives the mind something to focus on. Listening to this sound is an attentiveness-training technique, and enables us to practice mindfulness. The act of listening to the breath refines the breath and quiets the mind. By somewhat restricting the flow of air through the throat and across the larynx and epiglottis, we produce a constant flow, a fixed pattern.

As you establish this set pattern of breathing, the mind will follow. If the mind isn't paying attention, you can't do *ujjayi,* because *ujjayi* breathing doesn't happen by itself. You have to create it anew with each breath. So if your mind wanders off, the breath falls off. It's not easy for a beginner to focus on nothing. So the sound provides something for the mind to concentrate on.

When the breathing pattern is always shifting, the way it is in day-to-day life, we can see that breathing is a reflection of the mind's activities. In yoga, we are trying to bring the mind under the control of the breath and eventually the *prana.* So it is just the opposite of what we are used to. Yoga philosophy says that if you can learn to control the breath, you may one day learn to control the mind.

One of the ways to train the mind to pay attention to the breath is to give it something steady to focus on. If the configuration is always changing, the mind can't and won't follow. If the breath is erratic in the yoga practice, it is hard for the attention to stay fixed. So much of our early work in this practice is developing steadiness of the breath.

Another way to look at this might be to think of a wood-burning stove. To get the cleanest and most efficient burn, you want to establish a controlled flow of oxygen into the stove. If the flow of air is erratic, you will not get a clean burn. If the air goes in too fast, the wood burns up quickly, wasting energy. This would correspond to rapid shallow panting in the practice, which would dissipate energy and reflect strain and struggle. Instead of feeling energized after practice, which is the way you are supposed to feel, you would feel depleted. This is not correct.

If the air flow is too slow, there will not be enough oxygen to keep the fire going; and the fire will go out and the stove will get cold. This corresponds to lazy, insubstantial breathing. The mind wanders, the breath falls off, and the heat of the practice drops off. This condition could also show up in practice as yawning. Yawning means not enough oxygen. If you yawn in practice, it means you are not breathing correctly and/or you are not paying attention (or you need to stop practice and nap!).

Remember that mastering *ujjayi* breathing, like anything else, takes practice and patience. Don't be frustrated if you don't get it immediately. Making the sound on the exhale is a little easier to accomplish than on the inhale, so perhaps work with the exhale at first. In the beginning you may feel like you are trying to clear your throat or cough up congestion. This generally means you are trying too hard. Doing this breathing correctly doesn't irritate your throat. So relax. It will come.

Ujjayi breathing is a very exciting training method that is little understood and infrequently taught in yoga classes. It was one of the "secret techniques" that few people had the opportunity to learn unless they went off to India to study with a yoga master who spoke English or their native language, whatever that might be. Yet it is a technique with such powerful benefits that it should be accessible to everyone. It is an essential tool that you will find yourself using in every aspect of your life. People from my classes are always writing, calling, or coming up to me after practice to comment on the effectiveness of this breathing method and how it has helped them to raise mindfulness, birth babies, diminish stress, and appreciate life more fully.

the generation of heat 3

THE SUN SALUTATIONS

*While we practice conscious breathing, our thinking will slow down, and we can give ourselves a real rest.
Most of the time, we think too much, and mindful breathing helps us to be calm, relaxed,
and peaceful. It helps us stop thinking so much and stop being possessed by sorrows
of the past and worries about the future. It enables us to be in touch
with life, which is wonderful in the present moment.*

THICH NHAT HANH, *Peace Is Every Step*

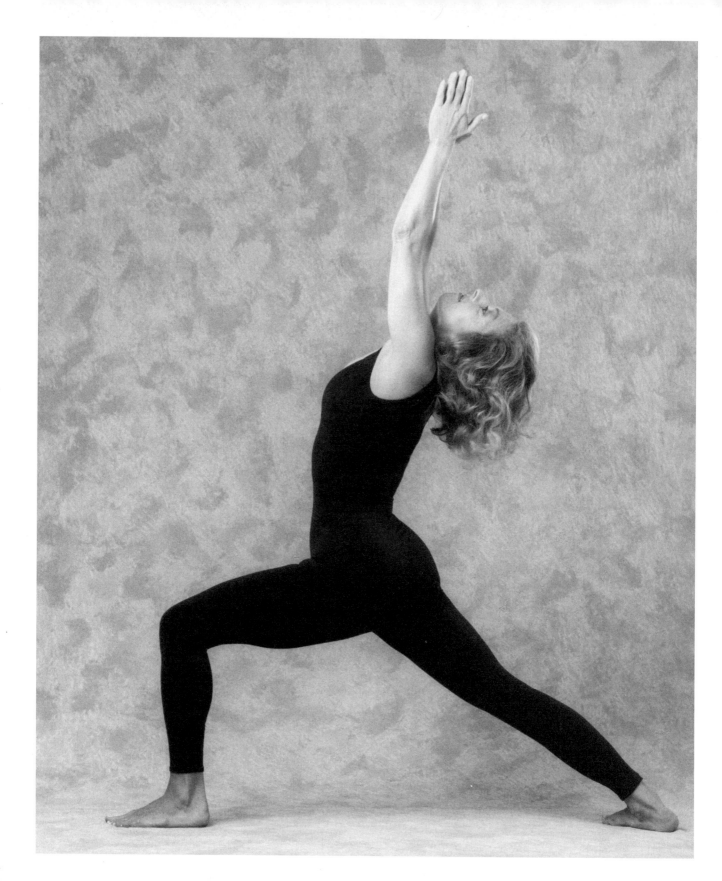

THE SUN SALUTATIONS

A COMPLETE WORKOUT

The first steps of the Power Yoga workout are the warm-ups, or Sun Salutations, as they are called (from the Sanskrit *surya namaskar,* which literally means "obeisance to the sun"). The Sun Salutations begin every practice and serve as the foundation for the entire form. They are a complete workout in themselves and act to loosen and heat up every joint and corner of the body. Like the complete Power Yoga form itself, their uniqueness lies in the fact that they are so comprehensive.

There are two sets of these Sun Salutations. The first is a grouping of nine positions and the second is a grouping of seventeen positions. In Power Yoga the spine is the structural core of all movement. The Sun Salutations begin the process of reawakening our awareness of the spine. Many of us, as a result of poor posture, injury, or specificity of training, have developed gross imbalances in the spine (which we will examine later in this chapter). Moving through the various positions of the Sun Salutations helps us begin to see the ways in which the range and freedom of motion of the spine has been restricted over the years, and to redevelop the natural agility of this remarkable backbone of the body.

If we were to analyze each step of the warm-ups, we would see how many different elements are included. We reach up and down. We stretch forward and backward. We use our arms to hold our weight. We use our legs to hold our weight. We contract the front of the body and the back of the body. We expand the front of the body and the back of the body.

Contraction and expansion are the hard and soft elements of Power Yoga. They are like action and rest. By first working a muscle, then resting or relaxing it, then working it again over and over throughout the form, the neuromusculature learns to distinguish between these two elemental conditions and to find its natural balance. Thus, the Sun Salutations begin the whole unique process of the Power Yoga workout, which is to contract and stretch, not only the same muscles sequentially, but opposing muscles simultaneously. This is one of the secrets to the unique success of this system.

HOT TO STRETCH

Compared with the effectiveness of the Sun Salutations, anything else you could think of to use as a warm-up would fall short. Jogging or a few rounds on an exercise bike, for example, would certainly wake up the legs and the cardiovascular system, but what about the upper body—the arms, shoulders, spine? Using aerobic sports as a warm-up will heat you systemically but will not provide the action/rest combination to all the muscle, or the range of motion-loosening to all the joints and connective tissues that need it.

Many of us attempt to stretch as a warm-up for our activities. But as Axiom No. 9 of the Power Yoga workout states, "Stretching does not equal warm-up!" You don't stretch to warm up muscles for activity. You have to warm up before stretching—or, in this case, before you start the *asanas,* or postures—and then work hard enough during your practice to keep the heat up. Remember Axiom No. 1 of the Power Yoga workout, which is, "You have to be *hot* to stretch"—not warm, not just out of a hot bath (although that helps), not "not cold," but hot from the inside out. Sweating. Stretching when you are cold or stiff is not only completely useless, it is dangerous. Stretching after an aerobic workout while cooling down is quite a bit safer than trying to stretch while you are cold, but it is still not particularly effective.

The totally unique premise here is that you are stretching only while the sweating mechanism is turned on. There are basically five elements that contribute to sweating and keeping the heat turned on during the practice: (1) *ujjayi* breathing, which was explained in chapter 2; (2) concentration, or "mindfulness," and (3) static muscular contraction, both of which we will begin to work with in this chapter; (4) *vinyasa,* or "flow," which refers to the connecting movement between the postures; and (5) *bandhas,* or internal locks or contractions, which we will learn about in chapter 4.

At first, learning all five factors seems a bit overwhelming. "How can I possibly think about breathing and *bandhas,* whatever they are, plus work hard, pay attention, and remember the connecting movement?" you might ask yourself. Getting a law degree, writing a thesis, composing a symphony, crocheting a quilt, painting a house, or painting the ceiling of the Sistine Chapel all seem a bit overwhelming, too, when we first have the idea to begin. But people get them accomplished.

Eventually these five components come together like a confluence of rivers, flowing together effortlessly, forming one focused stream of energy, and following the course directed by their banks. Now that you are about to begin the warm-ups, you will start to experience some of these components of the practice. Work with them one at a time, focusing on each singly as we work with it. Be patient.

TAKING THE PLUNGE

Take your time with this chapter. Give your attention to each position of the two Sun Salutations. The practice is built in small increments; any misalignment early in the form will be compounded later in the series. Therefore, start from the very first day to look for proper alignment, not perfection of the posture.

Often in a beginning class I will say, "What we are doing here is imposing order on chaos," with chaos representing lack of awareness, or "un"-consciousness that translates physically as some imbalance. In this practice we are *reconnecting* the body to consciousness. The emphasis here is not to force these techniques on tight, "unconscious" parts of the body, but rather to awaken the tight areas through mindfulness. Once we bring our attention inward and become aware of these limitations and blocks, we will start to refind our original and natural state of rhythm and balance. So, when I say that in this practice we are imposing order on chaos, what I mean is not that we are attempting to force a square peg into a round hole, but that we are slowly allowing the memory of our natural order and balance to awaken, penetrate the cells, and replace the disorder.

DON'T FORGET TO BREATHE

This all sounds great, you say, but how exactly do we "reconnect the body to consciousness" and "reawaken the tight areas"? You may be thinking, "Look, I move! I lift weights, run, bike, kayak, dance, play tennis, whatever, and all I get is tight. How is this movement alone going to 'reawaken' me when other forms of movement don't? How is it different?" Good question. *Astanga yoga* is based on the principle that changes in consciousness can be brought about by setting in motion currents of subtle forces in the physical body. So the first step is to make the body a healthy and fit vehicle for the movement and manipulation of these forces. The movement alone isn't going to set in motion these currents and reawaken you. What connects the body to consciousness is the breath, and it is the movement combined with *ujjayi* breathing that is the distinctive element of this practice.

In Yoga Swami Svatmarama's *Hatha Yoga Pradipika,* the ancient, classical Sanskrit text on yoga, it says that the mind is the lord of the body, and *prana,* or life force, is the lord of the mind (chapter 11, verses 29–30). Since *prana* is first experienced by us as breath, we notice that it is the breath that is acting as the bridge between the movement and our consciousness. So, as the breathing gets stronger, our awareness of the orderly arrangement of our body increases; as the alignment in the postures improves, the breath flows more easily and with more power. In a way, it's a catch-22. The breath has to be there for the postures and the postures have to be there for the breath. Which comes first? Another good question.

From my own experience, I can tell you they sort of evolve together. As the neuromusculature opens up and awareness or consciousness comes back into formerly tight or unconscious areas, the breathing becomes stronger, smoother, and more powerful. As the breathing develops and advances, the postures become easier and you will feel your body connecting back to its source, back to consciousness.

As the link between action and awareness, the breath is one of the most important elements of actually doing the *asanas,* or postures. It is used as a tool to enliven and facilitate the practice of the form. Eventually, each position of the Sun Salutation is accompanied by either an inhale or an exhale. But in the beginning you will have so much to pay attention to that just keeping the breath flowing evenly will be a major challenge. So if you aren't able to synch up the breath with the movement at the very first, don't worry. It takes a while for most of us.

THE RED FERRARI

Remember, the warm-ups are meant to be progressive. This means that you start very slowly and carefully, moving with great awareness—taking time to *feel* the tightness, the energy, the overall condition of your body. As you warm up, the movement starts to flow a little easier. Once you learn the basic alignment, and your neuromusculature familiarizes itself with the movement, your objective will be to link the breath and the movement together in a harmonious, orchestrated dance. It doesn't necessarily mean you get faster; you just get smoother.

Imagine a red Ferrari sitting in your driveway on a cold and snowy January morning. You need to drive it to work. What do you do? Most likely you go out and start it up easily, letting it warm up a bit before you drive off. What you don't do is go out, turn it over, stomp on the accelerator, and tear off down the road. If you want peak performance from your automobile, you warm it up progressively!

Keep in mind that the oil that lubricates the engine parts is practically frozen, sort of like the lubrication in your own body when you first wake up. You don't jump out of bed and race out the door at top speed—at least, most of us don't. We need time to wake up. But what I really mean is that we need time to warm up the oil in our engine and get it flowing. That is what the Sun Salutations do. They warm up and wake up the system—the cells, the organs, the muscles—and get the blood (oil) flowing!

DON'T ENVY FLEXIBILITY

As you work with the photos and instructions, be careful not to compare flexibility! For many of you it will take ten years to achieve the levels of flexibility seen in some of the postures. Don't envy flexibility. It is easy to be flexible if you sit around on your butt doing nothing. It is not easy to be flexible if you train. Training makes you tight, as I have explained. You have to work hard to get tight. So don't be embarrassed by tightness.

I can tell you from my own experience that it takes years of regular practice to develop one's suppleness. I didn't start out flexible, either. I was extremely tight in my shoulders, hips, thighs (both front and back), calves, and Achilles tendons. I was a majorette in high school and the New Jersey state champion in 1959 (ah, the sweet nostalgia of the good old fifties!). I trained like a fiend. The constant work with the baton, and the training for the competitions I entered, totally shut down the range of motion in my shoulders. Then I went on to become a cheerleader at Syracuse University for four years. We didn't exactly *train* in the early sixties, but we did practice for a few weeks before football season began and during the season. There were lots of big arm movements that further tightened the shoulder muscles. I also played lacrosse at Syracuse, which added another layer of tightness to my shoulders and introduced tightness in my hamstrings (muscles at the back of the thighs) from the running. I skied nearly every day for seven straight winters while living in Colorado, and skiing, like cycling or skating, strengthens and tightens the quads (front of the thighs). My calves and Achilles tendons were dramatically shortened from wearing high heels a lot in the late sixties. So when I started this yoga practice, I was pretty much a basket case in terms of flexibility.

GETTING STARTED

The practice of the Power Yoga workout begins with the directive to "bring the feet together." The entire practice is built on the feet and awareness of the feet, and I can tell you unequivocally that no external bodily part is less connected to consciousness than the feet! After telling thousands of people standing around in yoga classes over the years to come to at-

tention and bring their feet together, I can further tell you that compliance with this instruction is diverse and imaginative. If you want to get to know someone, check out their feet. Feet are astonishing. They are misused, abused, and neglected. Occasionally they are well treated, but more often than not they are ignored.

My husband, Thom, was a track-and-field All-American at the University of Houston, a school famous for its track-and-field athletes from the late sixties through the eighties. Thom went on to become a world-class runner and ran professionally until he was sidelined by Achilles tendon surgery in 1981. We met the following year and he started doing daily yoga practice. The doctors had told him after surgery that he would probably never run again. Yet a year later he won a race in San Francisco, and several years later he regained his national ranking.

Thom started teaching yoga with me in the mideighties after three years as the tightest but most dedicated, hardworking yoga student ever. Needless to say, he is pretty tuned into his feet, but most people aren't. Thom says that "because feet are the farthest thing from the brain, people tend to forget about them altogether, unless, of course, they hurt or stop functioning."

In biomechanical terms, feet can only do four things: they pronate (roll in), they supinate (roll out), they dorsiflex (pull the toes back), and they plantarflex (point the toes). All balance or imbalance in the way we stand or walk and run comes as a result of the interplay of these four movements.

Take your shoes off. Stand up and bring your feet together with the big toes, heels, and ankles touching. Is this possible? Can you touch your big toes, or do the big toes turn out as a result of bunions or bone spurs? Are your feet balanced or imbalanced? Imbalance in the feet or irregular bone structure can be the first indication of a potential for injury in training, especially in a sport that involves running, for example. Are your feet flat? Flat feet are an indication of excessive pronation, or inward rolling, and particularly in runners, will inevitably be accompanied by knee problems.

Many runners try orthotics (individually molded plastic foot supports that are inserted in shoes and change weight distribution and foot plant) to solve problems such as excessive pronation. The good thing about orthotics is that they change the contact point and the body alignment immediately, thus taking the stress off an injured area and allowing it to begin to heal. Yoga practice will do the same thing, only it takes a lot longer. Orthotics are a good, quick patch-me-up, and if you have an acute problem (i.e., pain) and need to run a race this weekend, orthotics can often get you through it.

But as a long-term solution to imbalance, I do not recommend orthotics. Over and over again I see people who become dependent on orthotics, and no sooner does one problem get solved than another surfaces somewhere else. The flaw in orthotics is that they treat the symptom, not the cause of the problem. If the cause is imbalance, propping up the weak spot can serve as a temporary solution. But a lasting solution requires correcting the structural imbalance, and this is most effectively done with your yoga practice. Ideally, *astanga yoga* would be prescribed along with every set of orthotics, slowly taking over the process of long-term restructuring begun by the orthotics. You would actually use your yoga workout to correct an imbalance like pronation, for example, by consciously and repeatedly shifting the weight toward the outside of your feet throughout practice, thereby developing and strengthening the arches.

So the first step is to take a look at your feet, get to know them, be aware how you stand, and deliberately attempt to balance the feet as you begin work in yoga. The weight of the body is distributed in three places in the foot—in the ball of the foot behind the big toe, in the ball of the foot behind the third and fourth toes, and in the center of the heel. Is a third of your body weight being supported at each of these points in the feet? Can you feel the weight distribution? Try shifting around, feeling the pressure in each of these three points. Then try to find balance. In the beginning, correcting an imbalance in the way you stand may feel very peculiar and not at all stable. But eventually, with

practice and awareness the new stance will become normal. A good analogy for this feeling might be to try brushing your teeth with the hand you don't normally use. In the beginning you would feel totally inept and awkward. However, if you kept at it, it would get easier and feel more customary. It's the same with changing the way you stand.

Bring your feet together, big toes touching. Your arms are at your sides. Relax the shoulders and roll them backward, slightly pressing the shoulder blades (scapula) toward one another. This will open the chest and lift the rib cage. This posture is called *tadasana,* or Mountain Posture (Figure 3.1). This is the starting and finishing point for all the standing

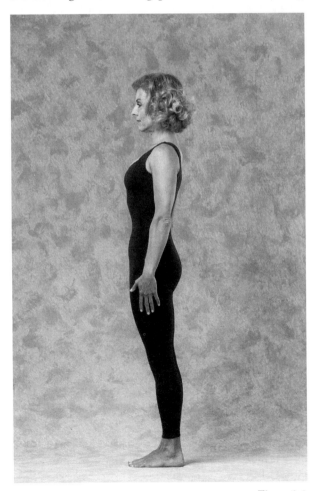

Figure 3.1

postures in chapter 4, and important to understand right from the start. In Figures 3.2 through 3.6 we show some of the postural and spinal imbalances that can exist due to tightness and/or weakness in a variety of muscles, and that can affect the form of Mountain Posture.

The first, Figure 3.2, shows a common misalignment of the spine called, simply, "forward head." This is probably the most frequent example of structural imbalance that I come across in my classes and workshops. It is most common in runners, both male and female, but is also prevalent in the general public and fitness community. It can be caused simply by poor postural habits, too much sitting or desk working, poor self-image, or years of unawareness. Correctly, the head should be at the top of the spine, as in Figure 3.1, not in front of it.

Forward head is often accompanied by the following irregularity. Figure 3.3 shows an exaggerated curve in the upper (thoracic) back. This condition is called *kyphosis*, an abnormal backward curvature of the spine resulting in a "hump" or exaggerated rounding of the upper back, and is often characterized by a caved-in appearance in the chest and accompanied by tight muscles at the front of the shoulders (pectorals) or front of the rib cage (inter-

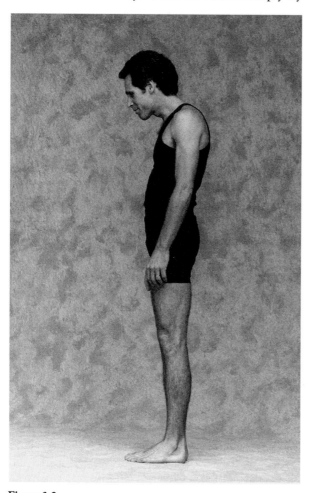

Figure 3.2

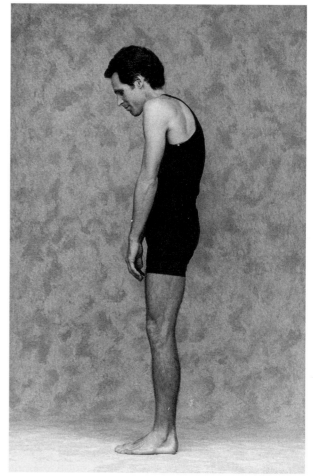

Figure 3.3

costals). It is a very typical condition in runners, cyclists, and skaters. In runners it can be caused by forward lean, the action of the arms, and probably most of all by the extreme tightening that happens at the back of the legs in the hamstring muscles. Generally, the better a runner and the longer she or he has been running, the worse the condition.

In skaters and cyclists, the rounding is caused by the overtraining of the "lats," the latissimus dorsi muscles, which are the big back muscles used when you chop wood, for example. These muscles are the lumbar flexors and the muscles that flex the lumbar or lower back. They are responsible for rounding or bending the back forward. They are paired with the lumbar extensors, the long, ropy muscles that go up the center of the back on either side of the spine (erector spinae) and straighten or lengthen the back. If you watch skaters or cyclists training, you can see how they spend hours bent over from the waist, pulling with the arms and pumping with the quadriceps, or thigh muscles. It is this type of specificity of training, or training for long periods of time at the same sport using the same muscles, that slowly forms the structural irregularities that we see in Figures 3.2 through 3.6.

In Figure 3.4 we see an exaggerated lower-back (lumbar) curve, or *lordosis,* the abnormal forward curvature of the spine. This is extremely common in runners and athletes who participate in running sports, as well as in skiers, cyclists, and skaters. It is generally associated with tight hip flexor muscles, in particular the iliopsoas and psoas muscles, and/or weak abdominals. As in kyphosis, this condition, when found in runners or other athletes, is generally proportioned in severity to the quality and quantity of training. For example, the higher the legs are lifted in running, the tighter the hip flexors become, so oftentimes the most elite runners have the most pronounced structural irregularities because of specificity and frequency of training. Figure 3.5 shows a combination of Figures 3.3 and 3.4.

Let's look at the effect of lordosis in another sport—say golf, for instance. Although playing golf doesn't actually cause lordosis the way running can, the constant hip-and-shoulder rotation of the golf swing, when loaded on to an exaggerated lower-back curve, *can* initiate back problems, such as inflamed, bulging, or slipped discs, and cause pain through pressure on nerves.

In Figure 3.6, we see a left/right asymmetry that can be found not only in the shoulders, as illustrated, but in the hips as well. Generally, when one shoulder is higher than another, I look for unequal muscular development, which may have been caused by playing a sport that predominantly uses only one side of

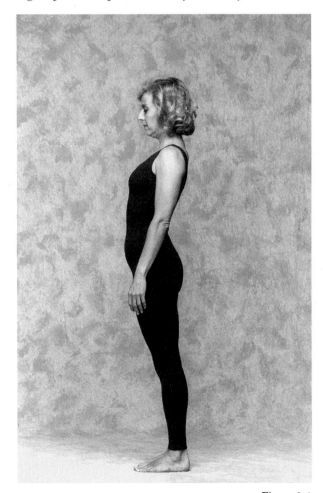

Figure 3.4

the body, such as tennis, squash, or racquetball. Unevenness in the shoulders can also result from an old injury, like falling on one shoulder while skiing, or falling off a bike onto one side. The resultant trauma tightens up, or shrinks, the injured area and causes lateral imbalance. After months and years this can show up as an irregular shoulder comportment.

The same things can cause hip asymmetry. Many of us have been to chiropractors who have told us we have uneven leg lengths. We feel distorted. But what the chiropractor may have neglected to tell us is that almost everyone has uneven leg lengths. Why? Do you generally stand on one foot? Did you crash into the catcher while sliding into home plate back in Little League or even just last spring? Remember that baby you carried on one side for a year? Living creates imbalance if we don't pay attention. Awareness of how you carry yourself can begin to even out the jagged edges.

Now that we have looked at some of the more common postural deviations we might have, and begun to have some awareness of the work we need to do, let's get started.

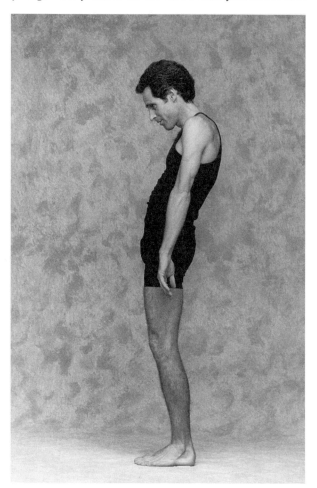

Figure 3.5

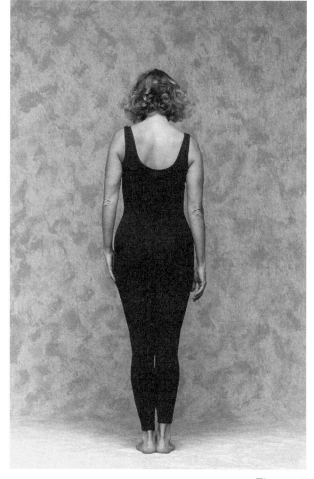

Figure 3.6

TIPS AND PRECAUTIONS

WHEN TO PRACTICE

It is best to practice either in the morning or later in the afternoon toward evening. In the morning our energy levels are generally higher than they are later in the day. It is also easier to concentrate, as the mind hasn't yet been assaulted by the stress and distractions of the day. But, on the other hand, our body is stiff and the postures may seem difficult. Regular practice, however, will diminish the stiffness, and the *asanas* will become easier.

When we practice at the end of the day, our body is more flexible and moves more easily, so the postures are easier and the practice seems "better." But our energy is generally lower and our concentration isn't as clean and clear.

Practice in the morning is energizing. It gives us vigor and focus to work more efficiently and enjoyably at our job. There is a feeling you have after practice (which I alluded to in chapter 1), that makes you feel as though the tough part of your day is over, and that anything else that happens, barring disaster, you'll be able to handle. Practice at the end of the day is relaxing. It removes fatigue from the day's strain and tension, clears out the cobwebs from the brain, and encourages a deep and peaceful sleep.

The important thing is to practice, whenever you can. I encourage people to find the time to do a *minimum* of fifteen or twenty minutes, four or five days a week. It makes a big difference in the effectiveness of the program and the rate of progress.

FOOD

Whenever you decide to do your practice, it is best not to have a bellyful of food. Always practice on an empty stomach. I generally recommend not eating at least three to four hours before practice, depending on the nature of the meal. Rice and veggies are digested fairly quickly and easily. A heavy meal might take half a day! If you feel that you need something before starting, you may want a cup of tea or coffee, or perhaps a bit of banana or apple for energy. Many of the postures increase intra-abdominal pressure and affect the internal organs. Practicing with food in the stomach might cause discomfort, dizziness, or nausea. It is also best that the bladder and bowels be empty as well.

COMMITMENT

Wellness and balance of the mind and body will not come about just because you decided to buy this book. You need to be strongly motivated to work on yourself and develop the discipline to practice on a regular basis. As I frequently tell people in our classes, "Signing up for the course isn't enough. Just coming to class isn't enough."

My husband, Thom, always tells people in class,

"Do you know what this will do for you if you just come to class once a week and that's all?" Then he waits for a minute while people ponder the answer. "Nothing!"

We encourage people to bring the same spirit to their yoga practice that they do to their other training. If you are preparing for your first triathlon, for example, you don't just run or swim or hop on your bike when the weather is nice. You have to train regularly, whether you feel like it or not. Jon Kabat-Zinn relates in *Full Catastrophe Living* what he tells patients at his stress clinic with regard to their practice: "You don't have to like it; you just have to do it. When the eight weeks are over, you can tell us whether it was of any use or not. For now just keep practicing." I love that!

For me, making time for regular practice is one way of reminding me of the first *anga,* or limb, of *astanga* yoga. Remember as I explained in chapter 1, the first limb is *yama.* There are five *yamas,* and the first of these is *ahimsa,* which means "nonviolence," or "reverence for life." (The *yamas* are sort of the ethical tenets of the practice, and along with the five *niyamas,* which I explain later, are like the Ten Commandments of yoga). When I make time for my practice each day, I feel as if I am consciously attempting to practice reverence for myself, which is a good place to start and definitely makes it easier to extend this practice of nonviolence to the rest of the planets' inhabitants.

The other four *yamas* are *satya,* which means "truth"; *asteya,* or "non-stealing"; *aparigraha,* or "non-accumulation, non-greed"; and *brahmacharya,* which literally means "to walk with God," and which I define as "walking with your own sense of Higher Consciousness." The discipline of creating space for my own work on myself helps me to be more aware of all the *yamas.* It helps to simplify an ever increasingly complex life and makes it easier to follow ecologically sound principles like "don't accumulate a lot of stuff," and "don't take what isn't yours," and "tell the truth"—you know, simple stuff that your grandmother used to tell you. This all helps me to

tread more lightly and consume less. How amazing that such an ancient system would contain such applicable truths for an overburdened planet and its overconsumed resources, eh?

So it is important to find a way to keep yourself motivated to practice. Often, as is the case with many of our clients in classes, people are motivated by their desire to return to their running or dancing or golf or whatever. They are injured and have had to cut back or quit exercising. They have been to a half-dozen doctors and nobody has been able to solve their problem yet. Now they are excited by the fact that they have in their hands a technique that may enable them to solve their problem themselves.

However, finding the time to practice takes a little effort and thought. For many of us, already feeling maxed out in terms of time constraints, being told that we need to set aside more time five days a week to do something else is in itself stressful. As you make your wellness and wholeness a priority, you will find it becomes easier to protect your practice by creating a special place and time in which to work on yourself.

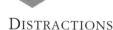

DISTRACTIONS

Work barefoot, in a clean space that is free of obstacles and distractions. Make this place as comfortable and uniquely your "practice place" as possible. Obviously, if you have a huge house in the country, it may be possible to set aside one room just for your practice, with a few motivational photos or art pieces or anything else that offers incentive to be present, mindful, and attentive. For many of you who live in small city apartments, you might need to be a bit more creative in designing your practice environment. Perhaps you might use one object—such as a vase of flowers, a piece of music, a trophy, a photo, or something representative of your goals for yourself—to help create the mood, in a Pavlovian sense.

It's best not to have to look at the phone, your desk, the vacuum cleaner, the cookie jar, the coffeemaker, etc. All of these material objects can suddenly loom up as important items for your immediate attention, which makes it difficult to stay focused on your practice. I cannot tell you how easy it is to be coming upon a difficult posture, see the vacuum cleaner, and decide that it's time to clean house.

I unplug my phone when it's time for my practice. This is not always easy, especially when I am expecting an important or exciting phone call. But I tell myself that without my regular practice, without taking the time to work on myself and tune my own instrument, I am not as mindful and whole a human being as I would like to be and certainly am not providing the example that is necessary to be effective as a teacher of a discipline.

BATHING

It is important to be clean for practice, particularly if you are working in a group or class situation. If you have a choice of bathing before or after practice, it is probably better to bathe before. When you first start this training, you may notice a strong or unusual body odor. This is not uncommon among people just beginning yoga practice. The practice starts to cleanse and detoxify the body in unique ways, and old toxins stuck in the body for days or even years will begin to be dislodged. So you will probably want to shower after as well.

After three to six weeks, the odor should be gone, depending, of course, on your diet. Meat eaters have a much stronger body odor than vegetarians do. Yet even persons who have been vegetarians for many years may notice strange and unpleasant odors emanating from themselves when they first begin practice, as the old vestiges of meat are cleansed from the body. Eventually, when your practice becomes regu-

lar and strong, and if your diet is pure, your sweat will be heavy but odor-free. The sweat will, however, make your body a little sticky, so you might want to rinse off before bed.

I like to take a hot shower or bath before practice—especially in the morning, as it helps to warm and loosen up the body. But more importantly, I like to be clean.

The second limb of *astanga yoga* is *niyama.* There are five *niyamas,* or "observances," as I explained in chapter 1, and the first is *saucha,* which means "purity" and refers to cleanliness of the mind and body. (The other four *niyamas* are *santosha,* which means "contentment"; *tapas,* which means "to burn" mental and physical impurities through your practice; *svadhyaya,* or "study of spiritual books"; and *Ishvara-pranidhana,* which literally means "surrender to or worship of God," or we might say, respect for a higher universal energy.)

Cleanliness of the body is essential for well-being, both physical and mental, and is an important element of correct yoga practice. I generally make a generic announcement in class about cleanliness: Be aware of how you smell. Many people aren't! And men and women are unaware in different ways. Always wear clean clothes. If you have only one set of yoga workout clothes, *always* wash them before you wear them again—and that includes undergarments!

WATER

If you observe an animal, any animal (except maybe a camel), over a period of twenty-four hours, you will notice that it drinks water frequently. Not tea, coffee, cola, or Perrier, but water. Everybody needs water. The absolutely first thing I ask people who come to me for nutritional consultation is, "How much water do you drink every day?" I've found many people don't drink enough water, and often not *any* water! This is an invitation to disease and imbalance.

Water is essential, not only for life, but for balance between the two primary intra- and extracellular minerals in the body, potassium and sodium, and for proper functioning of the organs and systems of the body. Water must be drunk daily, on an empty stomach and in large quantities. What is a large quantity? I start off the day with a liter or quart bottle. It's not easy. It's not fun, I'll be honest. I don't drink much coffee anymore, but water still doesn't taste nearly as good to me as a cup of coffee made from freshly ground, freshly roasted beans with a third of a cup of half-and-half. But . . . let's face it, caffeine takes its toll, like fat or sugar. I don't care how many studies they do hyping the positive effects of caffeine on training. The bottom line is that caffeine is hell on the adrenals and the liver. If you want good health, you limit your intake of caffeine or don't use it at all. One cup of coffee a day isn't too bad, but if you are a woman with a high risk of developing fibrocystic breasts, for example, it's important to know that if you don't use any caffeine, you may prevent or reverse the condition. So we all make our choices.

You will lose a tremendous amount of water from the body through sweating while doing this practice. If you do not replace this fluid, you are at risk of dehydration. Therefore, you must drink water. Not right before practice, not during, and not for at least thirty minutes after practice.

This means drinking water on a regular basis. Always drink water on an empty stomach. Do not drink it with or after meals. This dilutes the digestive process and diminishes the absorption of nutrients gained from the food you eat. Tea and coffee and bubbly water don't count as water. Anytime there is anything in water besides H_2O, the body treats it as food, and it requires effort on the part of the body. The nice thing about water in the body is that it goes straight through, flushing out the system, without requiring much work from any of the component parts. It is extremely cleansing. One good way to tell if you are drinking enough water is by the color and odor of

your urine. If it is dark yellow and strong in smell, you are not drinking enough water. Unless you ate asparagus the night before, your urine should not be strong-smelling. One good way to tell how much water to drink is to keep drinking until your urine is clear and odor-free. This is best done first thing in the morning when the stomach is empty and there is no digestion going on to divert or slow down the process. End to end, the whole operation shouldn't take more than an hour. Drink water. Develop the habit.

WOMEN'S CONDITIONS: MENSTRUATION AND PREGNANCY

Back in the old days in India, and I'm not so sure that this still isn't true there today, a Brahman yogi would barely even touch or teach a woman, much less one who was menstruating or pregnant! So the provisions that *asana* practice should not be done by menstruating or pregnant women were set down by a patriarchal society. I can actually think of several contemporary *hatha* yoga books that very explicitly say that women should "not practice *asanas* during menstruation," and further that "practicing *asanas* during menstruation may cause cramps and excessive bleeding." These particular books were written either by men or by female disciples of male Indian gurus directing American yoga ashrams (religious communities). My guess, in the case of the women, is that this is what they have been taught by their male gurus, and not something they have observed from their own practice. Since the postures demonstrated in these same books are rather sloppy, I would further conclude that none of these "authors" have a particularly strong *asana* practice.

Moreover, nothing could be further from the truth, according to my particular experience. I doubt if many women have done more strenuous and intense *hatha* yoga training than I have done since 1980. From my own experience I can tell you that, for me, doing strong *asana* practice before, during, and after menstruation is extremely beneficial and reduces cramping and symptoms of premenstrual syndrome. Regular strong practice, barring any medical problems, should eliminate cramps altogether. I *do* find that the rate of flow does increase for the first day or so, but the duration of the menses is decreased. The bleeding is quite heavy for two days and then it is over, which in my opinion is natural, healthy, and preferable to dragging out the whole ordeal for seven or eight days.

When occasionally I might feel a bit tired the first day or two of the cycle, I simply take it easy and shorten the practice somewhat, then have a long rest afterward. However, what works for me may not work for you. Listen to your own body, and if it says to take a few days off during menstruation, then that should be your final word.

The inverted postures should not be done while menstruating, as they reverse the natural downward gravitational pull of the menstrual flow from the body. You don't want this discarded blood-lining from the uterus to flow back into the body, so don't stand on your head, or do a shoulder stand, a hand stand, or any of the upside-down postures while you have your period.

As far as what to do when you are pregnant, nothing can be more wonderful for your heart, head, and body while carrying a child than doing yoga. It is absolutely the best form of exercise you can do, particularly the aspect of the breath work. I have files of letters from many, many women who have been students and gone on to be mothers, who say they used *ujjayi* breathing while giving birth because it totally surpasses all the other breathing techniques commonly taught. But ideally, the practice should be started *before* you become pregnant, or at least during the first or second month. After that point, you would need to proceed very slowly and carefully under the guidance of a skilled prenatal yoga therapist.

Some postures like Bound Angle Posture and Seated Angle Posture are excellent for the lower back at all times. Other postures, like back-bending, or even Face Up Dog in the Sun Salutations, should be eliminated or modified after the third or fourth month, as back-bending stretches the front of the body, and after the fetus begins to develop, such bending should not be done. But a carefully supervised pre- and postnatal yoga program is an excellent way to maintain fitness and health and to help ensure a happy, healthy baby.

BREATH AND GAZE

Keep in mind that during this practice, all breathing will be through the nose only; the mouth is kept closed. This particular method is called *ujjayi* breathing, as explained in detail in chapter 2, and is intended to help keep the mind steady and quiet. Another key aspect of the practice and also a means to help keep the mind smooth and focused is the *drishti,* or gazing point. Every posture in this practice has a gazing point. Sometimes the gaze is up, sometimes at the tip of the nose or straight out past the end of the nose, and sometimes to the side. In more advanced yoga practice, the *drishtis* are also more advanced. Technically, there are nine *drishtis.* Instead of just "up," the gaze might be at the point between the eyebrows. Or instead of "out," it might be directly at the center of the nose.

Generally, the gaze is simply in the direction the head is going. Gazing will improve the vision by exercising the eye muscles and the optic nerve, while increasing the blood flow. The important thing is to practice keeping the eyes focused on one point. Eventually, this will help lead the mind to be steadfast and still.

As we all have experienced in trying to have a conversation with someone whose eyes are darting around, it's a fairly safe assumption that you don't have their full attention! While I was working on the second draft of this book, I received a note from a woman in one of our classes that perfectly illustrates what wandering eyes can do to the mind. Her note read in part: "I had been feeling sort of sorry for myself, wondering why everyone else got to be married and have children except me. There I was struggling with Extended Hand-to-Toe Pose, still feeling sorry for myself and looking around to see how everybody else was doing. All of a sudden I heard Thom's [my husband, who was teaching the class] voice ring out: 'Don't look around to see where everyone else is at. *It won't help.'* I realized in a flash that that was true about everything in life. I felt so much better. Now I know why I love this yoga so much."

As you stand at attention, listen to the sound that you have learned to make with the *ujjayi* breathing and keep the gaze steady out in front of you. This attention on the breath and the gaze begins the whole process of the practice of developing the concentration. Don't fidget. Attempt to be still and just stand and listen to your breath for thirty seconds. Every cell of the body should be focused and ready to begin practice.

CONTRAINDICATIONS

There are a few conditions that preclude the practice of certain postures. These cautions and provisions will be listed individually under the particular postures that are contraindicated for various conditions. In general, inverted postures (upside-down positions like a headstand or shoulder stand) should not be done by persons suffering from high blood pressure, detached retina, glaucoma, pressure in the ears, obesity, back pain, spinal injuries, or dizziness. Also, if you have recently undergone surgery or have any serious physical illness or disease, it is imperative that you check with your physician before beginning this practice.

I work one-on-one with many people who are seriously ill, so it is truly possible, as I said in chapter 1, to start the Power Yoga practice at any age in any condition. Nevertheless, these persons are under close supervision, both by me and by their medical doctor.

Warm-up or Sun Salutation A

SURYA NAMASKARA A

Mountain Posture, or *Tadasana*

Bring the feet together, arms at the sides, as we saw in Figure 3.1. The chest is lifted, gaze is steady, straight ahead, with the chin tucked slightly in toward the chest. This is Mountain Posture, as already described—or "attention position." In Sanskrit, the command for attention is *sama-sthiti*. *Sama* means "same," "even," or "equal" and *sthiti* means "state," "condition," or "stability." Thus, *sama-sthiti* means "standing still and straight." Throughout the practice, there will continually be the command of *sama-sthiti*. This means to return to Mountain Posture or attention position.

Position 1

Inhale (Figure 3.7). Bring the arms straight up over the head, placing the palms together. Look up. Lift the kneecaps by tightening or flexing the thighs (quadricep muscles). Reach up as strongly as possible, lengthening the torso and lifting the rib cage. Don't arch the back or lean back.

Note: The lifting of the quadriceps muscles is what is called a "static contraction"—a tightening of a muscle without accompanying movement in the associated limb. A static contraction is the "hard," or sun, aspect of this practice. It takes energy and requires fuel to accomplish. Thus, it creates heat. Static contractions are an *extremely important* element of the practice and, as mentioned earlier in this chapter,

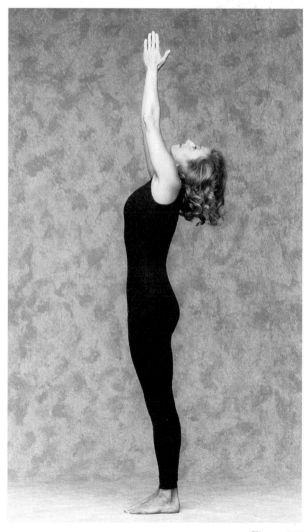

Figure 3.7

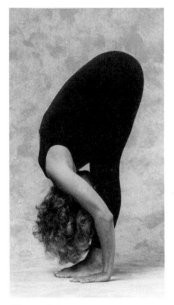

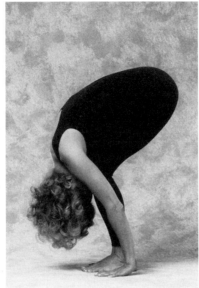

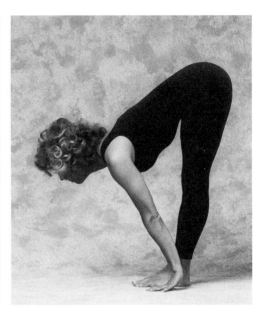

Figure 3.8   Figure 3.9   Figure 3.10

one of the five components of creating heat and keeping the sweating mechanism turned on. This procedure of static contraction will be referred to frequently throughout the book, and discussed in more detail in the next chapter.

POSITION 2

Exhale (Figure 3.8). Bring the palms to the floor, and tuck the head into the knees. Look toward the navel. For those persons with very tight hamstrings or lower-back problems, you must bend your knees here (Figure 3.9). Also, see the following section on modifications and/or problems.

POSITION 3

Inhale (Figure 3.10). Look up, lifting the chest and extending the back. More advanced or flexible readers will work with the legs straight as in Figure 3.10. However, most beginners will work with the knees bent (Figure 3.11).

POSITION 4

Exhale (Figure 3.12). This position is actually a posture called Four-Limbed Stick Posture (*Chaturanga Dandasana—chaturi* means "four," *anga* means "limb," and *danda* means "stick"). Walk the legs back, make the body stiff like a plank, and slowly lower the body to the floor as in a push-up position. The elbows are tucked in at the sides. Try to hold the body off the floor. If you cannot hold a push-up, put your knees down as you lower yourself to the floor. This will make the "push-up" easier and enable you to build up your upper-body strength so you can eventually do the position as shown in Figure 3.12. Look straight out in front of you.

POSITION 5

Inhale (Figure 3.13). This position is called Upward-Facing Dog Posture, or Face Up Dog (*Urdhva Muka Svanasana—urdhva* means "upward," *muka* means "face," and *svana* means "dog"). Turn the feet so the toes are pointed, as in plantar flexion

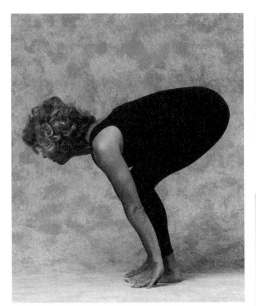

Figure 3.11

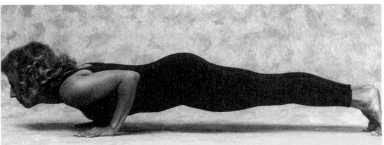

▲ Figure 3.12

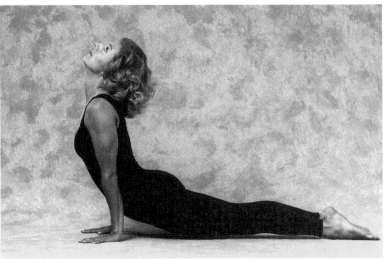

▲ Figure 3.13

position, and lift the body up onto the hands and the top of the feet. If this is too much work to begin or too much pressure on the lower back or the tops of the feet, keep the knees on the floor (Figure 3.14). Look up and back toward the ceiling or wall behind you.

Note of caution: This position will be extremely difficult for persons with tight feet or ankles. It can also create lower-back distress if done *incorrectly*. **Do not allow the back to sag or the shoulders to hunch up around the ears.** This will compress the lower back and can cause lower back discomfort. When done correctly, the lower back should not be uncomfortable. *If you have limited upper-body strength, tight feet or ankles, or lower-back problems, keep your knees on the floor (Figure 3.14) and see the section on modifications that follows.*

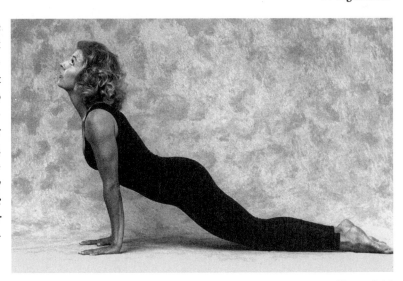

▲ Figure 3.14

POSITION 6

Exhale (Figure 3.15). This position is called Downward-Facing Dog Posture (*Adho Muka Svanasana*—*adho* means "downward," *muka* means "face," and *svana* means "dog"). Turn your toes back under (dorsiflex position) and push up and back into an upside-down **V** position, or as it is also called Face Down Dog. Your feet should be parallel and about ten to twelve inches apart, lined up with your hip bones, and your hands should be about the same distance apart, lined up with your shoulder blades. Make sure to flatten your palms and spread the fingers out evenly and push down on the heels. Look back "up" toward the navel. Keep the head relaxed.

Note: Don't worry about having your heels touch the floor. Most people's heels, especially in the case of runners, will be several inches off the floor. It took me about two years to get my feet flat on the floor.

TAKE FIVE COMPLETE BREATHS IN THIS POSITION.

While you are learning the movements, you will have plenty of work to do, and it will be difficult for you to pay attention to your breathing. However, in this position, as you hold for five breaths, you are going to have to pay attention to your breath in order to count the number of breaths. Try to begin here to listen to your breath as you count.

POSITION 7

Inhale (Figure 3.16). Step your feet, one at a time, back up to your hands. Look up. Lift the chest and extend the back. This is the same posture as Position 3. Make sure your feet are together, big toes touching. Most of you will be bending your knees, as in Figure 3.11, but don't squat. Only bend as much as necessary to get your hands on the floor.

POSITION 8

Exhale (Figure 3.17). Tuck your head into the knees and flex the back. If the back of your legs (hamstring muscles) are very tight, you must still bend your knees. This is the same move as Position 2. Look at the navel.

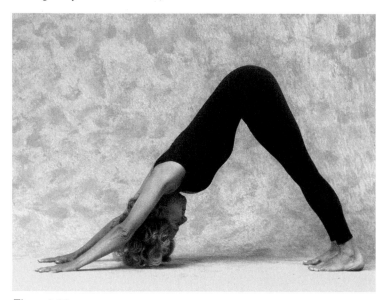

Figure 3.15

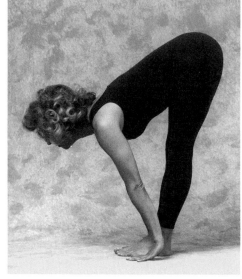

Figure 3.16

POSITION 9

Inhale (Figure 3.18). Come all the way back up to standing, arms straight up over the head, palms together. Look up, lift the kneecaps by tightening or flexing the thigh (quadricep) muscles, lift the rib cage, lengthen the torso and *strrrretch* up. You should feel and look as if you were being drawn up to the ceiling by a string attached to your middle fingers and connected through your spine to a point between your feet. I call the strength aspect of this move a "power lock." This means serious muscular output, in this case a blazing force of strength ascending through the arms all the way to the fingertips. This is the same as Position 1.
Sama-sthiti—Exhale, return to attention position.

This is where active rest occurs between repetitions. Active rest means that you are able to recover but you don't collapse. You should maintain "attention position." The mind stays focused. You don't have a vacation here. By maintaining the concentration between the warm-ups, you are maintaining the heat. It might be puzzling as to just how concentration affects heat. But the moment you aren't concentrating on what you are doing, you will see that the heat drops off. It takes concentration to hold the static contractions and to keep the breath going, for example. In fact, mindfulness is really the underlying component of all four of the other contributors (*ujjayi* breathing, effort or static muscular contraction, *vinyasa,* and *bandhas*) to the heat factor. Since each of them is a mindful activity—in other words, they must be done consciously—they don't happen if we aren't concentrating.

Attempt to do at least three repetitions of Sun Salutation A. If you are having any difficulties, look over the following for specific suggestions.

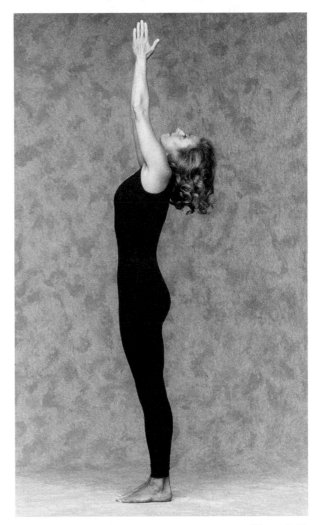

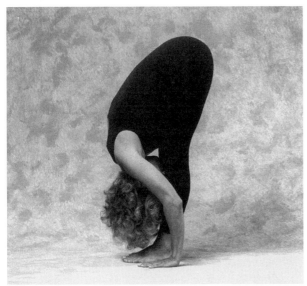

Figure 3.17

Figure 3.18

MODIFICATIONS FOR TIGHTNESS OR INJURY

The most common limitations that generally are associated with the Sun Salutations are weakness, tightness, or injury in the shoulders, neck, wrists, lower back, knees, feet, or ankles. Very often people will come up to me just before a class and say, "I just had arthroscopic surgery. Can I do this?" Or after a class they might say, "My wrists hurt. Is this good for me?" The answer to both of them is yes. And not only can they do it and is it good for them, but they desperately need to be doing it as well.

If you are coming into this practice with an injury, it is very important that you start slowly and pay careful attention to correct alignment. The practice *will* work for you if you don't overload yourself and you don't do things wrong. If you have a torn rotator cuff (shoulder injury), tendinitis in the wrists or Achilles tendon, a recovering sprained ankle or dislocated shoulder, back problems, knee problems, shin splints, or any number of hundreds of other injuries, this system will help you to recover. But you have to increase the work load on the recovering area *slowly*.

FOUR COMMON MISTAKES

There are four things that people frequently complain of in class, and all four are related to incorrect alignment as well as weakness or tightness.

One, the shoulders hurt. If your shoulders hurt while attempting to do the push-up, the most probable cause is weak upper-body strength and an attempt to compensate by hyperextending the shoulder on the descent into the push-up position. This is *not* correct form. When dropping into the push-up, you must avoid sagging between the shoulder blades into the lower back. This is bad for the back as well as the shoulders. If you can't do a push-up, put the knees down on the floor to take some of the weight off the arms. This will make the push-up easier and less stressful. Work to keep the torso stiff and touch chest to floor first.

Two, the wrists hurt. If your wrists hurt after a few repetitions of Sun Salutation A, it is most probably because they are weak. With practice they will get stronger. Do a little practice and work on them a bit every day. Rub them, rotate them, ice them, but keep doing the warm-ups. If your wrists hurt you, you particularly need to be doing this. So ease into it slowly until the wrists get stronger. I have had many clients over the years with severe arthritis in the wrists, but their wrists have become mobile and pain-free after weeks and months of practice.

Very often the problem results from extreme tightness in the back of the legs (hamstrings) or back. Consequently, the weight is pitched forward onto the wrists in Face Down Dog Posture, and the wrists need to do more work and support more weight than they normally would in this position. This can be another reason why the wrists might bother you after a couple of repetitions of the Sun Salutations. What can help you in the beginning if there is a lot of tightness in the back of your legs is to bend your knees slightly in Face Down Dog. This will enable you to press backward toward the thighs and get the back straighter and the weight off the wrists.

If the tightness is in the back, the problem is a little trickier to deal with. You might practice the following, as shown in Figure 3.19. Place your palms on the back of a chair or a wall in front of you, about shoulder-width apart and slightly higher than your head. Walk your feet back away from the wall until your arms are straight. Your hips should be directly over the feet and your back should be straight, not rounded. Then press the chest and shoulders toward the floor. Do not bend the arms. This will open the chest, shoulders, and upper back. Practice this every day until Face Down Dog gets easier.

Three, the lower back hurts. If you have chronic back pain or even occasional pain as a result of training, injury, or stress, then you are very susceptible to the negative effects of doing Face Up Dog (Position 5) wrong. If you have lower-back discomfort after doing a few warm-ups, then this is invariably because of weak or incorrect upper-body work in Face Up Dog position. Frequently, people in class will unconsciously allow themselves to sag in this position, and then complain of discomfort in the lower back. To avoid sagging into the lower back, lift up the chest, using the shoulder cap (deltoid) muscles, and put the knees down as shown in Figure 3.14.

Four, the feet hurt. Generally, the position that brings on the most complaints about the feet is Face Up Dog, where the feet are in the plantar flexion stretch. If the feet or ankles are very tight, especially from running (whether running while playing lacrosse and soccer or running in marathons), the ability of the feet to plantar flex (or point) might be severely limited. If this is the case for you, then this position is going to be difficult and uncomfortable. The position is meant to stretch the tops of the feet, not jam all the weight onto the front of the toes. A way to check your own plantar flexion is to sit on your feet with your toes pointed. The normal position is to have the tops of the feet flat on the floor, but "normal" isn't necessarily "average". If the front of your legs are not flat on the floor all the way from the knees to the toes, you should practice this position every day (provided it doesn't bother your knees), using cushions or carpet to ease the discomfort until it gets easier.

In the meantime, until you open up the tops of the feet somewhat by using the preceding method, keep the toes turned under (dorsiflexed) for the Face Up Dog position, as they are in the push-up and in Face Down Dog. After a few weeks, you can start to work the feet in the plantar flexion (pointed) position.

ADDITIONAL TIPS

Face Up Dog and Face Down Dog positions are very good for strengthening weak or injured knees because they alternately stretch and contract the hamstrings and the quadriceps, plus the shin and calf muscles, the major muscles that hold the knees in place and in alignment. This begins the process of putting the legs and knees back into correct alignment. Pay particular attention to the feet here. Work to make them parallel, balanced between supination and pronation, and as symmetrical as possible.

If the back of your legs are very tight—in addition to the heels being off the floor, which is okay—the heels may inadvertently turn out in a pigeon-toed stance, which is not okay. This generally happens unconsciously as the body tries to get around the hamstring stretch, which may frequently feel a little uncomfortable at first. Watch for this and make sure that your feet stay parallel in Face Down Dog position.

Another imbalance to keep an eye out for that frequently occurs in the feet in Face Down Dog position is pronation. You can spot it in your own posture simply by looking at the feet. Do the ankles cave in

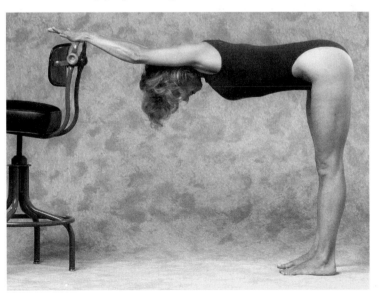

Figure 3.19

toward one another? If they do, you can begin immediately correcting this weakness by shifting the weight and pressing more on the outside edges of the feet. This will create more supination, or outward roll, and if repeated every time you practice, will slowly correct and strengthen this imbalance.

LEARNING THE "JUMP BACK"

Once you have learned correctly each of the individual positions within Sun Salutation A, and can roll through the nine positions without stopping to think what comes next, then you are at the point where you can link the breath up with the movement and learn the "jump back."

The jump back refers to the movement that connects Position 3 with Position 4. Up until this point you have been stepping the feet back into the extended push-up position. Once you can get your palms to the floor in Positions 2 and 3, you can begin to lean forward, put weight on the hands, and "jump" the feet back (instead of walking them back) into the push-up position.

There are two things that are important to watch for. One, you have to be careful to jump in control, and not donkey-kick the legs back, crashing on the toes. And two, when you land, you need to hold the torso firm, not letting the buttocks "boi-oy-oy-oing," or bounce up and down on the landing, thus stressing the lower back!

Now that we have spent some time working on the details of each individual position within Sun Salutation A, let's roll through it again, with the jump back (if you like), without stopping, and following the sequence as shown in Figure 3.20.

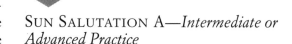

SUN SALUTATION A—*Intermediate or Advanced Practice*

Sama-sthiti—attention position

Position 1—inhale, arms up straight overhead. Legs and buttocks are power locked in static contraction. Gaze up. (Figure 3.20a.)

Position 2—exhale, palms to floor, nose to knees or as close as possible. This generally takes several Sun Salutations to get warm enough to accomplish. Some days it takes three reps, and some days ten reps still can't get you hot enough to touch your nose to your knees. (Figure 3.20b.)

Position 3—inhale, look up, lift chest, extend back (Figure 3.20c).

Position 4—exhale, jump back (Figure 3.20d).

Position 5—inhale, Face Up Dog, look up (Figure 3.20e).

Position 6—exhale, Face Down Dog (Figure 3.20f).

TAKE FIVE BREATHS.

Position 7—inhale, jump back up to the hands, land lightly, look up (Figure 3.20g).

Position 8—exhale, tuck nose to knees, look up at navel (Figure 3.20h).

Position 9—inhale, arms up straight, power up! (Figure 3.20i).

Sama-sthiti—Return to attention position.

This completes the first warm-up. This should be repeated at least three to five times at the beginning of every practice. Sun Salutation A is followed by Sun Salutation B.

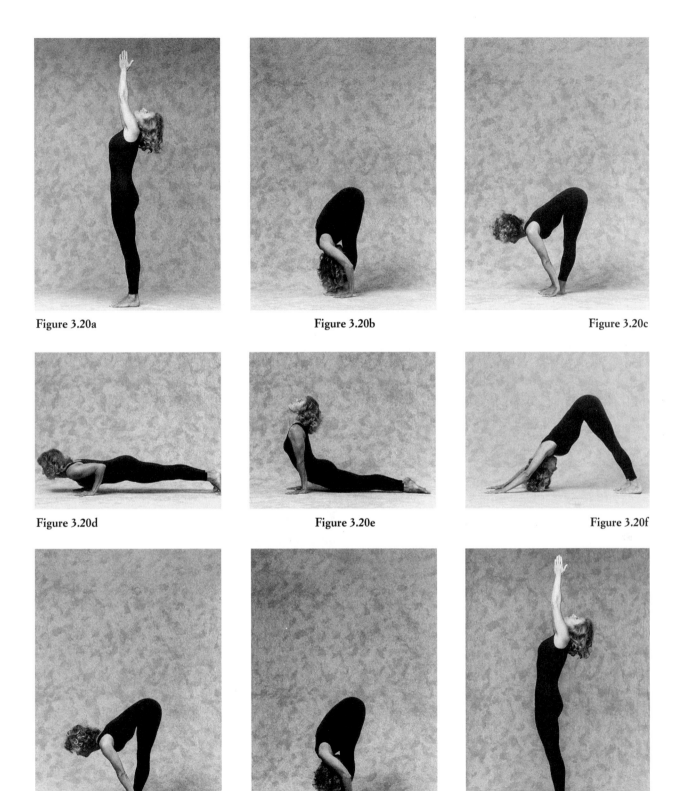

Figure 3.20a

Figure 3.20b

Figure 3.20c

Figure 3.20d

Figure 3.20e

Figure 3.20f

Figure 3.20g

Figure 3.20h

Figure 3.20i

Figure 3.21

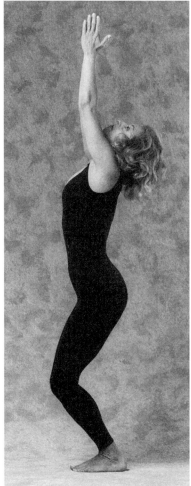

Figure 3.22

Figure 3.23

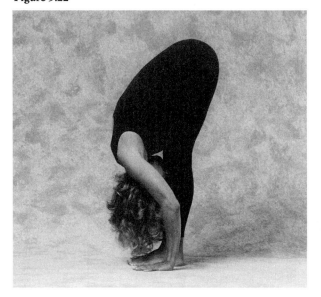

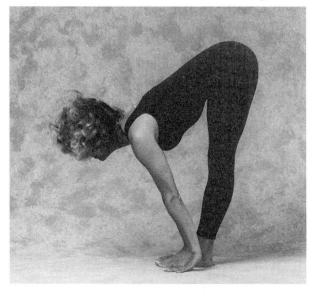

Warm-up or Sun Salutation B

Surya Namaskara B

Sama-sthiti—attention position.

Position 1

Inhale (Figure 3.21). Bend the knees, look up, raise the arms, and bring the palms together over the head.

Position 2

Exhale (Figure 3.22). Straighten up, then bend forward and take the palms to the floor. Bend the knees if you are tight or if you have lower back problems. Tuck head into knees. Look up toward the belly.

Position 3

Inhale (Figure 3.23). Look up, lift the chest, and extend the back. Knees are bent if necessary. In Position 2 and 3, try to align fingertips with toe tips.

Position 4

Exhale (Figure 3.24). Walk or jump the feet back into the Four-Limbed Stick, or push-up position. Look straight out in front of you along the floor.

Note: Remember to put your knees down as in Sun Salutation A if your shoulders hurt, your back hurts, or if you have not yet developed much upper-body strength.

Figure 3.24

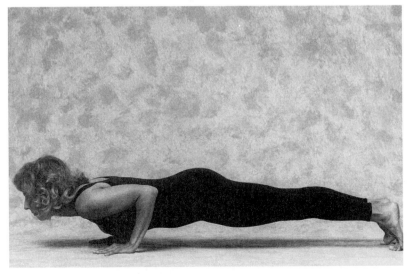

POSITION 5

Inhale (Figure 3.25). Face Up Dog.

POSITION 6

Exhale (Figure 3.26). Face Down Dog.

POSITION 7

Inhale (Figure 3.27). This position is called Warrior I

Posture (*Virabhdrasana I*—see chapter 4, Posture 11). Step the right foot up to a point between the hands. Pivot the back foot by turning the heel into the center line of the body and place the foot flat on the floor, toes angled slightly forward. Line the right heel up with the center of the left arch and make sure the right knee is bent directly over the right ankle. Bring the arms straight up over the head, palms together. Look up.

Note: If you are tight in the hips, you will be unable to step the foot all the way to the hands and do full Warrior Posture. In this case begin with a modified stance, determined by how far forward you can

Figure 3.25

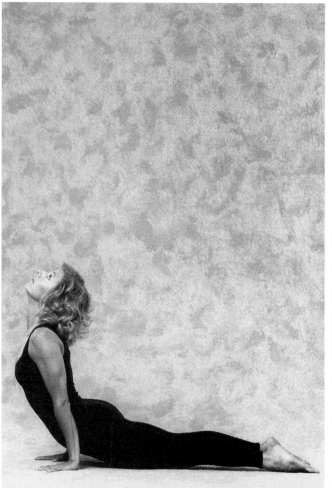

Figure 3.26

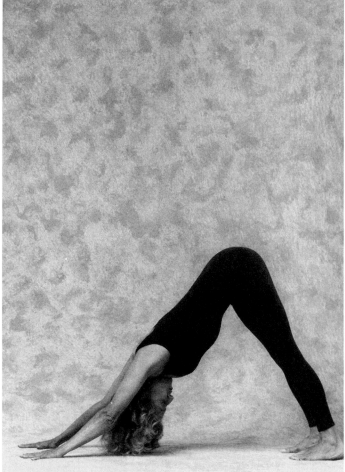

step the foot (Figure 3.28). As you become more proficient in the posture, you can begin to open up the stance to look more like Figure 3.27.

Don't hold your breath. Keep breathing while you are working to learn this and then simply begin the next move on an exhale.

POSITION 8

Exhale (Figure 3.29). Push-up position. Take your hands back to the floor, take your right leg back, and then drop down into the push-up position.

POSITION 9

Inhale (Figure 3.30). Face Up Dog. Pull shoulders back to open the chest. Keep buttocks firm. Look up.

POSITION 10

Exhale (Figure 3.31). Face Down Dog. Push shoulders through, but not past the straight-line plane running from the hips to the fingertips.

Figure 3.27

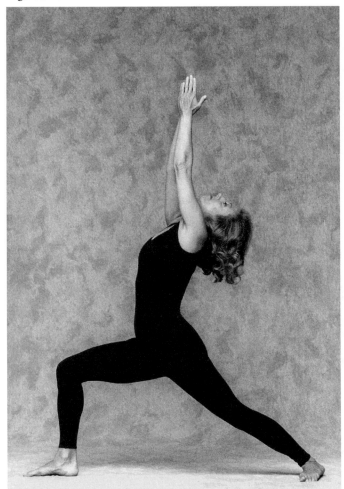

Figure 3.28

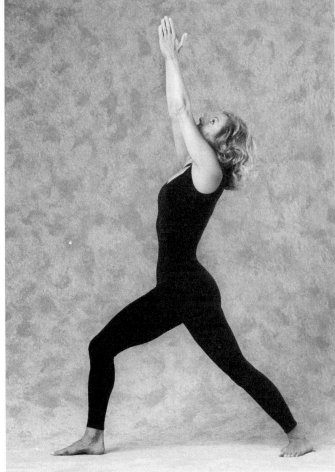

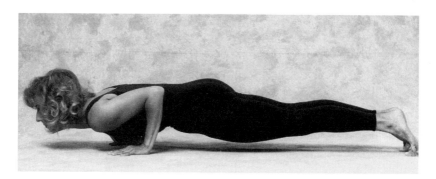

Figure 3.29

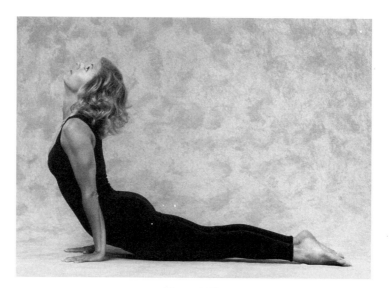

Figure 3.30

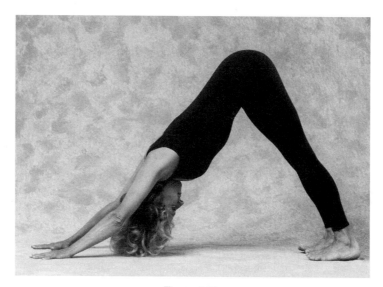

Figure 3.31

POSITION 11

Inhale (Figure 3.32). Warrior I, left side. Step the left leg up to a point between the hands, pivot the right foot, and place it flat on the floor. Raise up and bring the palms together over the head. Look up.

POSITION 12

Exhale (Figure 3.33). Push-up position.

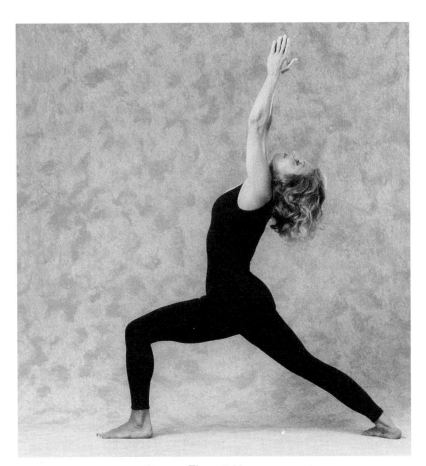

Figure 3.32

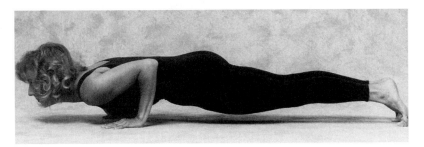

Figure 3.33

POSITION 13

Inhale (Figure 3.34). Face Up Dog. Stretch and open shoulders back, tighten buttocks.

POSITION 14

Exhale (Figure 3.35). Face Down Dog. Use thigh and shin muscles to push heels down. Flatten palms.

TAKE FIVE COMPLETE BREATHS IN THIS POSITION.

POSITION 15

Inhale, walk or jump the feet back up to the hands (Figure 3.36). Look up. Lift the chest and extend the back (Figure 3.37). Keep the knees bent if necessary or if you have lower-back problems.

POSITION 16

Exhale (Figure 3.38). Tuck head into the knees and flex the back. Bend knees if necessary.

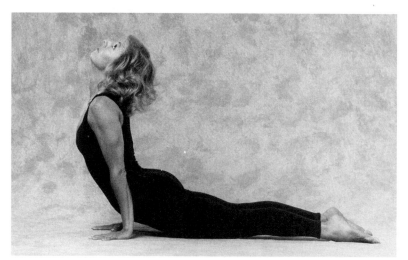

▲ **Figure 3.34**

Figure 3.35 ▼

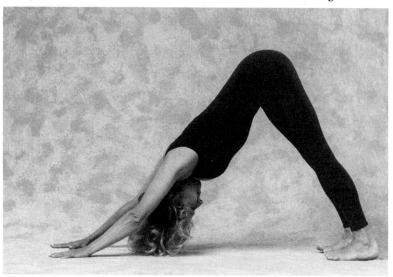

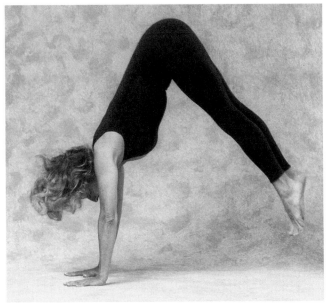

Figure 3.36

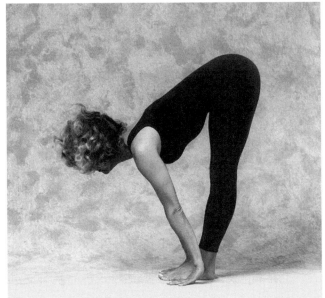

Figure 3.37

Figure 3.40

POSITION 17

Inhale, coming back to standing (Figure 3.39), arms up, palms together.
Look up (Figure 3.40).

Sama-sthiti—Return to attention position.

Figure 3.38

Figure 3.39

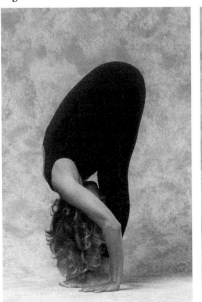

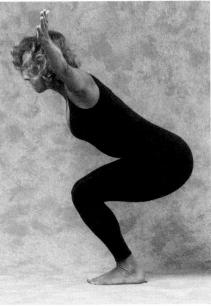

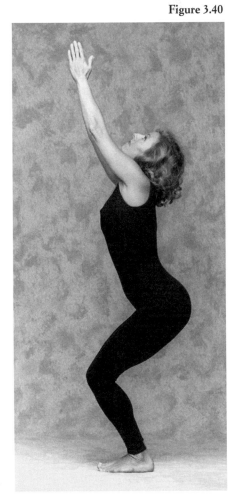

MODIFICATIONS FOR TIGHTNESS OR INJURY

Most of the problems in Sun Salutation B come in the Warrior Posture. If you are tight in the hips, which is a very common condition—particularly in cyclists, skaters, and runners, as well as in racquetball, baseball, and basketball players—the full Warrior Posture may be not only difficult, but impossible. You may have to begin with a shortened, or modified stance, because of limited range of motion in the hips (see Figure 3.28).

Whether the stance is shortened or full, it is important to pay attention to alignment of the knee. The knee must be held directly over the foot. What will often happen when there is tightness in the hips is that the foot can't step up as far as we would like it to go, so we allow the knee to keep going past the ankle into an exaggerated lunge. This is not great for the knees, and particularly not great for an injured, misaligned, or recovering knee!

Also watch to make sure your knee does not pronate, or cave in toward the midline of the body. This is most likely to occur in persons with tight groin muscles or in people with pronating or flat feet. This will be further discussed in chapter 4 as this position, Warrior Posture, is also the eleventh pose of the standing *asanas.*

Another mistake that often happens in the Warrior Posture is the position of the back foot. It should be flat on the floor and nearly perpendicular to the front foot (the toes are turned slightly forward). Often people are unaware of the position of their back foot. In class we can remind them to correct the alignment.

The reason that the back foot must press flat and angle in slightly is to protect the back knee from "torque," or twist, as the hips rotate forward. If the back arch is allowed to roll in or the foot to point out, or "away" from the posture, it can twist the knee. This is very bad for a healthy knee, and positively devastating for a weakened or injured knee.

This is a perfect example of how doing a posture incorrectly can mildly injure you. Granted, it isn't life-threatening, but the Power Yoga form is designed to be therapeutic and its practice is intended to solve problems, not create or aggravate existing ones. In class I have the opportunity to alert people to their unawareness and correct the problem right off the bat. Here in the book I can't jump off the page and help you or wave my arms until you get it right. But please pay attention to your alignment and, *if you have knee problems, pay extra attention while doing this posture.* Now that we have worked on each of the positions within Sun Salutation B individually, let's string them all together and practice them in succession with the breathing, as we did for Sun Salutation A. See Figure sequence 3.41.

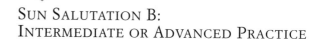

SUN SALUTATION B: INTERMEDIATE OR ADVANCED PRACTICE

Sama-sthiti—attention position.

Position 1—inhale, bend the knees, raise the arms over the head, look up (Figure 3.41a).
Position 2—exhale, straighten up, then bend forward, palms to the floor (Figure 3.42b).
Position 3—inhale, look up, extend the back (Figure 3.42c).
Position 4—exhale, jump back into *Chaturanga Dandasana,* or push-up position (Figure 3.42d).
Position 5—inhale, Face-Up Dog (Figure 3.42e).
Position 6—exhale, Face Down Dog (Figure 3.42f).
Position 7—exhale, Warrior Posture, right leg forward, arms up, look up (Figure 3.42g).
Position 8—exhale, back down into push up position (Figure 3.42h).
Position 9—inhale, Face Up Dog (figure 3.42i).

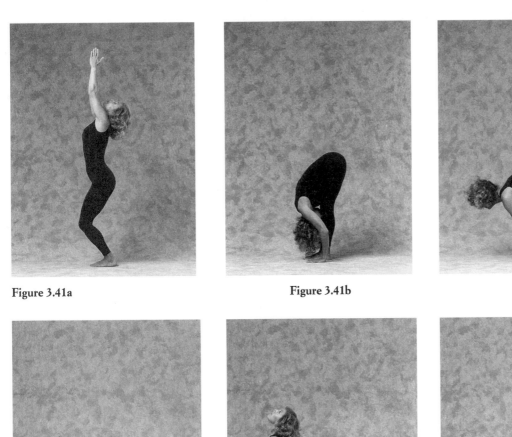

Figure 3.41a

Figure 3.41b

Figure 3.41c

Figure 3.41d

Figure 3.41e

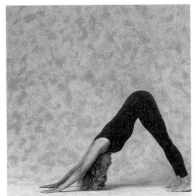

Figure 3.41f

Figure 3.41g

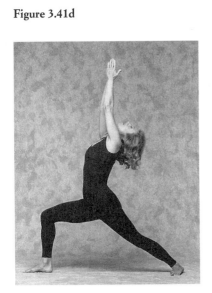

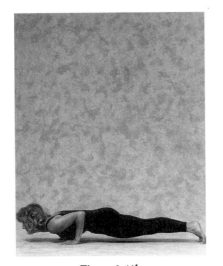

Figure 3.41h

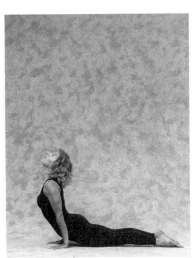

Figure 3.41i

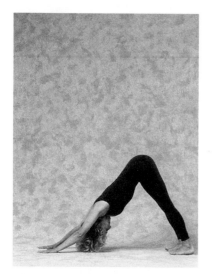

Figure 3.41j

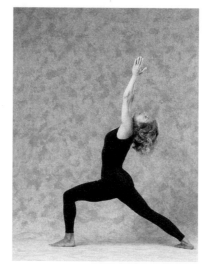

Figure 3.41k

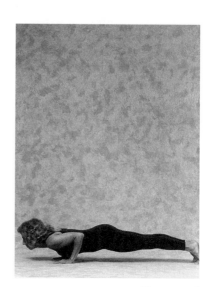

Figure 3.41l

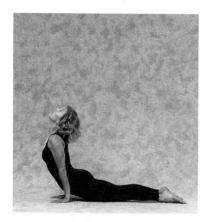

Figure 3.41m

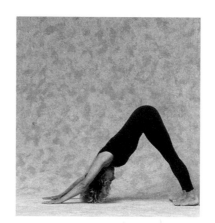

Figure 3.41n

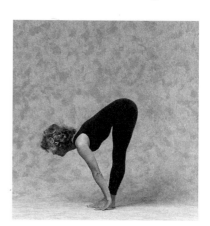

Figure 3.41o

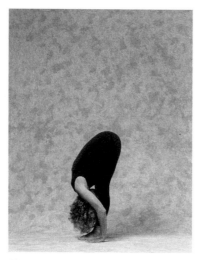

Figure 3.41p

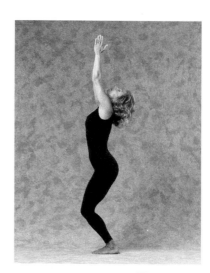

Figure 3.41q

Position 10—exhale, Face Down Dog (Figure 3.42j).
Position 11—inhale, Warrior Posture, left leg forward, arms up, look up (Figure 3.42k).
Position 12—exhale, back down into push-up position (Figure 3.42l).
Position 13—inhale, Face Up Dog (Figure 3.42m).
Position 14—exhale, Face Down Dog (Figure 3.42n).

Hold this position for five breaths.

Position 15—inhale, jump the feet back to the hands, inhale, look up (Figure 3.42o).
Position 16—exhale, nose to knees (Figure 3.42p).
Position 17—inhale, arms up, knees bent, look up (Figure 3.42q).

Sama-sthiti—return to attention position.

This completes the second warm-up. Practice the warm-ups until you can comfortably do between three and five repetitions of each set, Sun Salutation A *and* Sun Salutation B, without stopping. This might take anywhere from three to four weeks of regular practice, with "regular" meaning at least four times per week. The Sun Salutations are the foundation of the form. It is absolutely impossible to do too many. As a beginner working with my teacher, we would frequently do thirty minutes of just Sun Salutations. This work will help to prepare your stamina, concentration, and heat for the next chapter.

One of Thom's and my favorite workouts when we are really trying to get strong is fifty Sun Salutation A's and twenty-five B's, followed by Closing Sequence (every practice, whether just Sun Salutations or the complete Primary Series, ends with some version of Closing Sequence—see chapter 7), rest, and breakfast. Without the rest and breakfast, this takes a little under two hours. It's a hot workout. One of the purposes of doing a long sequence of warm-ups like this is to develop endurance and concentration. It's fairly easy to count three Sun Salutations. But in order to get up to doing thirty or forty, you really have to pay attention. The minute you space out, you lose count, and you know what that means? You have to start over!

One Sun Salutation A takes, on average, about one minute and twelve seconds to one minute and fifteen seconds. This means it takes about sixty minutes to do fifty repetitions. You could always go by time—do thirty minutes of warm-ups, for example, and estimate you did about twenty-five repetitions of Sun Salutation A. Although it's tougher to count the repetitions than to work by time, you should try to keep track of the count. It's better training for the mind! (This workout is not recommended for beginners. The number of Sun Salutations one does in any given practice should be increased slowly. I mention the workout here only to give you an idea of what is possible.)

Once you are comfortable with the breathing and the form, you will begin to study the first standing posture in the next chapter. For now, you will have to stop and do some reading, slowly learning the first postures in the Primary Series. But once you learn them, *the last exhale of Sun Salutation B will be followed by the first inhale of Standing Posture 1.*

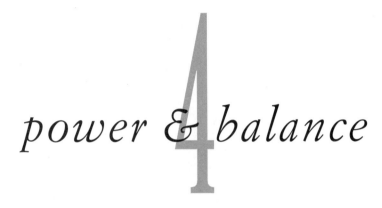

power & 4 *balance*

THE PRIMARY SERIES—STANDING POSTURES

Only when you can be extremely pliable and soft,
can you be extremely hard and strong.

ZEN PROVERB

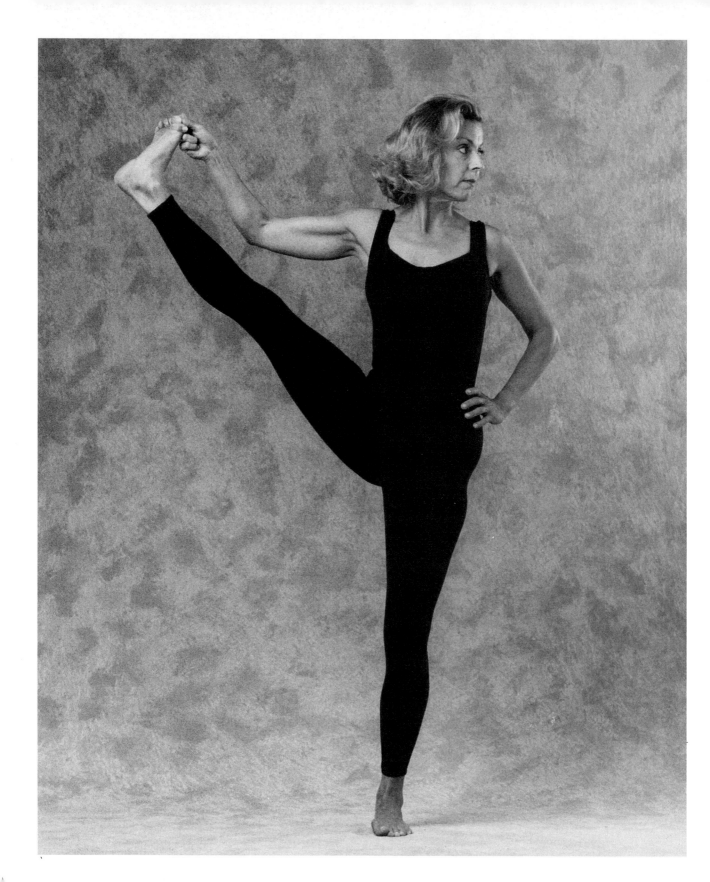

The Primary Series

Standing Postures

Hard and Soft

The Primary Series of postures of the Power Yoga workout, as given in the next three chapters, is an extremely sophisticated, logical, and orderly progression of movements. As I explained in chapter 1, the series is called *yoga chikitsa,* or yoga therapy, and is specifically conceived to therapeutically align the body and spine. The plan and purpose of the practice is to heal, strengthen, adjust, and balance.

Traditionally, the standing postures were intended to develop strength and power. They taught a person how to stand with a noble countenance and presence, self-assurance, and commitment. In our practice we will find that these poses require precise awareness of the play between hard and soft, contraction and letting go; they teach us to remain centered in the present moment. And being present, you will begin to notice how the various pairs of muscle groupings work together and come into balance for mastery of these postures. As philosophical as that might sound for a physical activity, you will see as you go along through this chapter that the times you lose balance are often the times when you have lost your concentration, and your mind has drifted off to something else, either past or future.

Kundalini Rising

As I explained in chapter 2, in yoga philosophy there are seven *chakras,* or energy centers in the body. The third, or *manipura chakra,* is located at the navel and roughly corresponds with our center of gravity. By keeping our attention rooted at this energy center when we begin to feel unsteady, we can literally activate a feeling of balance. The Japanese martial art term for this same center is called the *hara,* or "the place of power." You may also remember that the symbol for this center is a flame. By mentally "contacting" this place of power and "seeing" the flame we find there, we begin to feel the capacity we have to bring up the energy, or fire.

How do we keep attention focused on this *chakra*—or anywhere else, for that matter? In yoga, attention follows the breath. We direct attention by directing the breath. Notice that by using *ujjayi* technique and exhaling down into the *manipura chakra* (which is actually what we began experimenting with in chapter 2 with active exhalation), you can feel your attention going there as well.

Yoga philosophy says that the nature of *prana* is to flower, to rise and expand. With *ujjayi* breathing, we are learning to control this energy and force it down from the chest through the *nadis,* or "nerve" channels and link it to *apana,* an aspect and principal current of *prana* that circulates in the lower abdominal region of the body. The nature of *apana* is to contract and descend. Through the practice of the *bandhas,* which are internal muscular contractions that lift energy up from the lower abdomen, we are trying to bring *apana* up and link it to *prana*. The Sanskrit word *bandha* comes from the root *bandh*, which means "tie," "bond," "chain," or "lock." So what we are really trying to do is chain or tie these two energies together like two connecting wires, so that electricity can pass through. Once this connection is made, at the *manipura chakra*, it is possible to then direct this current to the base of the spine.

According to ancient yoga thought, it is here, at the first *chakra*—or *muladhara,* as it is called (*mula* means "root" and *adhara* means *base*)—that a latent divine energy called the *kundalini* lies slumbering. This dormant energy is traditionally depicted as a coiled serpent, soundly sleeping in the doorway of the first *chakra* and blocking the entrance to the *sushumna nadi*—the main channel up through the spinal cord. However, once the snake wakes up and the divine cosmic force is roused through yoga practices, this pathway is opened and the *kundalini* begins to ascend the *sushumna nadi,* through which life force flows, from the psychoenergetic center at the base of the spine (the lowest or first *chakra*) to the crown of the head (the highest or seventh *chakra*).

This energy flow can stop, sometimes for lifetimes, and sometimes for only an instant, at each *chakra* along the way. The practice of *astanga yoga* is intended to wake up this slumbering serpent blocking the pathway to higher consciousness and actively move energy up through the *chakras,* resulting in ever-expanding awareness and evolving consciousness.

Pretty image. But for our purposes for now, we are simply trying to get a little heat up so our hamstrings don't hurt so damned much when we stretch them! Only through the experience of doing the practice can you actually begin to understand in real terms what is meant by bringing up the heat and energy.

TURNING UP THE HEAT

With conscious powerful breathing, the breath becomes a generator for heat and energy. *The heat in the body must stay up for this work!* And the single most important contributing factor to the heat is the breath. The trick is to develop your concentration and endurance so that you can keep the yoga breathing going *consciously.* The awareness of the breath should be there at all times. If the mind drifts off to entertain itself, or spaces out, the breath becomes unconscious and shallow. Immediately you will notice that the energy falls back down and the heat drops off.

Another element contributing to the "fire of the body" is the *vinyasa,* or the "connecting movement," between the postures. In this chapter the connecting movement consists of the choreographed "flowing" from one standing posture to the next and then the coming back to attention position between each one. In the next chapter, however, when we begin the seated postures, the connecting movement is gleaned from Sun Salutation A. This means that between each posture, you do a portion of the Sun Salutations. It's like a musical bridge between verses of a song. In music, the bridge gives flow and continuity to the composition.

In *astanga yoga, vinyasa* links the postures together into one continuous form. It keeps the sweating mechanism turned on and helps to neutralize the body between postures. It has been a long time since I have done yoga without *vinyasa,* but I cannot imagine how anyone could ever stay warmed up enough to actually do the postures without using connecting movement (and breath)—except very flexible people who might need less heat.

According to the *Yoga Korunta, asana* should never be done without connecting movement. The *sloka* (verse), *vinya vinyasa yogena asana din nakareayet* ("Oh, yogi, don't do *asana* without *vinyasa*) is repeated frequently throughout the original manuscript. The word *vinyasa,* like most Sanskrit words, has a variety of meanings, and its specific connotation depends on the context in which it is used. It can mean (1) "movement," "position (of limbs)," (2) "arrangement" or "order," or (3) "putting together and connecting." When used with its root, *vinya* ("to put down in different places or spread out"), it tends to mean "don't put yourself down in different places or spread out (as in *asana* practice] without connection or arrangement." Whew!

I like the idea that the concept contains both the energy of dispersion (expansion) and the energy of organization (contraction), because this epitomizes the point of yoga—finding balance between putting down and grounding and pulling up and moving on. Thus, this "connecting movement" that links the postures will simultaneously take you out of one posture and into another, creating endless flow. Without this continuous work, sufficient heat and stamina cannot be built up to cleanse, purify, strengthen, and realign the body, and enough concentration cannot be developed to focus the mind—all the things yoga is supposed to do.

When you begin doing the standing postures in this chapter, you will start to feel for yourself how the this linking movement builds heat and acts as a bridge for the concentration and body to flow uninterrupted from one posture to the next.

OVERGROWN JUNGLE PATHS

This work can feel great, yet it can also be uncomfortable at times. It might be awkward for you because it begins a very deep untangling of inappropriately established neuromuscular pathways. These may be due to old injuries or postural and emotional irregularities, which are thus contributing to imbalance or chronic injury. Ever notice on a hiking trail in the woods how, if a tree falls across the trail, hikers will initiate a new trail around the tree? It's the same way in the body when there is an injury. The brain reroutes the messengers around the jammed-up place. Even though the injury may have happened twenty years ago, the body will continue its rerouting. Yet the original pathway is still there, under the overgrowth, waiting to be cleared of debris and returned to service.

You will learn to play the edge between pain and intensity. The deeper the breathing and the harder you work, the hotter you will get and the more intensity you will be able to tolerate. Conversely, the hotter you get, the more you can safely handle the "soft" work, or stretching. You will start to distinguish between real pain and just discomfort. Discomfort has to be pushed through with breath and fire in order to repair the faulty wiring and find freedom from chronic short-circuiting and injury!

The incorrect paths have to be redirected. It is hard work because it is like hacking your way through an overgrown jungle path with a machete. But we are not really ripping and tearing muscle fibers; we are slowly prying open these jammed-up paths and places, allowing the original route to be reestablished and the *prana*, or "life force"—the oxygen, the energy, the intracellular fluid—to flow back through these compacted areas (or "dead spaces," as I call them). We slowly untangle the fibers with the breath and the strength, separating carefully the cells and permitting the nutrients and life force carried by the circulatory system to reenter the spaces between the cells and bring healing and redevelopment.

Much of the discomfort is psychological. The memory of an old injury, for example, is still lodged in the tissue and fibers. Because of the intensity of the "soft" work, the focus tends to be on the stretch. In the beginning, it is hard to remain aware of the hard work, the strength work. But the more we are able to shift our focus to the strength, *or the contraction of each posture,* and let go of the resistance, the more effective we will become in keeping the sweating mechanism turned on, in enabling the stretch, and in actually realigning the body. Many of you will feel like iron. But remember Axiom No. 6 from chapter 1: "Even iron will bend if you heat it up."

The postures must be done with awareness, not with fear or machismo. The postures are organized in a logical sequence and each one prepares you, mentally and physically, for the one that follows it. Postures are *not meant to be done out of sequence or singly!* Athletes, especially since their time is limited, are always asking, "Isn't there just one stretch I can do, just one posture, that will solve this problem or that?" The answer is always no. This is a synergistic system. It is meant to be done as a complete training program.

If you, like me, have an old neck injury and are kept in balance and pain-free by a grouping of postures toward the end of the Primary Series, for example, then you must still do the entire sequence leading up to those particular postures. I have tried all the shortcuts. They don't work. It isn't the same. The heat isn't the same, the preparation of the body to do the healing work isn't the same, and the results are not the same.

I have a friend and longtime client who is a full-time and very talented triathlete. He has a packed training schedule, and when he isn't biking, swimming, or running, he's in the gym lifting weights, doing sit-ups, or out getting body work. He had chronic shoulder pain for over a year as a result of a tear in a tendon connecting one of the rotator cuff muscles to the shoulder joint. This was finally solved through surgery. Next, it was chronic lower-back pain as a result of thousands of hours on the bike and hundreds of workouts with weights, not to mention the twenty years prior to his triathlete career spent as a professional drummer. He spent thousands of dollars on massage therapy, physical therapy, and consultations with orthopedists and sports medical professionals.

While all of this was going on, he was beginning to look at yoga as a possible solution to his problems, and would occasionally come to class. I was always telling him to do more practice and he would say, "Well, I do the Sun Salutations and standing postures at home pretty regularly." I kept saying that it wasn't enough and that he should come to class five days a week and do the whole practice. So he would do a little yoga for a few days and there would be a little progress, but

then he'd go out and do fifty miles on the bike and his back would be killing him. He'd go off to his physical therapist, seeking (understandably) some relief from the pain. He'd tell his therapist that he had been doing yoga for months, and the therapist would then assume that the practice hadn't helped and tell him to stop his yoga. I would go crazy. "Don't tell your therapist you're doing yoga. You aren't doing yoga. You're fooling around with yoga."

The point is that the practice wasn't regular or complete enough to do what needed to be done. This guy was not going to be helped by a few Sun Salutations a few days a week. He needed the whole Primary Series every day for three months, minimum, just to get pain-free, and then every day the rest of his life to *stay* pain-free.

Just recently, after six months of regular practice, my friend said to me, "You know, I used to think you were crazy when you said I had to do this five days a week. I just couldn't relate to what this was going to do for me. But now that I'm there, I can see what you meant when you said I had to do it every day."

So, the point of this story is that you won't understand what you will feel like after three months of regular practice until after you do three months of regular practice!

The "perfect" human body, whatever that might be, with practice could do all the positions given in this book. The imperfect body will eventually be able to do them, too, but it will just take a little longer. Most of us are going to require modifications, dilutions, and adaptations of the postures until the imbalances and shortcomings are slowly, slowly corrected and changed. This takes time. If you are in a hurry, pitch this book in the fireplace now (or give it to someone you care about)! If, however, health and balance are a priority, then you must commit yourself to regular practice. If the postures are practiced incorrectly, as I have also said a few times now, they can cause injury or imbalance. That is why you cannot allow yourself to be in a rush to get through or complete this book. It should be read through once for an overview when you are beginning practice. Then read it again, chapter by chapter, as you are working your way through the form. In a way, it's like reading James Joyce's *Ulysses.* Not in a literary sense, of course, but in a logistical sense. You read it through once just to get familiar with the style and language. And then again to get the story. But unlike a novel, there is no end. There is no prize offered simply because you make it to the last page. The sole (soul) prize is the benefit of good health that comes about only from continuous practice. This prize is fleeting and must be earned every day as you work your way through the practice, pose by pose, breath by breath.

Fitness isn't something you acquire, like a material object that you put up on the shelf and forget about. It's something you work at every day for the rest of your life. Even when you win a road race, as my husband tells me, it feels great for a few minutes or a few hours. But what happens the next morning? You have to get up, do yoga, work out the kinks, and then put on your running shoes and head out the door like everyone else. The key to success in this system may be found in one word discovered in the ancient secret doctrine. *Sadhana,* or "the means to realization," is the path, the practice itself, that leads to self-mastery.

▼

STATIC CONTRACTION

There are eleven standing postures that begin the Primary Series. Each posture works and opens the body in a slightly different way, but as a group they continue and build upon the work of the warm-ups. One of the most important aspects of the standing postures is the work of the quadriceps, or thigh muscles. In the directions that accompany the illustrations, you will constantly see the reminder or directive to "contract" or tighten the thighs. For some people, especially those with tight hamstrings, this is extremely difficult to learn.

It isn't an automatic contraction, like the kind that happens in the biceps when you pick up a weight in your hand and then flex your arm up toward your chest. That kind of muscular contraction is called a *dynamic contraction* and happens automatically when you take a limb through a range of motion.

When you flex a muscle without moving a joint or limb, it is called a *static contraction.* In this yoga practice, tightening the thighs while standing still is an example of a static contraction, as I explained at the beginning of Sun Salutation A (see chapter 3). Another way to describe the action of the thighs is to say that you are using the thigh muscles to lift or pull up the kneecaps. It is important to understand that this is not the same thing as "locking" the knees. Locking the knees implies pressing back on the knee joint, and for people who have knees that hyperextend, locking the knees only aggravates the hyperextension. Think instead of lifting the kneecap up toward the hips. One effect of this action, repeated constantly throughout the standing postures, is the strengthening of the knees as a result of the balancing and building of the vastus medialus and vastus lateralus—two of the four quadriceps (thigh muscles) that hold the kneecap in place. Eventually, this will help to bring misaligned knees back into correct alignment.

You might want to take a break here for a moment and try it. Stand up and see if you can tighten the thighs so that the kneecaps lift up. Try to hold the contraction for five breaths. This takes constant vigilance. The thighs will not stay up there by themselves. You have to consciously hold them in contraction, and for some of you it will not be easy.

The emphasis on the contraction of the muscle opposing the muscle being stretched tends to shift your focus. Instead of thinking about the tightness or discomfort in your hamstrings, for example, you concentrate on tightening your quadriceps. I have used the thighs here as an example, but all through the standing postures and for the rest of the series, there will be *working,* or contracting, muscle groups opposing and enabling the stretch. You need to be aware of them and engage them—whether the work is to twist or extend, balance or bend.

This work has three effects when done in the postures: (1) it prevents overstretching of the opposing muscle, i.e., the hamstrings, and facilitates the stretch in a way that other types of stretching—for example, ballistic stretching (bouncing) or *static stretching* (holding a stretch) can't; (2) it provides heat, which also makes the stretch easier and more effective; and (3) it focuses the concentration.

The conscious contraction of a muscle group, particularly a large one like the quads, requires effort. Along with the *ujjayi* breathing, concentration, and the *vinyasa,* or connecting movement, the effort of the static muscular contractions is a very important contributing element to heat. Without it, you aren't "working" the posture effectively and the heat will not be there. The same can be said for all the static contractions in the form. In this practice, every posture involves a static contraction in some muscle group. This strength work generates heat and develops the flexibility. As Axiom No. 2 of Power Yoga stated in chapter 1: "Strength, not gravity, develops flexibility." It takes time and awareness to understand how to use the practice to develop your strength, but it comes. These first eleven postures will begin to teach you how to work in an *asana* and gain the most benefit from that effort.

▼

THE *BANDHAS*

There is one more aspect of the training that is unquestionably the most important part of the practice and yet the most subtle. We have talked about the effects of the breathing, the connecting movement, the concentration, and, last, the importance of effort, or the strength work. We have looked at contracting the thighs—a big, obvious muscle that we see every day and are fairly familiar with. Many of us had difficulty getting in touch with *this* muscle and quite a bit of trouble holding the contraction.

Now we are going to learn a more elusive contraction called a *bandha,* or "lock," in yoga terminology. Remember earlier in this chapter I defined the root word *bandh* as meaning "bond," "tie," or "lock." A *bandha* refers to a muscular contraction, literally a "lock," used to focus concentration, stimulate heat, and, ultimately, control the flow of *prana,* or the psychosomatic energy we call life force. There are two *bandhas* that are performed in this yoga practice: *mula bandha* and *uddiyana bandha.* The first, *mula bandha,* means "root lock." Root lock is the contracting and lifting of the perineum and the perineal muscle, which is located between the genitals and the anus. Reference to the perineum generally includes the vaginal and anal sphincter muscles as well.

Through the practice of *mula bandha,* or the lifting of the perineum toward the navel, we continue the training of the mind in attentiveness, begun by the other aspects of the practice such as the breath, the gaze, and the static muscular contractions. When we engage root lock, not only does it force us to be mindful of what we are doing, but we bring together the downward action of the deep *ujjayi* breathing with the upward muscular force of *mula bandha.* This meeting of *prana* and *apana,* according to the *Hatha Yoga Pradapika,* is supposed to stimulate a *nada,* or inner sound. Thus, through what at first may seem simply physical means, the student of yoga is able to tune into and become mindful of the inner "voice."

In more practical terms the practice of *mula bandha* is literally a static contraction of a muscle—a bit more subtle than that of the quadriceps, for example, but a muscular contraction nonetheless. This is strength work and produces heat. It takes concentration to practice *mula bandha,* because you can't do it unless you think about it or focus on it. So concentration is supporting the lock, which is supporting heat.

The second *bandha, uddiyana,* literally means "to fly up," and refers to the drawing inward and upward of the navel. This produces a corresponding action in the abdominals and creates a hollow under the rib cage. An effective little trick that will help you to get in touch with the movement of this *bandha* is to consciously contract the oblique abdominal muscles. You can do this by exhaling, and as you begin the exhale, tip the bottom of the rib cage in slightly toward the spine. As you do this, you will feel the muscles at your waist, just under the ribs, contract. These are the oblique abdominals. The movement of this *bandha* strengthens and tones the internal organs of the pelvic region, and since it is a strong muscular contraction, like root lock, it creates heat. One ancient yoga text states that "this *bandha* sends the life breath rising up into the body like a great bird soaring without effort." Again, for our immediate purposes we are also trying to bring up this same energy, only initially in the form of heat.

The *bandhas,* when applied together, help to assure proper breathing. Really, they are a combination of effort and concentration, requiring strength and attention. These *bandhas* take years and years of training to master and perform continuously during practice. But as my teacher used to say, "Without the *bandhas,* this practice is just gymnastics"—meaning that the *bandhas* place an emphasis on concentration and on personal evolution that sets this yoga practice apart from just doing physical exercise.

Although there will be a lot for you to think about in the early stages of this practice—the breathing, the form, the strength work, the alignment, and now the *bandhas*—it is important to develop the habit of holding the *bandhas* right from the start, even though they are a fairly advanced yogic practice. So now before you go on, spend a few moments doing *mula bandha* and *uddiyana bandha* root lock and abdominal lock.

Lift and hold the perineum. At first you may not exactly "feel" the contraction of the perineum. Practice contracting the anal sphincters and (for women) the vaginal muscles. This will engage the perineal muscle. Eventually, after much practice, you will be able to distinguish the perineal contraction on its own.

Now lift and hold the navel and abdominal area below the diaphragm. What happens as you continue to breathe? Well, up until now we have been doing beginners' breathing and allowing the belly to expand on the in-breath—which is what it does naturally when we are breathing correctly. Now, if we apply abdominal lock, where does the breath go? You should notice that the inward and upward lift of *uddiyana* drives the breath into the space that contains the lungs (thoracic cavity) and actually pushes out, or expands, the rib cage, working the muscles between the ribs (the intercostals). So not only are we creating heat with this lock, but with practice we will truly expand the capacity of our thoracic cavity, rib cage, and lungs and strengthen the respiratory muscles.

As the diaphragm contracts on the in-breath (or sun breath, as it is called in yoga), and flattens or descends somewhat into the abdominal cavity, it now pushes up against the *uddiyana* lift. This resistance strengthens the diaphragm, thus enabling it to draw in more air to the lungs as it contracts. When it relaxes and raises up underneath the heart, the action of *uddiyana* helps to push up the diaphragm and expel the outgoing, or moon, breath.

You will remember in chapter 2 that I explained the concept of "backward" breathing, where the abdominals tighten and pull in on the inhalation. If you were someone who discovered your breathing was very shallow and you had been breathing backward, you have hopefully been practicing correct breathing and have changed your breathing pattern since then. Now I am saying that you have to learn a new technique that will contract the belly again on the in-breath. Are you confused? What is the difference between incorrect, "backward" breathing and breathing with the application of *uddiyana bandha*?

The first and most important difference is that in most cases backward breathing is *unconscious.* The collarbone and shoulders are raised up and the ribs are lifted, drawing in the abdomen, which then pushes against the diaphragm and keeps it from expanding downward. The small upper part of the chest and lungs is used, but only a minimum amount of air enters the lungs. If you watch someone who breathes in this way, you will see how they unconsciously exert maximum effort for minimum return.

Second, the practice of *uddiyana bandha* is a *conscious* technique to develop deeper and more subtle control of the breath—or more specifically, in yoga terminology, *prana,* or life force. Before you can learn to *control* something, you need to know it fairly well. So people who may be aware that their breathing is limited, but other than that don't have much idea of what they are doing with their breathing, need to learn to expand the breath first and explore the potential fullness of the lungs before they attempt to learn an even more subtle and sophisticated breathing technique. That is why we learned initially to relax the abdomen on the inhalation. This is what we should be doing in our natural, everyday breathing, so as to allow the diaphragm to contract and draw in air without interference or restriction, thus experiencing the deeper capacity of the lungs.

"Well," you might say, "doesn't *uddiyana* also press up against the diaphragm when it is trying to expand, and keep it from doing its work?" Well, yes it does press against it, but now, in this case, it strengthens it. Because you are now working *consciously,* the abdominal lift and diaphragm are working against each other isometrically. Additionally, you are drawing up the abdominals and holding the lift for both the inhale and exhale. We can feel the two muscular actions meeting and strengthening one another.

A less tangible but just as real function of the *bandhas* has to do with the energizing of the nerve "channels," or *nadis,* and the unblocking of the *chakras.* In yoga philosophy there are five aspects of the *prana* (life force) in the body. These are referred to as the five *vayu,* or winds: (1) *prana,* or the ascending breath that issues from the heart and circulates in the chest area of the body; (2) *apana,* or the descending breath that circulates in the lower abdomen and controls the functions of elimination; (3) *samana,* or the breath localized in the abdominal region and connected with digestion; (4) *udana,* literally the "up" breath that dwells in the thoracic cavity and is responsible for speech and the ascent of attention in higher states of consciousness; and (5) *vyana,* or the diffuse breath circulating in all the limbs.

The two principal *vayu,* or currents, that interest us at this point are *prana* and *apana,* both of which I have already mentioned. Through the action of the two *bandhas,* these apparently opposite *vayu* will come together. The point at which they meet is the place where you feel *uddiyana bandha* pressing against the descending diaphragm. This coincides with the *manipura chakra,* which you may remember from chapter 2 and earlier in this chapter. Here, according to yoga philosophy, the two "winds" are fired and energized by a crystal jewel, *mani.* Once merged they complete a circuit that will then enable this energized, awakened power to enter the spine, or the *sushuma nadi*—literally "most gracious channel" in Sanskrit, and which you may remember is the main energy path up the spine. This energy then ascends through the sequential *chakras,* unblocking the potential of each center and bringing higher levels of awareness to the practitioner. From each of these energy centers, the *prana,* or energy can move out the efferent channels to peripheral areas of the body that may need balancing (either stimulating or calming) energy.

Now, I love this stuff. You might not be so keen on it. But admit it—it's a lot more fun imagining setting fire to a magical energy current that has the capacity to move us toward self-fulfillment than to simply grunt along, focused on how tight we are or what a stressful day we have had. Anyway, that's why we do the *bandhas*—from the most basic reason, heat and concentration, to the most esoteric, self-realization, with the side benefit of increased lung capacity!

GENERAL GUIDELINES

As you work through each chapter, it is important that you try to get a sense of the rhythm and sequence of the postures. When I was learning the form from my teacher, Norman Allen, the first day I did practice, all I did was Sun Salutations. The next day I repeated the

Salutations. The first week all I did was Sun Salutations, increasing the repetitions slowly. The second week I did five Sun Salutation A's and five B's, and then added one or two standing postures. The following day, I would repeat the Salutations and the first two standing postures, then add one or two more. Every day, I would go to practice and repeat what I did the day before, every few days or weeks adding a little bit more. As I was going through the sequence, if I ever forgot or skipped a posture, Norman would make me go back to the beginning and start all over. One result of this was that I learned the Primary Series. Backward, forward, and sideways. I don't ever need to "think" about what posture comes next. My body just automatically goes into it.

Guidelines to keep in mind as you begin the practice are as follows:

1. Balance the weight evenly on both feet for all postures.

2. Keep the breath flowing. Don't ever hold your breath. The script for the breath is written as it eventually flows with the movement. But it will take time and practice to coordinate the two correctly. So while you are learning, breathe!

3. Work the breath. Inhale and exhale as deeply as you can, consciously exercising the diaphragm with each breath. Listen to the breath constantly and practice mindfulness. Try to match the inhale to the exhale in strength, duration, depth, and sound.

4. Try to coordinate the duration of a connecting movement with the duration of the accompanying breath. So, as you finish a descent or an ascent into or out of a posture, the movement and the breath will be ending together.

5. Keep the head and neck aligned.

6. Pay close attention to the "hard" work in each posture, or the contraction of the muscle opposing the stretch. Keep the thighs contracted and pulled up.

7. Don't be sloppy. Sloppy practice isn't going to do anything. Learn exact alignment and then temperature control. If there isn't enough heat, and the alignment is not exact, the work of the movement will not steer the body toward balance, increased energy, and health.

8. Pay attention to alignment of the feet. If the feet are sloppy the whole posture will be sloppy. Sloppiness is unconsciousness.

9. Spend a few seconds, at least, of every minute concentrating on the *bandhas*. Perhaps once you get into a posture and you have the feet correct, the alignment pretty good, the head and neck lifted and extended, and you are concentrating on the muscular contractions like keeping the thigh muscles pulled up, you might add one more task: Pull up the perineum and abdominals and then try to hold the whole thing together for a few breaths.

10. Practice the *vinyasa*. This means practice coming into and out of the posture according to the form, beginning and ending with Mountain Posture, or attention position (the *sama-sthiti* command). As much as possible, given space limitations I have tried to illustrate the movement in and out of the postures. In some cases it is obvious and I have chosen to show only the posture itself, leaving you to glean the connecting movement from the text. In other cases, where the *vinyasa* might not be so obvious, I have tried to illustrate the movement with sequential photographs.

THE POSTURES

1

BIG TOE POSTURE: *PADANGUSTHASANA*

Pada means "foot" or "leg." *Padangustha* means "the big toe."

TECHNIQUE

Sama-sthiti—attention position.

Preparation: Step or jump feet six to eight inches apart. Feet are parallel and approximately lined up with the hip bones.

Inhale, bend over, grab big toes with first two fingers, lift head, extend back, look up.

Exhale (Figure 4.1), fold at hips, using arm muscles (biceps) and shoulder muscles (deltoids) to pull torso into thighs. Work with straight legs. Contract thigh muscles, lifting kneecaps. Don't round the back. Gaze out between legs. Listen to the breath.

Beginners' Modification: Bend knees.

Note of caution: Standing forward and bending with straight legs is contraindicated (or not recommended) for anyone with any kind of back problems or injuries or with very tight (short) hamstrings. If you have lower-back problems or pain, or are extremely tight in this posture, you must work with your knees bent!

THIS IS BIG TOE POSTURE—HOLD FOR FIVE BREATHS (FIGURE 4.1).

Inhale, lift head and chest, look up, extend the back. *Go directly to . . .*

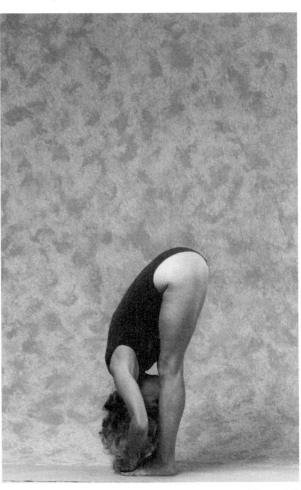

Figure 4.1

2

HAND UNDER FOOT POSTURE:
PADAHASTASANA

Pada means "foot" or "leg." *Hasta* means "hand." In this posture the feet are placed on top of the hands.

TECHNIQUE

Exhale, let go of toes from last posture and place palms under feet, with toes to wrists, and back of the hands facing the floor.

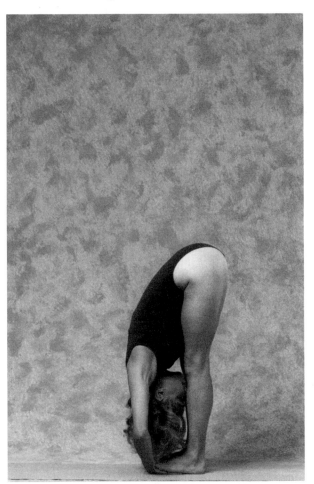

Figure 4.2

Inhale, head up, lift the chest, gaze up. Arms straight, knees bent if necessary.

Exhale (Figure 4.2), fold at the hips and use arms to pull torso into thighs. Gaze straight out through legs. Work with straight legs, kneecaps pulled up and thighs working throughout. Place weight *slightly* forward on balls of feet to enhance calf stretch. This is a counter pose to the hand/wrist position of the Sun Salutations, so it is important, to receive the full benefit in the wrists, that you place the hands all the way under the feet. Attempt to hold the *bandhas*—both root and abdominal lock throughout.

Note of caution: Be careful not to lean too far forward, for obvious reasons. As you become more advanced, you can increase the forward pressure on the hands.

> *Beginners' Modification:* Work with knees bent throughout the posture until you return to standing. In the posture, try to press the chest into the thighs while extending the back.

THIS IS HAND UNDER FOOT POSTURE—HOLD FOR FIVE BREATHS (FIGURE 4.2).

Inhale (Figure 4.3 sequence), lift chest, look up, extend back, and straighten arms.

Exhale, bring hands to hips.

Inhale, stand up, lift thighs, squeeze shoulder blades together, look at ceiling (basically, tighten back of body to act as counter pose to forward stretch).

Exhale—Sama-sthiti, return to attention position.

Note of caution: If you feel dizzy coming up from this or any standing forward-bending posture, it is most probably due to low blood pressure, low blood sugar, dehydration, or just the redistribution of blood flow. Simply stand still in the halfway position until you regain equilibrium, then continue up to the standing position. Do not look up during the closing inhale. If dizziness persists, stop practice and consult your doctor.

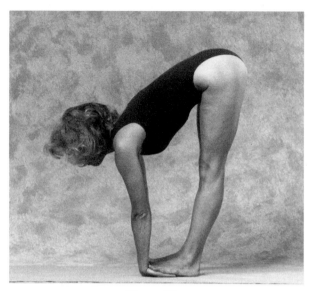

Figure 4.3a

Figure 4.3b   **Figure 4.3c**

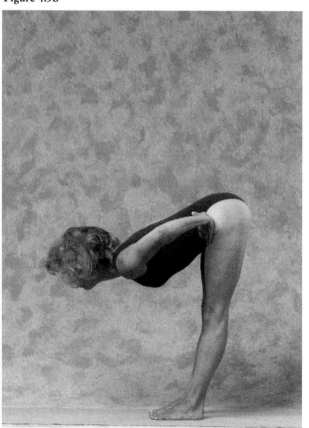

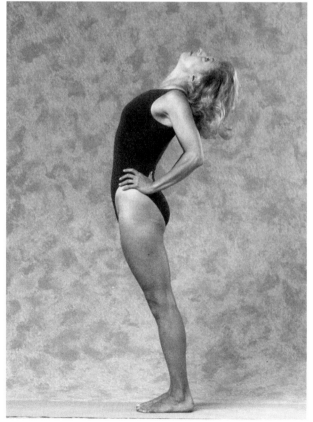

3

EXTENDED TRIANGLE POSTURE: *UTTHITA TRIKONASANA*

Utthita means "extended." *Tri* means "three." *Kona* means "angle." Thus, this is called Extended Triangle Posture.

TECHNIQUE

Inhale as you jump or step your feet three feet apart. (If working on a mat, turn ninety degrees to right so you are still going long way on mat). Turn right foot out ninety degrees. Turn left foot in thirty de-grees, or slightly toward your right. The heel of the right foot lines up with the arch of the left foot. Extend arms out. Flex right thigh! Make sure right knee points in *same* direction as right foot!

Exhale (Figure 4.4 sequence), bend to the right, keeping arms, shoulders, and hips aligned in a vertical plane. Grab big toe with first two fingers. Look up at left thumb. Hold right thigh contracted. Do not bend knees. Left hand and arm are straight up toward ceiling. Head, arm, hand, torso, and legs are in one plane (Figure 4.5).

Figure 4.4a

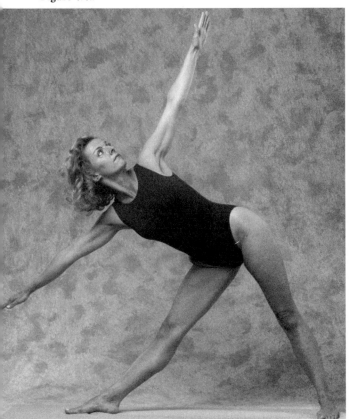

Figure 4.4b

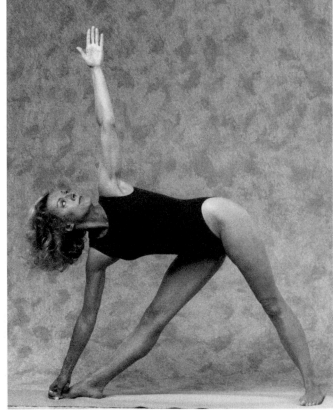

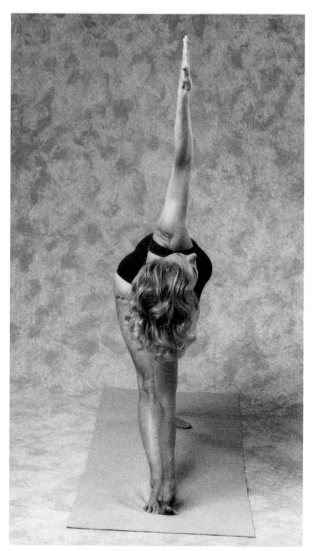

Figure 4.5

Inhale (Figure 4.8 sequence), come up with arms out straight from the sides, *reverse feet exactly,* with left foot now turning out ninety degrees and right foot turning in thirty degrees.
Exhale, repeat posture to left side.

HOLD FOR FIVE BREATHS.

Inhale, come up with arms straight out to the sides, reverse feet again, with right foot turning out ninety degrees and left foot turning in forty-five degrees this time.
Go directly to . . .

Figure 4.6

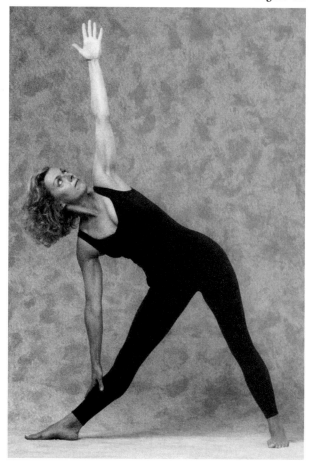

Beginners' Modification: Take hand to ankle or shin (Figure 4.6). Keep right kneecap pulled up, or thigh flexed with right kneecap pointing the same direction as the right foot. Keep head in line with spine. Do not let the head hang. Use neck muscles. Look up at left thumb.

THIS IS EXTENDED TRIANGLE POSTURE—HOLD FOR FIVE BREATHS (FIGURE 4.7).

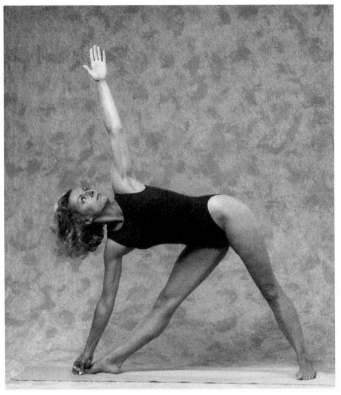

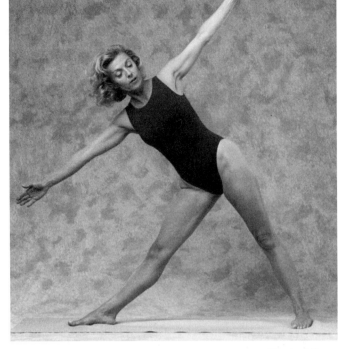

Figure 4.8a ▲

Figure 4.8c ▼

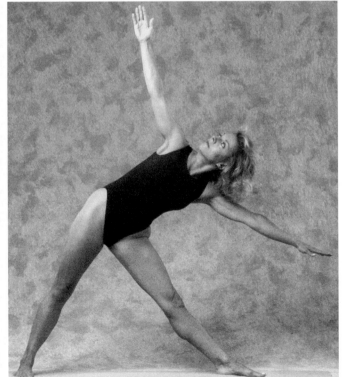

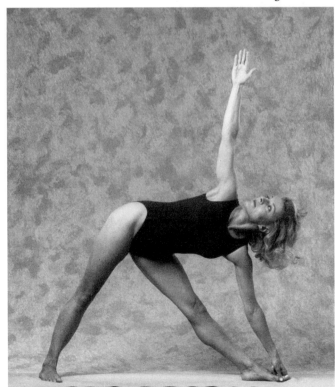

4

REVOLVED TRIANGLE POSTURE: *PARIVRTTA TRIKONASANA*

Parivrtta means "revolved" or "turned around." *Tri* means "three." *Kona* means "angle." This is therefore the turned over—or Revolved Triangle Posture.

TECHNIQUE

Exhale, rotate torso, reach out with left arm (Figure 4.9), and place left hand flat on floor on inside or medial portion of right foot. When this becomes easy, increase twist and hamstring stretch by placing hand on outside or lateral portion of right foot. Press down into hand and extend (work) back muscles. Hold head in line with spine and fix gaze on a point beyond the hand. Keep right thigh flexing, or lifting into groin. Do not bend knees (Figure 4.10).

Beginners' Modification: Take both hands to knee, shin or ankle. Do *not* bend knees (Figure 4.11). Keeps shoulders and hands level with one another and equidistant from the floor. Concentrate on strength (thigh contracting, lifting). Look at toes. Once hands reach the floor without bending knees, move to the advanced posture.

Note of caution: Contracting the thigh muscle is not the same as "locking" and/or hyperextending the knee. If you tend to have hyperextended knees, be

Figure 4.9

Figure 4.10

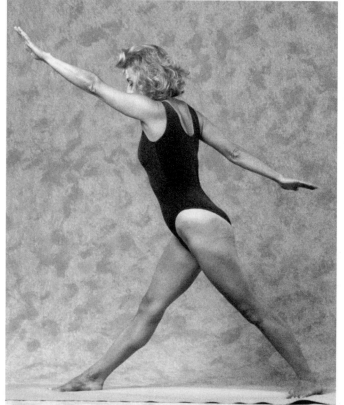

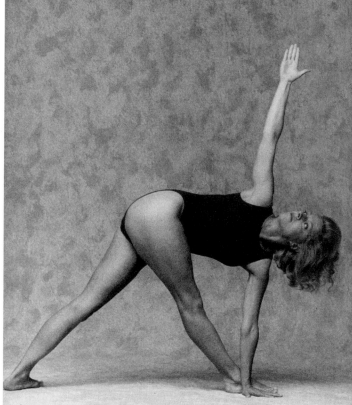

careful not to go over the edge from "lifting" into "locking back."

THIS IS REVOLVED TRIANGLE POSTURE—HOLD FOR FIVE BREATHS (FIGURE 4.10 OR 4.11).

Inhale, come up, pushing off with toes, thighs, and hands, swing through with arms out to sides, just as you did in the connecting *vinyasa* for the previous posture, *reverse feet exactly,* with right foot turning in forty-five degrees and left foot out ninety degrees.

Exhale, rotate torso and reach out, this time leading with the right arm, *repeat posture to left side.*

HOLD FOR FIVE BREATHS.

Figure 4.11

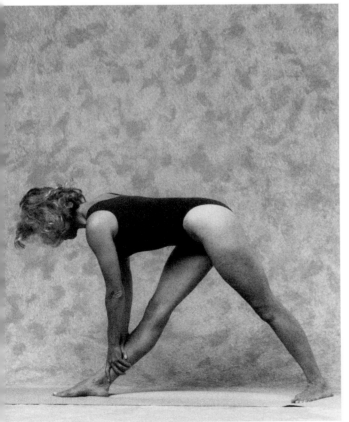

Inhale, push off, come back up, swing through with arms out to sides, face front, square off feet.

Exhale—Sama-sthiti, jump or step back to attention position.

5

EXTENDED SIDE ANGLE POSTURE: *UTTIHITTA PARSVAKONASANA*

Uttihita means "extended" or "stretched out." *Parsva* means "side" or "flank," "lateral." *Kona* means "angle."

TECHNIQUE

Inhale, jump or step your feet four feet apart, with feet parallel. Extend arms out to sides. Turn right foot out ninety degrees and left foot in thirty degrees. Right foot and knee points in direction of extended hand.

Exhale, descend into the posture by bending right knee over right ankle (Figure 4.12 sequence). Place right hand to outside or lateral side of right foot. Reach over left ear with left arm. Look up to left hand. Tuck chin into armpit. Hold root lock and abdominal lock. Be aware of the working muscles in the arms, legs, back, and torso. One straight line should be formed by your hand, down through the arm, the lats, hips, leg, and outside edge of the foot (Figure 4.13).

Beginners' Modification: Place right hand to inside or medial side of right foot (Figure 4.14). Reach straight up to ceiling with left arm. Keep shoulders in straight line. Look up.

Note of caution: Keep head aligned with spine. Do not let the head hang. This can be stressful on a mis-

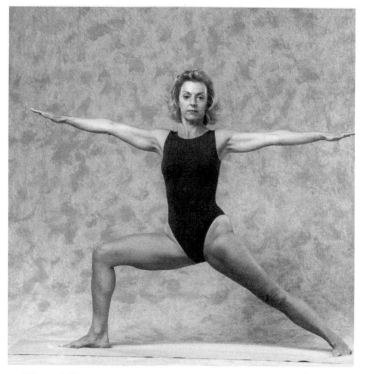

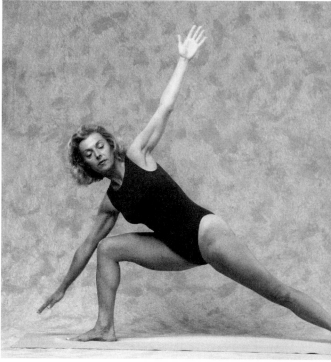

▲ **Figure 4.12a**

Figure 4.12b ▲

▼ **Figure 4.13**

Figure 4.14 ▼

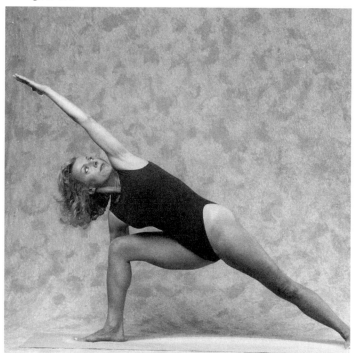

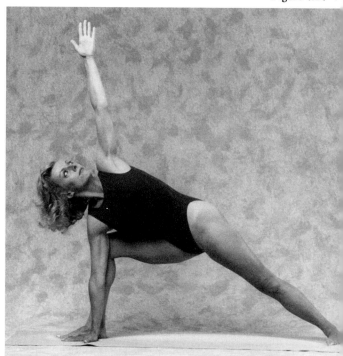

aligned spine. Also, do not let knee extend past the ankle. This can be slightly stressful on the knee, particularly an injured or misaligned knee.

THIS IS EXTENDED SIDE ANGLE POSTURE—HOLD FOR FIVE BREATHS (FIGURE 4.13 OR 4.14).

Inhale, come up with arms straight out to the sides, *reverse feet exactly,* turning right foot (toes) in toward the left foot thirty degrees and the left foot out ninety degrees.
Exhale, repeat posture to the left side.

HOLD FOR FIVE BREATHS.

Inhale, come up with arms straight out to the sides, square off feet (turn them parallel), face front.
Exhale—Sama-sthiti, jump or step back to attention position.

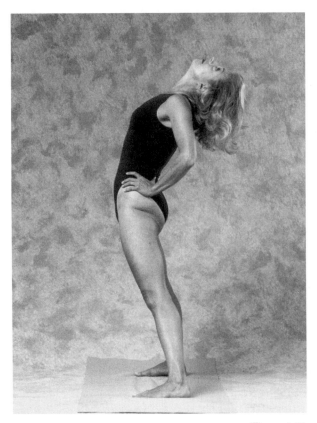

Figure 4.15

6

EXPANDED LEG INTENSE STRETCH POSTURES A–D—*PRASARITA PADOTTANASANA A–D*

Prasarita means "spread out" or "expanded." *Pada* means "foot" or "leg." *Uttana* means "intense stretch." This means that the legs are in an expanded position and then stretched intensely.

EXPANDED LEG INTENSE STRETCH A

TECHNIQUE

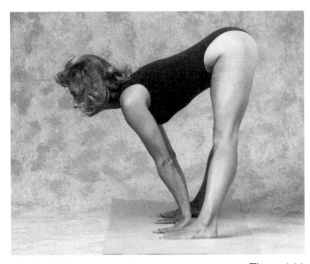

Figure 4.16

Inhale, jump or step your feet 3 1/2 to 4 feet apart with feet parallel, toes pointing forward. Hands on hips. Look up, squeeze shoulder blades together, and stretch back, but keep pelvis tucked under. Contract thighs (Figure 4.15). Hold *mula* and *uddiyana bandha,* root and abdominal lock, throughout.
Exhale, fold forward at the hips, placing hands on the floor. Head up. Arms straight (Figure 4.16).

Beginners' Modification: Reach as far forward as necessary to take hands to floor, as in Face Down Dog. Do not bend knees. Keep head up. *Do not go further.* Don't round the back in an attempt to "look" flexible. If your hands don't reach the floor, keep them on your hips and hold this position as your posture until the hamstrings open up enough to allow your hands to reach the ground, as in Figure 4.16.

Inhale, again, head still up.
Exhale, fold forward at hips. Do not round back. Use inner upper arm (biceps) as well as shoulder and abdominal muscles to "pull" torso toward thighs and into the stretch. *Keep thighs working!* Hold *bandhas.* Gaze is straight out through legs, past the end of the nose (Figure 4.17).

Note: This is a good posture to develop awareness of the oblique contraction in the abdominal lock. As you exhale into the posture, press the rib cage down and in slightly. This activates the oblique abdominal muscles, as we first practiced earlier in this chapter. Attempt to be mindful of this contraction not only in this posture but throughout. In most instances, it helps to lengthen and decompress the lower back.

THIS IS EXPANDED LEG INTENSE STRETCH A— HOLD FOR FIVE BREATHS (FIGURE 4.17).

Inhale, lift head, look up, lift chest (Figure 4.18).
Exhale, hands to hips (Figure 4.19).
Inhale, stand up, look up, squeeze shoulder blades together, thighs still holding firm (Figure 4.20).
Exhale, relax, and look front.

▼

EXPANDED LEG INTENSE STRETCH B

TECHNIQUE

Inhale, stretch arms out to sides.
Exhale, hands on hips.
Inhale, look up, squeeze shoulder blades together, contract *bandhas* (beginners tighten buttocks).
Exhale, fold down, keeping back in extension. Then pull into stretch with abdominals and back muscles, or lats (lumbar flexors). Although back is "flexed," it is not excessively rounded! Remember the perineal and abdominal locks. Now you can

Figure 4.17, front view

Figure 4.17, side view

Figure 4.18

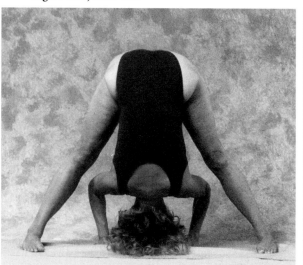
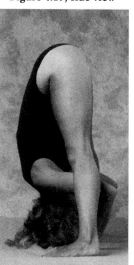
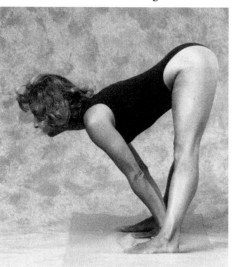

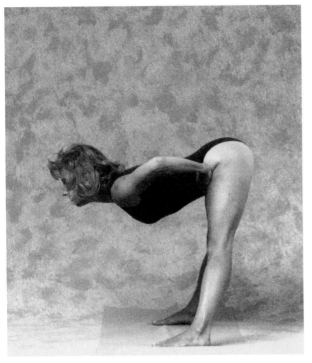

Figure 4.19

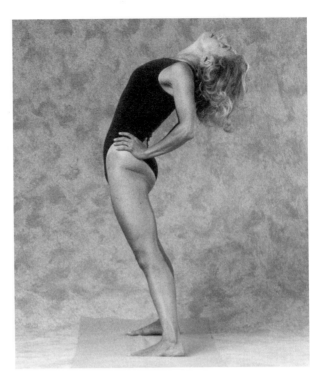

Figure 4.20

actually "feel" the contraction of the oblique abdominal muscles under your fingers where they are placed on your waist. Use the fingertips as feedback detectors here to aid mindfulness of this contraction. Gaze straight as in A (Figure 4.21).

Beginners' Modification: Do not round back or hunch shoulders. Keep head up. Look straight out to front.

THIS IS EXPANDED LEG INTENSE STRETCH B—HOLD FOR FIVE BREATHS

Figure 4.21

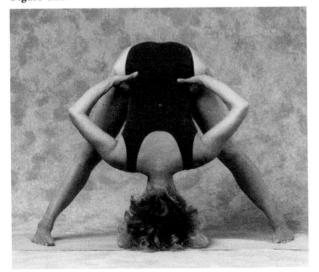

Figure 4.21, side view

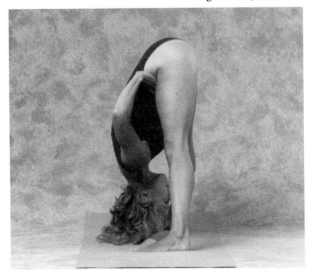

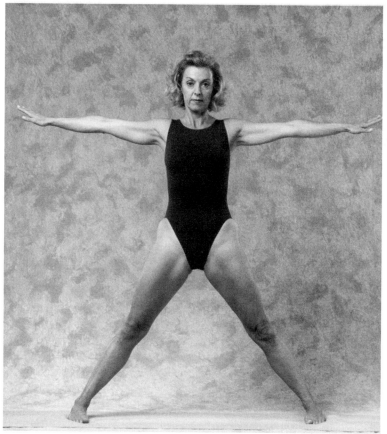

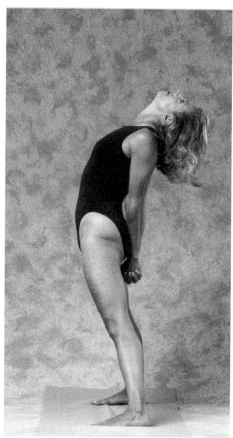

▲ Figure 4.22

Figure 4.23 ▲

▼ Figure 4.24, side view

Figure 4.25 ▼

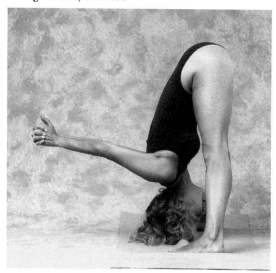

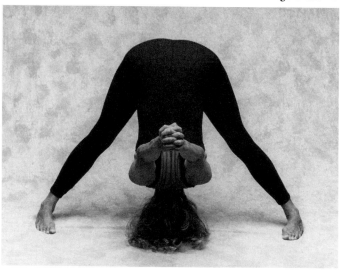

Inhale, look up, lift chest, start ascending.

Exhale, continue coming up.

Inhale, look up, stretch back, tighten shoulder blades, thighs *still* lifting.

Exhale, relax, look front.

EXPANDED LEG INTENSE STRETCH C

TECHNIQUE

Inhale (Figure 4.22), extend arms out to sides.

Exhale, clasp hands and interlace fingers, then press wrists, forearms, elbows, and upper arms together; open shoulders and press back, contracting the shoulder blades together.

Inhale, stretch back, look up, hold the *bandhas* (Figure 4.23).

Exhale, fold forward (Figure 4.24), keeping hands clasped and arms strong. Bring arms over head, go as far as possible. Use strength. Hold locks. Gaze is straight through legs (Figure 4.25).

Beginners' Modification: Try to lift arms off back, toward ceiling. Use your strength. Keep head in neutral position so you don't compress the front or the back of the neck. Look straight.

THIS IS EXPANDED LEG INTENSE STRETCH C—HOLD FOR FIVE BREATHS (FIGURES 4.24 AND 4.25).

Inhale, head up, look up, lift chest.

Exhale.

Inhale, come back to standing with hands still interlaced, contract the shoulder blades together, stretching open front of shoulders. Look up. Thighs are still working!

Exhale, release hands, and place on hips. Look straight.

EXPANDED LEG INTENSE STRETCH D

TECHNIQUE

Inhale, hands on hips, look up, squeeze shoulder blades, contract quads, hold *bandhas.*

Exhale, bend over, grab big toes with first two fingers.

Beginners' Modification: Grab backs of legs with hands, do not bend knees, keep back straight.

Inhale, head up, look up.

Exhale, using arm muscles (biceps), chest muscles (pectorals) and back muscles (lats), pull torso to-

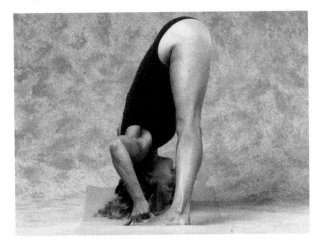

▲ **Figure 4.26, side view**   **Figure 4.27** ▼

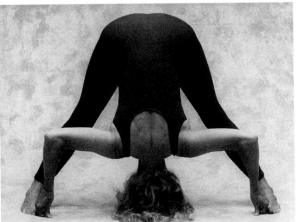

ward thighs (Figure 4.26 and Figure 4.27). Try to pull torso through legs, using arm and abdominal muscles. Remember the locks, including the upper or oblique aspect of abdominal lock. Gaze straight out.

Beginners' Modification: Flex elbows and pull with arms, but keep chest lifted and back in extension. Look out straight.

THIS IS EXPANDED LEG INTENSE STRETCH D— HOLD FOR FIVE BREATHS (FIGURES 4.26 AND 4.27).

Inhale, look up, lift chest.
Exhale, hands to hips.
Inhale, come up to standing, look up, stretch back.
Exhale, Sama-sthiti—jump or simply step your feet back together, returning to attention position.

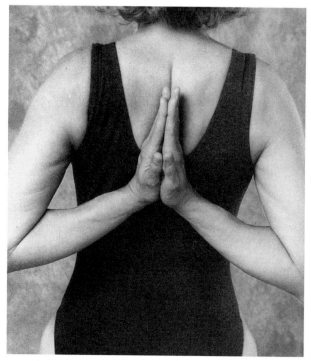

▲ **Figure 4.28**

7

INTENSE SIDE STRETCH POSTURE: *PARSVATANASANA*

Parsva means "side" or "flank." *Uttana* means "intense stretch." What I always figured this meant was an intense stretch while turned to the side. The intensity here is in the hamstrings!

TECHNIQUE

Inhale, jump or step your feet three feet apart, arms extended out to sides, right foot turned out ninety degrees, left foot turned in forty-five degrees
Exhale, place palms together behind back in "prayer" position.
Tip: Start with palms together and fingers pointing down, then invert the hands (Figure 4.28). Turn hips and torso ninety degrees to the right.

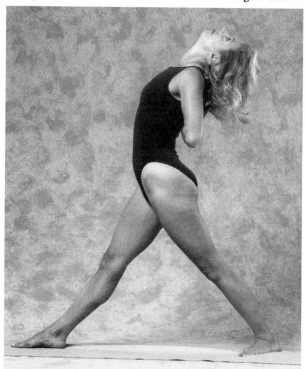

Figure 4.29 ▼

Beginners' Modification: If you wrestled in high school or college, ever lifted weights, or have an old shoulder injury that limits your range of motion, then this position may be difficult. Instead, fold your arms behind you and try to grab the elbow of the opposite arm with your hands.

Inhale, look up, lift chest, and open shoulders, stretch back (Figure 4.29).

Exhale, fold down over right leg, chin to shin (Figure 4.30). Hold *bandhas,* press on outside of back foot and inside of front foot, keep hips level. Gaze up and out at big toe.

Beginners' Modification: Keep back straight, head up, chest lifted, and find balance as you see Thom doing in (Figure 4.31). Keep eyes steady and use toes to help with balance. Don't round back in attempt to get head to shin. Face up and out.

THIS IS INTENSE SIDE STRETCH POSTURE—HOLD FOR FIVE BREATHS (FIGURES 4.30 OR 4.31).

Inhale, come all the way up on one breath, look up, stretch back.

Exhale, reverse feet exactly, changing direction as in previous postures.

Inhale, look up again, stretch back.

Exhale, repeat to left side, take five breaths.

Inhale, come all the way up on one breath, look up, stretch back, rotate torso back to center, square off feet.

Exhale. Sama-sthiti, return to attention position.

Figure 4.30

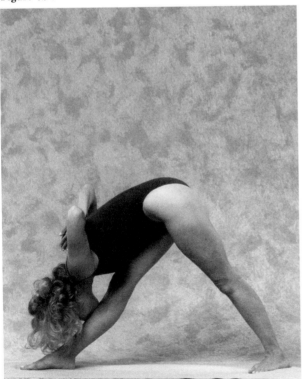

Figure 4.31

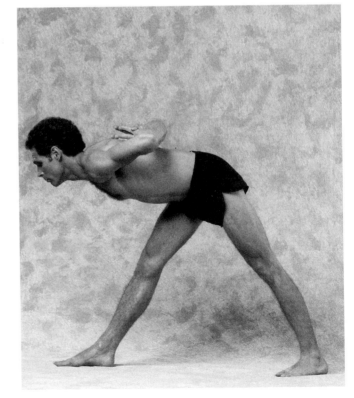

8

EXTENDED HAND TO BIG TOE POSTURE— *UTTHITTA HASTA PADANGUSTHASANA*

Utthitta means "extended" or "stretched out." *Hasta* means "hand." *Pada* means "foot," in this case, and *padangustha* means "big toe."

Helpful hint: Since this is the first of the standing balancing postures, it might take some practice before you will learn to stand comfortably on one foot. Use the gaze and the breath. Picking a point with your eyes and then riveting your gaze on that point is helpful in maintaining balance and developing concentration. Using the breath to ground and center yourself also helps to keep you balanced.

TECHNIQUE

Note: Some of the illustrations for this series show both the left and the right sides. To avoid confusion, follow directions, and as with all postures, practice the right side first. Figure 4.43 on page 116 shows the complete sequence for the right side from start to finish.

Inhale, take big toe of right foot with first two fingers of right hand (Figure 4.32), extend leg, and lift right leg as high as possible (Figure 4.33). Place left hand on hip. Keep right hip level with left hip. If this is as much as you can do without losing your balance, use Figure 4.32 or 4.33 as your posture for five breaths until balance gets easier and you can go on to the next level.

Exhale, bend over, and try to touch your chin to your shin while lifting leg up to meet chin (Figure 4.34).

Figure 4.32

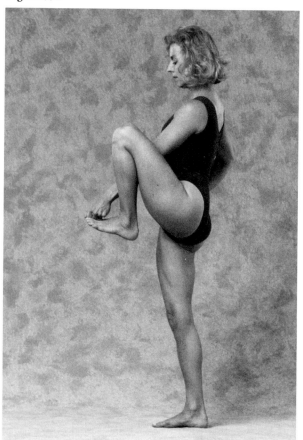

Figure 4.33

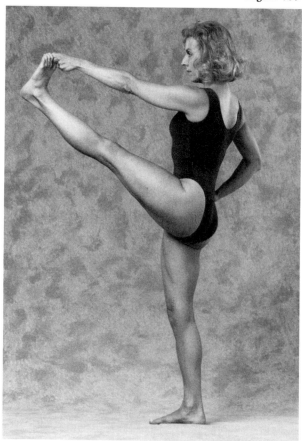

Gaze straight. Do not round the back to attempt to take head to knee. Keep the chest lifted and bend at the hips, keeping the back extended.

Beginners' Modification: Mastering the completed posture, as you see in Figure 4.34, takes a bit of practice, especially for those of us with tight hamstrings or hips. Start with the following modifications and get these down before you begin to work on extending the leg. *It's better to do the modifications with dignity and grace than to be hopping around in flail state attempting the more difficult posture.*

Inhale, hands on hips, bend knee and lift right leg, and practice standing on one foot. Knee should be up as high as possible, yet maintaining balance. Foot is dorsiflexed (toes pulled up) and directly under knee (Figure 4.35).

Exhale, take your five breaths in this position. After practicing this position for several weeks (and following with the knee-to-chest position in Part B), you will eventually be able to reach down and grab the toe, extending slightly. Eventually you will be able to extend fully. Pick a point in front of you, gaze at it, and don't change your gaze! Go to Beginners' Modification for Part B.

THIS IS EXTENDED HAND TO BIG TOE POSTURE, PART A—HOLD FOR FIVE BREATHS (FIGURES 4.32, 4.33, 4.34, OR 4.35). CONTINUE TO PART B.

Figure 4.34

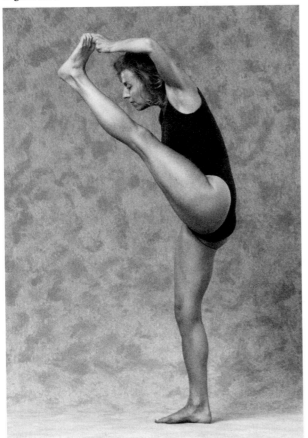

Figure 4.35

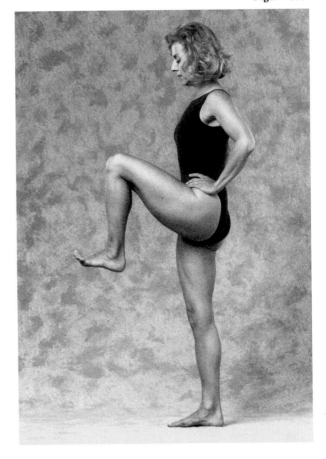

Inhale, look up, straighten torso (Figure 4.36).
Exhale, open right leg out to side. Keep torso straight and hips level. Gaze to the left (Figure 4.37).

Beginners' Modification:

    Inhale, grab right knee with both hands. If you have knee pain or injury, hold leg behind the knee.

    Exhale, pull knee to chest, use arms to pull knee in, keep standing leg pulled up, rib cage lifted, shoulders down (Figure 4.38). Take your five breaths in this position. This is a great posture for lower-back pain or tight hip flexors. Don't lean back. The tendency to lean back can be caused by tight hip flexor muscles.

THIS IS EXTENDED HAND TO BIG TOE POSTURE PART B—HOLD FOR FIVE BREATHS (FIGURE 4.37 OR 4.38).

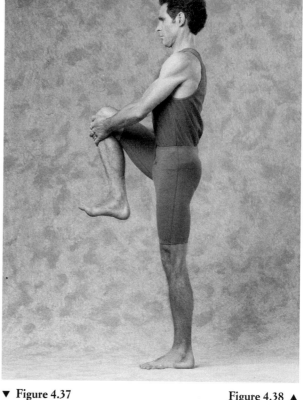

▼ **Figure 4.36**

▼ **Figure 4.37**   **Figure 4.38** ▲

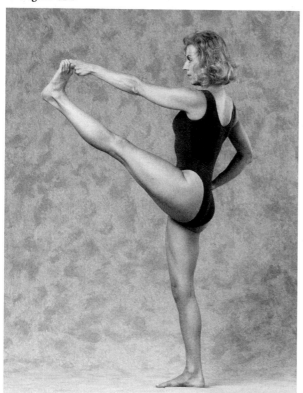

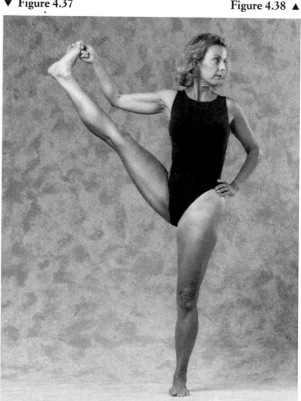

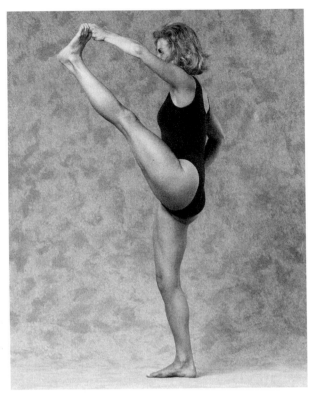

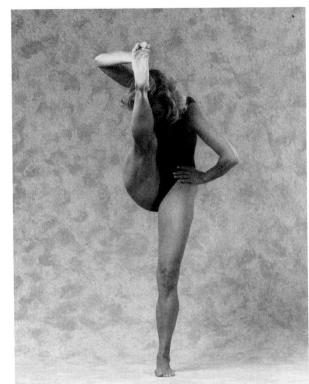

Figure 4.40 ▲

Figure 4.42 ▼

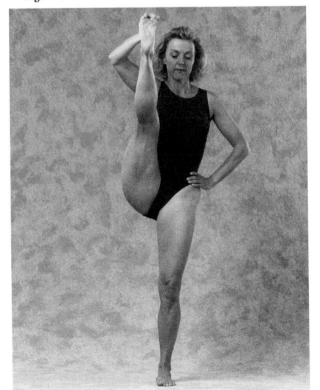

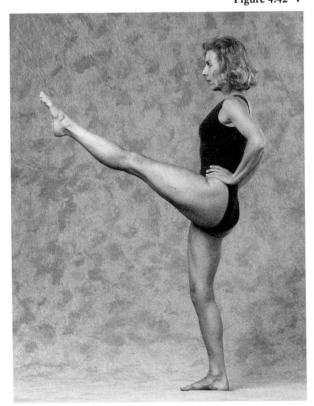

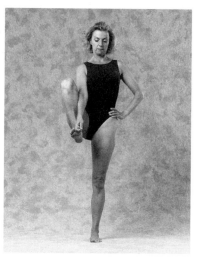

Figure 4.43a

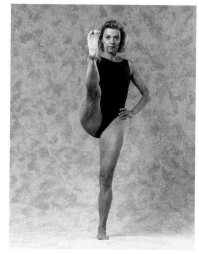

Figure 4.43b

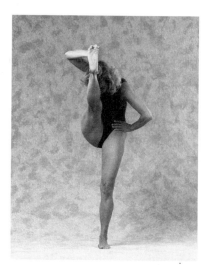

Figure 4.43c

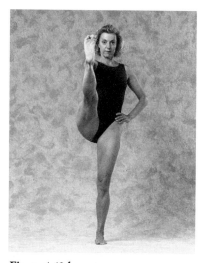

Figure 4.43d

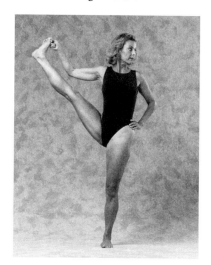

Figure 4.43e

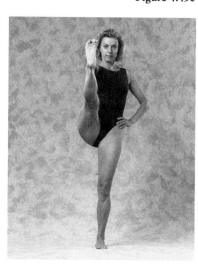

Figure 4.43f

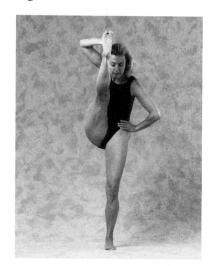

Figure 4.43g

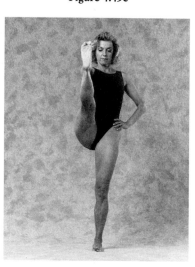

Figure 4.43h

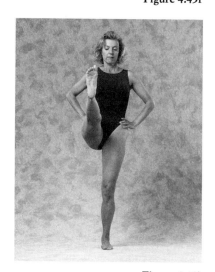

Figure 4.43i

Inhale, look front, swing leg back to front (Figure 4.39).

Exhale, bend over, pull shin to chin, elbow bent (Figure 4.40).

Inhale, head up, torso straight (Figure 4.41).

Exhale, release toe, hold leg straight out for three breaths (Figure 4.42), then *sama-sthiti,* return to attention position.

Note: For those practicing the *Beginners' Modification,* simply hold the position for five breaths, and on the following exhale return to *sama-sthiti.*

Helpful Hint: Since the complete routine of Extended Hand to Big Toe Posture is a somewhat intricate mixture of posture and *vinyasa,* you might wish to work with each move individually at first. This makes it a little easier to learn the alignment of each movement and find the balance. Once you are somewhat familiar with each piece of the sequence, you can practice putting them all together with the breathing (Figure 4.43). Figure 4.43, shown on the opposite page, is a composite of Figure 4.32 through 4.42 (except for modifications), and helps to show the flow of the complete sequence of movements (left to right, top to bottom).

Repeat instructions for left side.

9

STANDING BOUND HALF LOTUS POSTURE: *ARDHA BADDHA PADMOTTANASANA*

Ardha means "half." *Baddha* means "bound" or "caught." *Padma* means "lotus." *Uttana* means "intense stretch."

This is the first of a number of postures where one limb or part of the body is "bound," or compressed by a particular position. As one limb, for example, is bound off, the blood supply circulating in that limb is actually squeezed out and the incoming circulation to that part of the body is reduced. Consequently, the rest of the body then experiences a forced increase in blood supply. Once the sides are reversed or the counter postures are done, the situation is reversed. Now the blood is pushed into the part where it was previously squeezed out.

This control over circulation seems to create a very strong presence for cleansing and healing, and seems to be one of the unique benefits of the yoga discipline. It is important to keep the breath going during the bound postures. This way, the heat stays up for the compressed joints, and the circulation that *is* still moving in the bound body part is sufficiently oxygenated and flowing.

Note of caution: This posture incorporates the famous "lotus" position. This is a perfectly safe posture and continues the range of motion work for the hips, begun by the prior standing postures. However, this posture is one of a small group of yoga postures that have developed something of a bad reputation over the years in sports medical circles, primarily because there can be a high risk of injury if they are practiced incorrectly by someone with a weak or injured knee.

What occasionally happens is that someone will attempt a particular posture, like Standing Bound Half Lotus Posture, do it wrong, and get injured. Let's say they "tweak" something, or the next day the knee hurts a little. Off they run to their orthopedist or sports medical doctor and say, "Oh, I got injured doing yoga!" Great! They don't bother to explain that they got injured doing yoga *wrong!*

The "expert" then goes off to write an article about the bad, or "contraindicated," yoga postures. The irony about these articles is that they are never written by anyone who knows anything about yoga. In a way these articles are helpful, because they do alert the general public to the postures that have potential to injure people if they do them wrong. But there is nothing inherently "wrong" with this system of yoga or any or its postures. The only thing that can be wrong is doing the postures incorrectly or doing the form incompletely. The important thing to remember is that in this form there is an *order* to the postures and that they must be done in the precise sequence given. There is also correct and incorrect form within the sequence. This means correct alignment.

This particular posture is a hip opener, not a knee stressor. Do not force the knee in any circumstances to move or "open." It can take up to two years or more to "bind" or grab the foot behind the back with the hand, especially if you are coming from a strong athletic background and are tight in the hips. Work patiently.

If you are just coming back from arthroscopic surgery, move very cautiously! This range of motion work *is* therapeutic, but you must increase the compression in the joint *very, very slowly* and progressively. At first, just barely bend the knee. Each day slightly increase the closure of the knee, which is a hinge joint and meant to fold in half. This work will help you to regain full range of motion in the knee. If you have a knee injury involving any of the tendons or ligaments surrounding the knee, the same rules apply. Work slowly and progressively. And breathe!

TECHNIQUE

Inhale, bring right leg up at angle.

Exhale. There are three levels of options here:

> *Beginners* (Figure 4.44): Hold right foot with both hands. Gaze straight at one point. Use gaze, locks, and breath to keep balance. Take your five breaths in this position.

> *Intermediate* (Figure 4.45): Reach around your

Figure 4.44

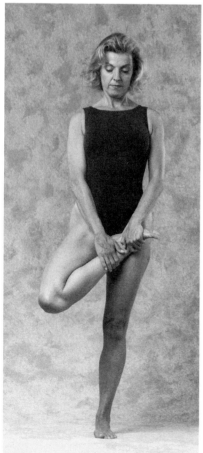

Figure 4.45

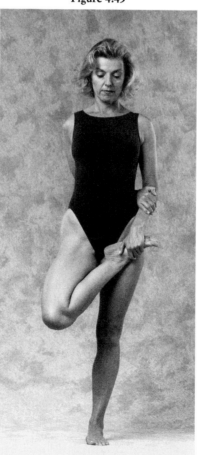

Figure 4.46

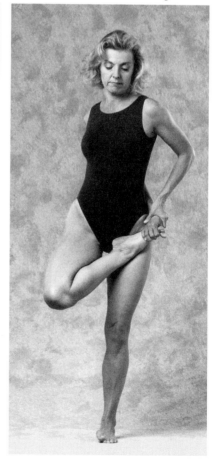

back with your right hand and grab your left forearm, which is holding the right foot. Hold gaze steady out in front of you, perhaps at floor. Hold locks.

Advanced (Figure 4.46): Reach around your back with your right hand and grab your right foot over the top of the foot, as shown in the close-up (Figure 4.47). This is called "binding" the hand and foot. Hold locks.

Inhale.

Beginners and Intermediate: Hold in position.

Advanced: Reach left arm in air (Figure 4.48).

Exhale.

Beginners and Intermediate: Hold in position.

Advanced: Fold at hips and take left palm to floor alongside foot (Figure 4.49 and 4.50). Try to bring nose to knee. Gaze out past the end of the nose.

Note of caution: Do not attempt to bend forward unless you are "binding," or holding foot. Binding must precede forward bending. The knee is not in correct alignment to take forward pressure until the hip is open enough to allow binding. *Bending forward without binding can cause knee injury!*

THIS IS STANDING BOUND HALF LOTUS POS-TURE—HOLD FOR FIVE BREATHS (FIGURES 4.44, 4.45, 4.46, 4.47, 4.48, 4.49, OR 4.50).

Inhale.

Beginners and Intermediate: Continue to hold in position.

Advanced: Look up.

Exhale, all levels hold.

Inhale.

Beginners and Intermediate: Hold in position.

Advanced: Come back up to standing, pushing off with hand and the toes, and using the leg muscles to return to upright posture.

Exhale, release and place foot back on the floor.

Sama-sthiti, return to attention position.

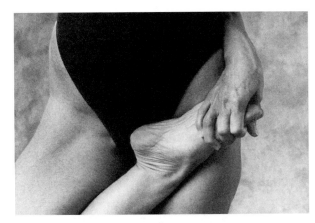

▲ **Figure 4.47**

▼ **Figure 4.48**   **Figure 4.49** ▼

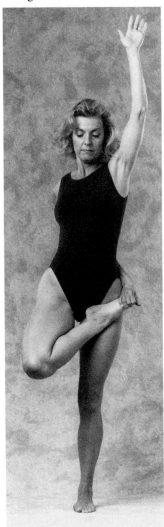
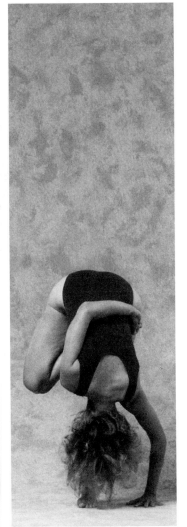

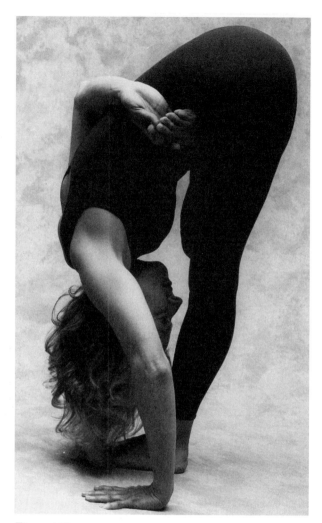

Figure 4.50

Note: Any of the positions illustrated from Figure 4.44 through Figure 4.50 may be used as your working posture. As you progress, you will slowly move further through the sequence until you accomplish binding and forward bending.

Repeat instructions for left side.

10

FIERCE POSTURE: *UTKATASANA*

Utkata means "fierce" or "powerful."

TECHNIQUE

Note: The opening *vinyasa,* or connecting movement, for this posture corresponds to the first six movements of Sun Salutation A.

Inhale, arms up, palms together.
Exhale, palms to the floor.
Inhale, head up.
Exhale, walk or jump back.
Inhale, Face Up Dog.
Exhale, Face Down Dog.
Inhale, step or jump the feet to the hands, bend knees.
Exhale, keeping knees bent, and remaining in as "deep" a tuck position as possible, bring arms up over the head, palms together, look up (Figure 4.51). The dual effort here is (1) to lift *up* with the chest *using* the back muscles while trying to straighten the arms, pointing the middle fingers directly at the ceiling and pressing the palms together, and (2) to sink the buttock bones *down* toward the floor.

Important note: If you are feeling any compression in the lower back, you will probably notice that you have forgotten to hold the abdominal lock, especially the contraction of the oblique muscles. Strongly working the obliques, by pressing downward and in on the rib cage slightly, will completely remove any stress in the lower back.

THIS IS FIERCE POSTURE—HOLD FOR FIVE BREATHS (FIGURE 4.51).

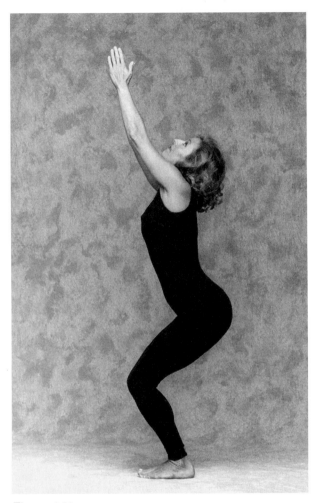

Figures 4.51

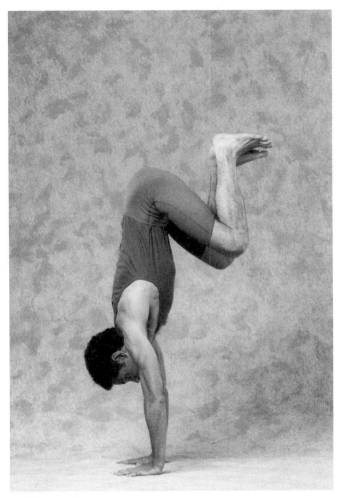

▲ **Figure 4.52**

Figure 4.53 ▼

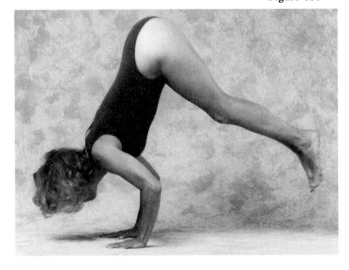

Inhale, take palms to floor, keep head up.

    Advanced: If you are feeling real adventurous and want to work on extra upper-body strength, you can try the advanced "take it up" as Thom does here in Figure 4.52.

Exhale, jump back (Figure 4.53).

Inhale, Face Up Dog.

Exhale, Face Down Dog.

Go directly to . . .

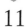

11

WARRIOR I POSTURE: *VIRABHDRASANA I*

Vira means "hero," and Virabhadra was a powerful mythical hero created from a lock of hair torn from the head of Shiva, the god of destruction in the classic trinity of Hinduism. The other two gods forming the triad with Shiva are Brahma, the god of creation, and Vishnu, the god of preservation. Shiva is the Hindu personification of the static, masculine form of the divine, and his "destructive" power symbolizes the essential breaking down of the ego personality so that it becomes pervious to divine light.

TECHNIQUE

Inhale, step right leg up to a point between the hands. This is the same position as in Positions 8 and 11 in Sun Salutation B. Beginners should follow the same procedure as given in chapter 3 for these movements.

Exhale (Figure 4.54), bring arms up over head, palms together. Head is back. Look up.

Note: Make sure that the right foot points directly forward and the toes of the back foot are pointed slightly into the posture. The back foot should remain flat on the floor, with the arch lifted. Keep the right knee directly over the right ankle, making certain you do not allow the knee to pronate. Work to

Figure 4.54

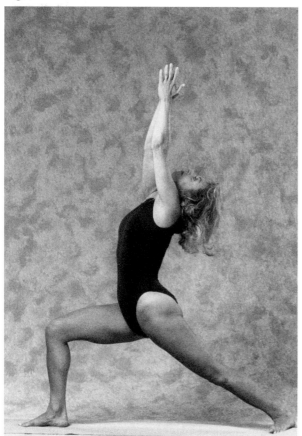

Figure 4.55

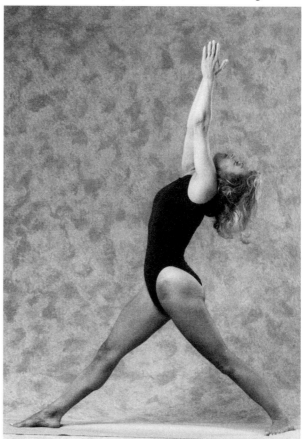

square off the hips and shoulders to the front. *As in the preceding posture, any compression in the lower back can be avoided or eliminated by focusing strongly on abdominal lock, especially the upper part of the* bandha, *which is the contraction of the oblique abdominal muscles.*

THIS IS WARRIOR I POSTURE (right side)—HOLD FOR FIVE BREATHS (FIGURE 4.54).

Inhale, straighten right leg (Figure 4.55), then turn the right foot in and the left foot out (turn around 180 degrees).
Exhale, bend left knee over left ankle, *repeat posture to left side.* Look up (Figure 4.56).

HOLD FOR FIVE BREATHS.

Go directly to . . .

12

WARRIOR II POSTURE: *VIRABHDRASANA II*

TECHNIQUE

Inhale, swing right arm down and back and left arm down front (Figure 4.57), bring the arms into the

Figure 4.56

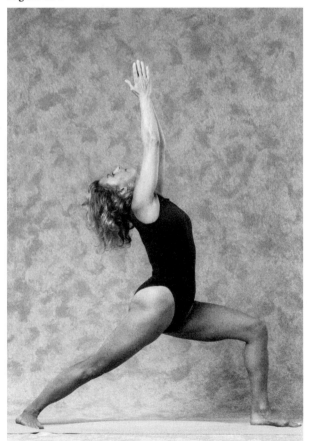

Figure 4.57

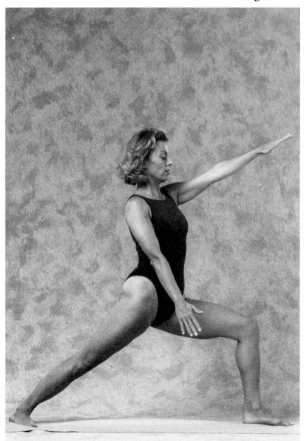

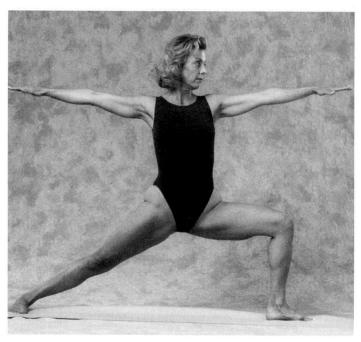

▲ **Figure 4.58**

same plane as the legs. Gaze out over fingertips of left hand. Hips and shoulders shift ninety degrees to the right (from facing front in Warrior I Posture), but stance of legs does not change (Figure 4.58). The wider the stance, the more intense the work of the thighs. Eventually the front thigh is parallel to the floor as the hips sink. Advanced practitioners, however, should be careful not to go too wide and lose form, looking sloppy. *Keep back foot flat on floor.*

Beginners' Modification: Stance will be somewhat shorter than for the advanced posture, because of tightness in hips and groin as shown in Figure 4.59 to the right side. Be careful not to let knee lunge past ankle. This can be stressful on the knee.

This is Warrior II Posture (Left Side)—hold for five breaths (Figure 4.58 or 4.59).

Figure 4.59 ▼

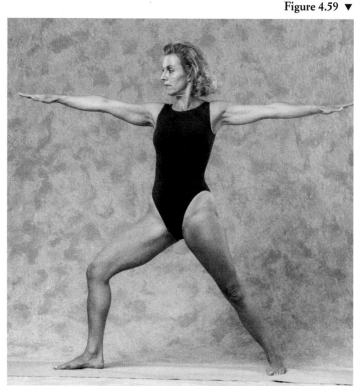

Inhale, straighten left leg (Figure 4.60), reverse feet as for Warrior I *vinyasa.*

Exhale, descend, or bend right knee over right ankle. Gaze out over fingertips of right hand (Figure 4.61). *Repeat posture to right side.*

Hold for five breaths.

Inhale, take hands to floor alongside right foot (Figure 4.62).

Exhale, jump back (Figure 4.63) into the Push-up position (Position 4) of the Sun Salutation (Figure 4.64).

Inhale (Figure 4.65), Face Up Dog.

Exhale (Figure 4.66), Face Down Dog.

Inhale, bend the knees, and "jump," butt up into air, as high as possible. Practice this jumping-up move every time you do a Sun Salutation or *vinyasa,* as it may take some time to get it. This will develop your arm strength and prepare you for Handstand Pose later in the book. Then on the way "down" from the jump-up, cross the feet, slide them

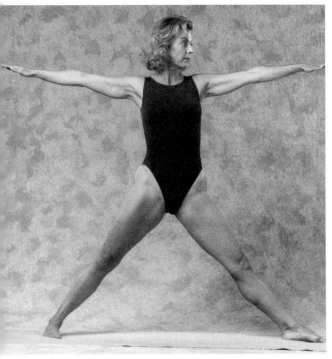

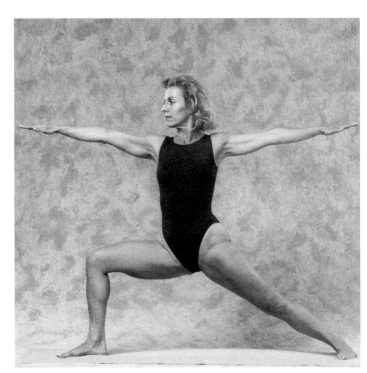

Figure 4.60

Figure 4.61

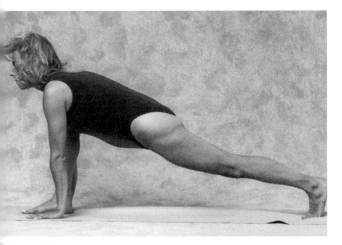

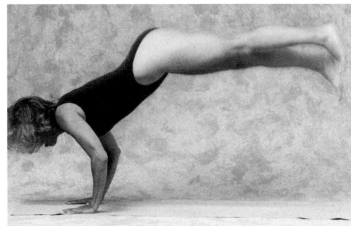

Figure 4.62

Figure 4.63

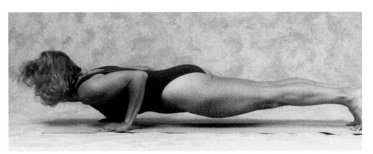

Figure 4.64

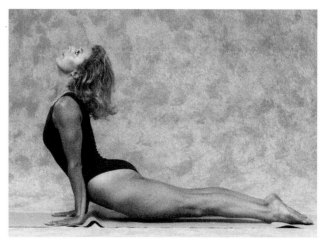

Figure 4.65

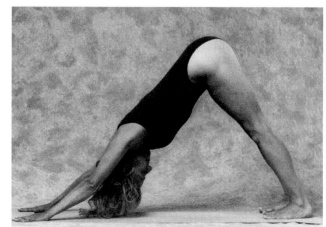

Figure 4.66

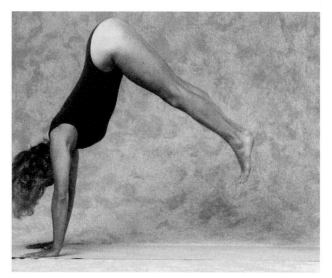

Figure 4.67a

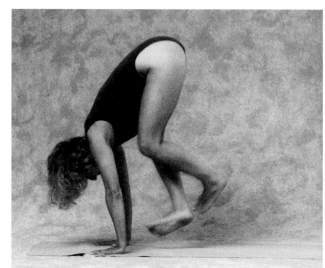

Figure 4.67b

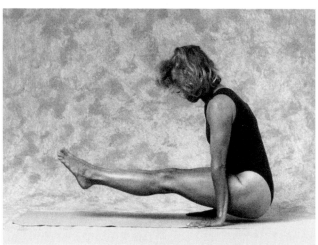

Figure 4.67c

through the hands, try to hold yourself off the ground as you straighten your legs, and then sit down (Figure 4.67 sequence). This *vinyasa* movement is called the "jump through." It is explained in detail in the next chapter after the first posture.

THIS COMPLETES THE STANDING POSTURES.

HOW LONG BEFORE I GO TO THE NEXT CHAPTER?

Spend three to four weeks learning and practicing the sequence of postures in this chapter before you go on to chapter 5. *Once you know the form thus far by heart, go on,* and add to your practice by starting the first five postures of chapter 5. This will take you through Single Leg Forward Bending A (*Janu Sirasana A*). This is a logical grouping of *asanas,* the last three being variations of Single Leg Forward Bending. They all work to open the hips and hamstrings.

Then, just as you now go from the warm-ups directly into the standing postures in your practice, so you will go directly from the last posture in this chapter to the first posture in the next chapter. How much time it takes for you to progress to this point in your practice depends on a number of factors, and

they will not be the same for everyone. Some people will learn and become comfortable with chapters 3 and 4 in a matter of weeks. Others may take several months or longer. Take as long as you need, but do practice regularly.

HOW DO I END PRACTICE?

Remember, every time you practice, whether it's just Sun Salutations or the complete Primary Series, you need to end with some version of the Closing Sequence in chapter 7. This is the group of postures that completes the restoration of structural, biomechanical, and biochemical balance to the body.

As a beginner, if you are ending your practice at this point, always follow Warrior II Posture (the last posture in this chapter), with the Modified Closing Sequence. This basically involves lying down, bringing your knees to your chest and rolling around a bit. But you should check out the specifics in chapter 7. Also remember, as I mentioned on the first page of this chapter, that this is therapy. If your back did not bother you when you began practice, it should not bother you when you finish practice. If for some reason it does not feel relaxed, the Modified Closing Sequence is aimed to alleviate any discomfort.

strength & surrender

5

The Primary Series—Seated Postures I

A political victory, a rise of rents, the recovery of your sick or the return of your absent friend,
or some other favorable event raises your spirits, and you think good days
are preparing for you. Do not believe it. Nothing can bring you peace
but yourself. Nothing can bring you peace
but the triumph of principles.

Emerson, "Self-Reliance"

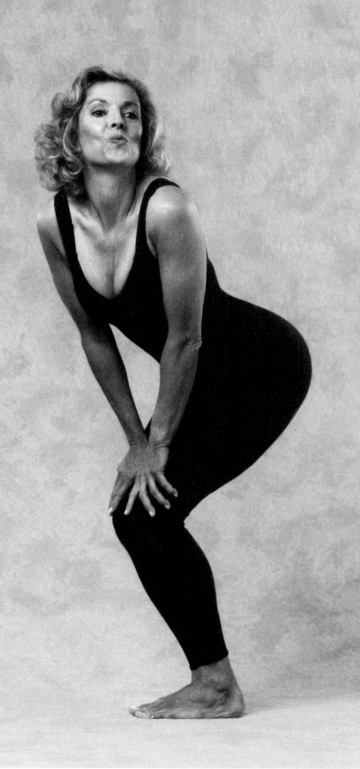

THE PRIMARY SERIES

SEATED POSTURES I

YOGA THERAPY

It is at this point that the *yoga chikitsa,* or yoga therapy, begins to deepen its effects. Although many of you have already begun to markedly notice your residual stiffness in some of the standing postures, especially in the back of the legs, the tightness developed over years of training can get downright discouraging and "discomfortable" about now. The very first seated posture, like the first standing posture, tells you in pretty clear language how tight (or flexible) you may be in the back of the body.

The encouraging news is that if you continue to practice with earnestness and regularity, the body changes. Not only do the hamstrings get longer and more flexible, but your mind seems to become more flexible, too. The rigidity and resistance locked in for so long begin to dislodge. A not-uncommon occurrence after a few months of practice is for a person to begin crying during practice. No, it is not from the pain! I guess the best way to describe it is in the words of one of the students, Genie, a woman in her early forties who had been coming to class for many years: "I had just come out of forward bending and was lying down waiting to begin Closing Sequence. The music [occasionally played at the end of class for Relaxation Posture, the very last pose in the practice, and used for cooldown, rest, and meditation] had started and the heat was coming on again. The radiators started banging, and I couldn't tell what was radiator and what was on the music tape. Slowly it all seemed interconnected. Suddenly I thought I felt my father [this student's father had died several years before] standing behind me, as if he were dancing. I felt

happy and relieved and started to cry. I didn't sob or anything, but it was a very deep crying, from the very depth of my heart."

After years of watching hundreds of people go through very real emotional release and catharsis as a result of what superficially seems to be strictly physical work, I can tell you unquestionably that the practice not only liberates the tightness and restriction of physical injuries and training, but the constraints developed from years of emotional pain or trauma as well.

You cannot work day after day on "opening" the muscles, cells, joints, and connective tissue without affecting the nervous system and the emotional condition. The emotions have to be stored somewhere. Yes, they are in the mind, but from my observations they are just as assuredly in the cells, even the DNA. Memory of every nanosecond of your life is in the DNA. There is physical storage on the hard drive somewhere deep in the mind's computer bank. Memory just doesn't float around in the ether somewhere. It has form and is comprised of bytes linked into kilobytes and megabytes. However, we can't always access our own memory as easily as we can the computer on our desk. Sometimes it gets stuck or buried or covered over with other information. If it was painful memory, it seems to become insulated, like a physical injury does by scar tissue. These little insulated pockets create blocks, detours, and limitations. To go the distance, we need to blast through and open them up. When the system is realigned and free of a lifetime of blocks, only then can we function at full potential.

As you stretch out and lose rigidity, you will notice

the unfolding suppleness begin to carry over into your day-to-day work. As you slowly train the mind to focus on the breath, you will notice an increased ability to concentrate in other aspects of your life. You may see your talent for conflict resolution improving. You may begin to yield where you used to resist. And you may begin to stand firm where you used to consistently acquiesce. So when I say that the yoga therapy begins in earnest, I don't just mean putting the spine in line.

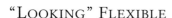

"LOOKING" FLEXIBLE

A lot of people "fake" forward bending. By rounding the back and straining to get the head to the knees, people can try to "look" flexible. This is not only incorrect yoga, but dangerous. This chapter will teach you absolutely the *only* correct way to do forward bending safely and effectively. The downside of doing it correctly, for many of you the first time ever, is that in the beginning you will feel a lot less flexible, because you can't cheat. This means dealing with the ego straight on. The ego, of course, wants to demonstrate how good it is at this work. I see it in classes all the time, particularly in classes where people can look around and compare themselves with others! It becomes a competition. "Oh, my God, I'm not the stiffest person in class, am I?"

Looking flexible in forward bending generally involves hunching the shoulders, rounding the back, collapsing the front of the body, dropping the head, and totally compressing the entire cardiopulmonary space! I actually know of an instance where a very well-known runner and client of our program in New York City was seriously injured doing a "stretch and reach" test for an exercise physiologist at a local health club. The runner was sitting with his legs outstretched, trying to reach his toes, and straining to "perform" well or score high on the test results. In

reaching forward, pressing down, and collapsing the front of the body, the downward pressure of the shoulders on the rib cage actually popped a piece of connective cartilage off the rib cage.

There are two points to this story: One is to illustrate that very few of us know what correct form is when we are attempting to stretch. This particular runner who tore cartilage had been in classes for years and should have known about not rounding the back when forward bending. But often we just don't get it. We can't exactly see ourselves from the back, and we may be so used to the way the "rounding" feels, that it may indeed feel straight to us. We are eager to make progress, especially when scoring is involved. Old habits are very hard to eliminate and change. It takes time and patience. Often we need to learn the hard way to really get the teaching.

The second point is to illustrate the power of the ego. We have a lot invested in our tightness. It represents, for most of us, some kind of accomplishment. Now, we have come to the point where it is beginning to get in our way, to limit us. Hmmm. We have to begin to change our way of thinking.

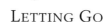

LETTING GO

Traditionally, in yoga literature, the forward-bending postures—especially Intense West Stretch, or *Paschimotanasana,* the first posture in this chapter—are said not only to quiet the mind and teach "surrender" (meaning to give up limitations), but to conquer ego and develop the *siddhas,* or yogic powers like clairvoyance, psychic energy and communication, and altered states of consciousness.

By conquering the ego, we should be clear here that we are talking only about the negative aspects of the notion of ego, the "inner enemies" such as false pride, arrogance, wrong knowledge, conceit, and narrow-mindedness. Indeed, in order to make headway in these forward-bending postures, one must learn to let go. If you resist the stretch and hang on to the old pathways, the work will be more painful and less effective.

Letting go of the ego means letting go of the tightness. The density of the tightness has clouded the sensitivity of the pores, of the skin, of the tissue. The ability of the *prana* to circulate through the tissue and bring energy to the area is limited. The yogis would say that this density obscures the sensitivity of the "aura," or the energy body around the physical body, as well. As we give up holding on to the old patterns, both physical and psychic, the clouds begin to dissipate, and clairvoyance, or "clear seeing," for example, gets stronger.

I like to think about becoming more clairvoyant when my hamstrings are screeching at me on a Monday morning yoga practice after a weekend of running, hiking, biking, or whatever. It helps soothe the intensity! Anyway, it's a nice thought, and there is no question that after many years of yoga practice, people do become more perceptive. But for now, back to the issue at hand: tightness that has ceased to become fun or fashionable. We are too tight and it's getting in our way.

Macho Muscles

It is important to remember that there is a difference between strength and tightness. You don't have to be tight to be strong! Look at dancers and gymnasts. It has always been my contention that the still often-held notion in the world of sports, particularly professional sports like football and baseball, that flexibility is equal to weakness is just plain erroneous! Tightness will eventually *limit* strength, and I think more coaches and trainers are slowly coming to see this.

We see scores of people come to our classes from weight-lifting programs, for example. After years or sometimes even only months of lifting, there is no question they have developed strength; however, the problem is that they have also dramatically reduced their range of motion as a result of the bulking and tightening of the muscles. Consequently, they can't access this strength effectively because they can't move anymore!

So whether it's lifting weights or playing college football that causes the tightness, the muscles are eventually held by the autonomic nervous system in a state of suspended semicontraction. Over time, this weakens and exhausts them, making them increasingly susceptible to injury. The result can be tears in the muscle tissue. The strength of the contracting muscle overpowers the flexibility of the opposing muscle, and r-r-r-rip! Sports injury! So while to the general public this massive tightness may give the impression of power, in reality this is an example of muscles in a continually contracted and weakened state that are at an ever increasingly high risk of injury.

I am sure many professional sports teams have tried "stretching" programs of one sort or another, only to end up with injured athletes or with a feeling of wasting valuable training time. Other teams may actually practice a bit of stretching here and there. They bounce a little or push against a wall for a few minutes, but then go and lift weights for three hours. Most professional athletes I have spoken with have failed to see much in the way of tangible results from traditional stretching routines. Additionally, since stretching represents the "soft" aspect of training, it is often still regarded, even today, as too feminine and not something that should be practiced by real men.

Stand Firm or Surrender

Perhaps you are one of the fortunate few who aren't feeling tight as you begin forward bending. Maybe you have always been flexible. For you the issue will be maintaining the static contractions in the postures and developing strength with the connecting movements. So whether you need to develop strength or flexibility, or both, the same challenge exists for everyone: balancing the hard with the soft. Learning where and when to hang on, stand firm, and where and when to let go, surrender. Where are we tight, narrow, oblivious, unaware? Where are we loose, sloppy, overflowing, and unfocused?

Once yoga practice begins, strength and flexibility reach new levels of refinement. Resistance breaks down (and I mean resistance to growth and change, not resistance to disease), and lightness comes. For a professional offensive tackle, perhaps, lightness isn't exactly a goal. But I would certainly imagine it to be a goal of a quarterback, and for most of the rest of us.

Using the practice, we continue to develop our awareness of balance, not only balance between strength and flexibility, but more subtle forms of balance, such as between overstimulation and lethargy. By paying attention to the breath-synchronized movement of this form, you will begin to tune in to this tension or looseness and take control of reeducating the mind and the muscles, and reestablishing the neuromuscular pathways.

THE THREE *GUNAS*

If you have been doing regular practice up until now, you are probably beginning to see some small progress. Let's say that you have slightly developed your body awareness and are somewhat more conscious of what is going on in the cells and tissues surrounding your brain. You may begin to notice variations in the way you feel from day to day when you do your practice. Some days you may feel blazing, other days you may feel terrible. Yes, this is very normal. But what causes these shifts? you may ask. Regular practice helps you to figure out these shifts in energy and their causes.

Did you train hard the previous day? Did you rest? Did you get enough sleep? Did you eat early? Or late? Did you eat enough? Too much? What did you eat? Did you eat well? Or poorly? Did you have a couple of glasses of wine? Did you have a high-stress day? Was it a full moon? New moon? All of these factors can affect the way you feel in practice. The more regularly you do practice, and the longer you have been doing it, the more you will be able to tune in to these various influences and analyze their effects on your mind and body.

In yoga philosophy, there are three *gunas,* or qualities of consciousness or energy: *rajas, tamas,* and *sattva. Rajas* has the power of projection and is the quality of activity. *Tamas* has the power of veiling or obscuring the real nature of things and is the quality of darkness and inertia. *Sattva* has the power of purity and calmness, and is the quality of illumination. Everything we do, say, think, imagine, eat, drink, or involve ourselves in is a combination of these *gunas,* according to yogic thought.

Tamas is an attribute of inertia, idleness, apathy, and ignorance. When this *guna* predominates we can sit around too much, become idle or bored. We feel sluggish. The mind vacillates, mistaking delusions for reality. *Rajas* is the attribute of mobility. It makes a person energetic, tense, overheated, and willful. We might sit around and engage in too much chatter, gossip, get too worked up or too stimulated. We are unsteady, fickle, easily distracted. Attachment, desire, and greed are caused by its power. This quality could be considered an aspect of evolution—the driving desire to move forward.

Sattva is the illuminating quality that leads to mental serenity, clarity, and the divine. Those of us in whom this *guna* is dominant are fearless and pure. We are generous and self-controlled. We pursue the study of self. We are nonviolent, truthful, and free from fickleness. We might engage in activities that bring harmony and balance, like biking in the country or hiking through the mountains, or listening to melodious music or reading uplifting literature.

Food can also have these three qualities. White

flour, for example, is *"tamasic"*—lethargy-producing. It provides a lot of calories in the form of simple carbohydrates, like sugar, but zero nutrient value, also like sugar. Thus, unless the calories are burned off immediately through an equivalent expenditure of energy output (like aerobic training), the excess is stored as fat. White flour can make you sleepy or heavy-feeling. The body requires considerable energy to push fiberless white flour through the intestinal tract.

Sugar, which starts out in the body as *"rajasic,"* or stimulating, also becomes *"tamasic"* as it passes through, and creates lethargy or stagnation. Meat, like sugar, starts out *"rajasic"* and becomes *"tamasic"* as the system struggles to digest and eliminate the great chunks of dead, processed flesh we ingest. Spicy foods such as Indian or Mexican dishes can be—are—*"rajasic"* and cause heat and stimulation.

As you become more regular and sensitive in your practice, you will begin to notice the effect that the food you ate in the preceding twelve hours has on the quality of your energy level and on the way you feel during practice. I know that I can always feel the effects of sugar, for example, during practice. It makes my muscles very stiff and increases the level of uncomfortableness enough so that the next time, I usually think twice about eating any sugar when I have to face practice at six the next morning.

I think it works that way in most bodies. Most people don't notice because it takes practicing the same time every day, for weeks and months, to tune into the subtle effects of food, emotion, etc., on the body. Pizza or any white-flour product (like bagels or hard rolls, for example) tend to make me feel very lethargic.

The best food choices, therefore, are the *"sattvic"* foods, such as whole grains, legumes, nuts, vegetables, and fruits. These foods have always been the mainstay of the yogic diet and bring balance and nutrients to the body and mind. A good *"sattvic"* meal always is appreciated the next day during practice. It digests effectively and is easy to eliminate in the morning before you begin the workout.

Too much *tamas* can mean tiredness, lethargy, exhaustion. Too much *rajas* can mean overexcitement, sleeplessness, hyperactivity. This practice works on clearing out the toxins, stress, training, discomfort, disease, or whatever else might be the causes of these imbalances. Slowly, slowly, *sattva,* or harmony, is reestablished—not only in the body, but in the mind as well.

THE POSTURES

1

INTENSE WEST STRETCH POSTURES A AND B (FULL FORWARD BENDING): *PASCHIMOTTANASANA*

Paschima means "west" or "hinder" and refers to the backside of the body. *Uttana* means "intense stretch." This posture is the basic forward bending of the series and I often refer to it, for simplicity, as *Full Forward Bending.*

This posture begins a long series of variations on forward bending, all of which stretch the back of the body, especially the back of the legs (hamstring muscles). It is essential to continue the emphasis begun in the standing postures on the contraction of the front of the thighs (quadriceps muscles). Remember, without this simultaneous strength work to balance the stretch, it isn't Power Yoga.

TECHNIQUE

Preparation: Sit with legs outstretched (Figure 5.1), chest lifted, back straight, palms flat on floor (if possible), with fingers forward, chin level to floor, thighs contracted, feet dorsiflexed (pulled back). This is a *working* posture. It is sometimes called in yoga *dandasana,* or stick posture. We use it here as preparation of the back for forward bending, in order to develop the awareness of extending the back. This action strengthens the middle back muscles, which first reach out in the forward bend and then relax in

order to stretch forward. You should be able to work hard enough in this posture (as in *all* postures) to keep the sweating mechanism turned on. This means not only being aware of and in conscious touch with the breath but also with the working muscles—those opposing the muscles being stretched—as well.

Note: If you are either very tight in the back or the back of the legs, or both, you should work to open the shoulders and straighten the back. You might try placing a pillow under your seat and bending your knees slightly. Also, you may wish to have a training partner place his or her feet on your lower back and push slightly, giving lift and support to your back (Figure 5.2).

Figure 5.1

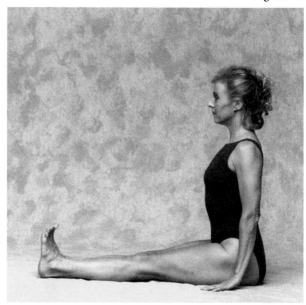

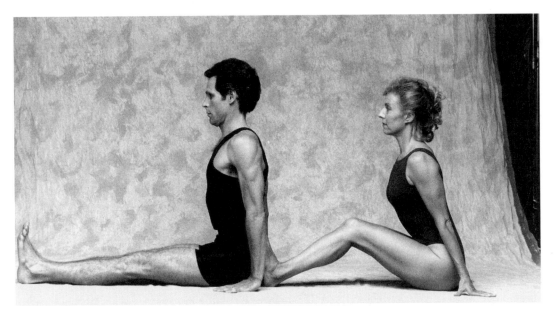

Figure 5.2

THIS IS STICK POSTURE, OR PREPARATION FOR IN-
TENSE WEST STRETCH—HOLD FOR FIVE BREATHS
(FIGURE 5.1).

Inhale.

Exhale, reach forward and grab your big
toes with the first two fingers of each
hand. If you cannot reach your toes,
grab your ankles or shins (Figure 5.3).
If you cannot reach that far because of
extreme tightness in the back of your
legs, *bend your knees* and then take
hold of your ankles or feet. *Keep your
feet and knees together.* **Do not round
the back!**

Inhale, straighten arms, lift chest, length-
en back and spine, contract thighs
and shins, head up, look up. This is
the position that extends or strengthens the middle back muscles.

Exhale, bend elbows, use the inner arms
(biceps) to pull the torso toward
thighs. First touch belly and rib cage to
thigh bone, then chest to leg, and last,

chin to knee (Figure 5.4). Hold *bandhas,* listen to
breath. Keep thighs contracted and elbows up.

Now the middle back muscles are being stretched
by the forward bend, although you should not allow
the back to round. Work to keep the extension alive,

Figure 5.3

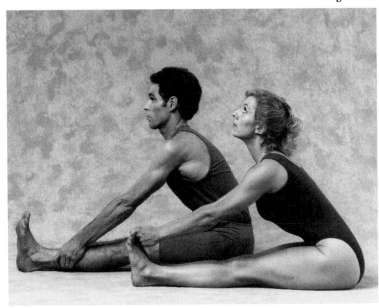

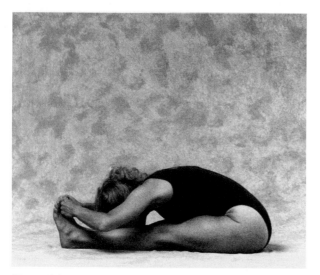

Figure 5.4

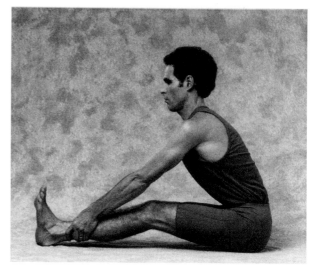

Figure 5.5

then relax just enough to feel the stretch in those same muscles. Gaze out past the end of the nose toward the toes. Notice how the muscles in the front of the body are working and those in the back are stretching.

> *Beginners' Modification* (Figure 5.5): As you reach forward, back off slightly so that you leave room to bend elbows slightly and pull with arms. You can work with legs straight or knees bent. Don't round the back, collapse the chest, look down, or hunch shoulders up around the ears. Keep head in line with spine.

THIS IS INTENSE WEST STRETCH POSTURE A— HOLD FOR FIVE BREATHS (FIGURE 5.4 OR 5.5).

Inhale, head up, straighten arms.
Exhale, take sides of feet with hands (Figure 5.6).
Inhale, again, head up.
Exhale (Figure 5.7), fold at hips, same as in West Stretch A, use arms and abdominals, pulling torso toward thighs. Bend knees if necessary.

THIS IS INTENSE WEST STRETCH POSTURE B— HOLD FOR FIVE BREATHS (FIGURE 5.7).

Inhale, head up, straighten arms.
Exhale, release posture.

Note: This is the first encounter with the floor *vinyasa,* or connecting movement, between the seated postures. Although in the standing postures we have already linked postures together with connecting movement, once we get to the seated postures, the connecting movement changes somewhat and is taken directly from Sun Salutation A. Basically, what we will be doing is half a Sun Salutation or technically half a *vinyasa.* This means that you are taking a sequence of moves out of the Sun Salutation and using it as connecting movement to link the postures.

What happens is that after the last exhale of the posture, you begin the first inhale of the connecting movement. In this case, for example, after you take the fifth exhale of forward bending, you start the first inhale of *vinyasa.* The first move is to "take it up," or lift yourself up off the floor into a position that is actually called *lolasana. Lola* means "to quake or dangle," so this posture is called Quaky Pose. You then swing this tucked or "dangling" position back through your hands and jump back into Position 4 of the Sun Salutation, or the push-up position (see illustrated sequences). Position 5, Face Up Dog, and Po-

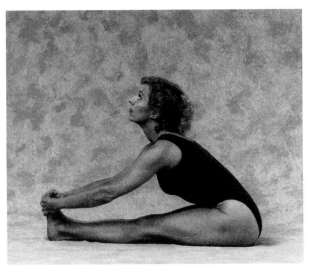

Figure 5.6

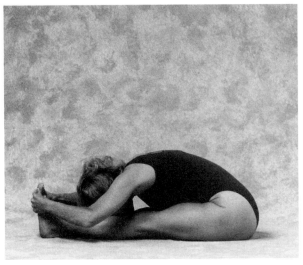

Figure 5.7

sition 6, Face Down Dog, follow. From there you jump back through your hands and return to a seated position.

This movement will be repeated over and over between every posture for the rest of the Primary Series, so we will give some attention to it here. For some of you, just rolling over your feet will be a major production. For others, perhaps more flexible, it will be less of a chore. For a rare few, extremely strong in the abdominals and flexible, lifting yourself up off the floor into Quaky Pose, swinging through, and jumping back will be no problem.

It takes a lot of abdominal strength to do this, and if you have weak or underdeveloped "abs," this method will slowly strengthen them.

Inhale, "take it up" (Figure 5.8).
  Beginners (Figure 5.9 sequence): Bend your knees, cross your feet, push yourself over your feet, as illustrated.
  More Advanced (Figure 5.10 sequence): Bend knees, cross feet, place hands flat on floor, and lift yourself off the ground. Swing the legs back and through.
Exhale, walk or jump back into your push-up position (Position 4 of the Sun Salutations).

Inhale, Face Up Dog.
Exhale, Face Down Dog.
Inhale, jump forward through legs.

Note: This move is the reverse of the jump back. Now you are attempting to jump forward "through" your legs to a seated position, as we did at the end of the last chapter after completing Warrior II Posture.

Figure 5.8

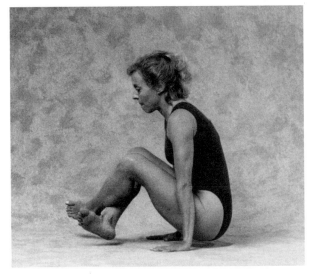

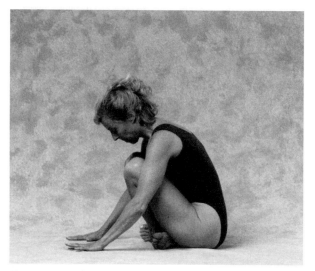

Figure 5.9a

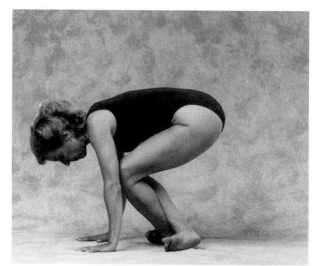

Figure 5.9b

The trick is to jump up with the hips as high (Figure 5.11) as possible, then cross and tuck the legs up underneath you and swing them through. The jump-through motion obviously requires full range of motion in the shoulders and strength in the arms and shoulders, but most important, it takes a lot of strength in the abdominals.

At this point, if you were to jump back to standing and complete the Sun Salutation, then start another Sun Salutation and continue back through to Face

Figure 5.10a

Figure 5.10b

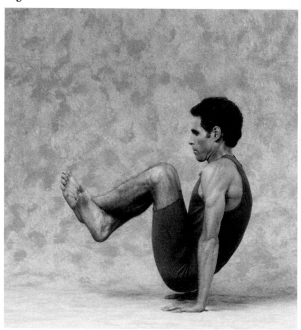

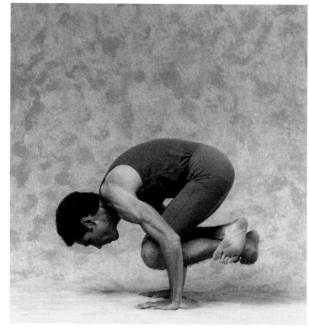

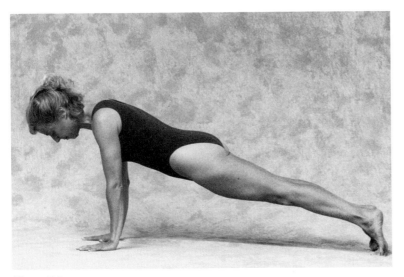

Figure 5.9c

Down Dog again, and *then* jump back through your hands, this would be called a full *vinyasa*, or a complete round of the Sun Salutation. Using full *vinyasas* between postures is a great way to keep heat up and build strength and endurance, and is actually the

Figure 5.11

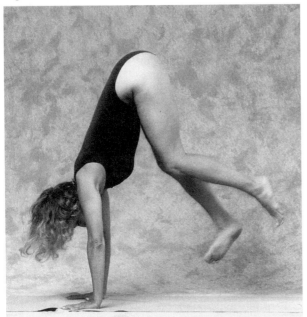

"correct" traditional form. However, since it takes a lot of time, full *vinyasa* is not customarily done, and we don't usually do them in our classes or our own practice except occasionally for extra heat.

Beginners: Bend your knees, take a little hop, cross your feet, land between your hands, sit down, and straighten your legs out in front of you.

More Advanced: Bend your knees, jump as high as possible, cross feet, hold yourself up and swing through (touch down between hands if necessary), pull legs through arms, and extend legs in front (Figure 5.12 sequence).

Exhale, as you land on the jump through.

2

INTENSE EAST STRETCH POSTURE— *PURVOTTANASANA*

Purva means "east," or "the front of the body." *Uttana* means "intense stretch." It is interesting to me that here, at the very beginning of the Primary Series, we have Intense West Stretch followed by Intense East Stretch, two counterposes setting the tone for the rest of the series, right off the bat stretching a particular set of muscles and strengthening another, then reversing it.

TECHNIQUE

Inhale, place hands one foot behind you on the floor. With fingers pointing toward buttocks, lift the tor-

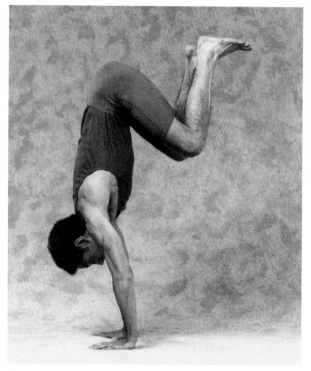

Figure 5.12a

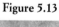

Figure 5.12b

so, hips, and thighs up, drop head back, look back (Figure 5.13).

Exhale, push up into posture! Notice how the muscles in the front of the body are now stretching and those in the back are contracting.

Note of caution: If you have pain, misalignment, or discomfort in the neck in this position, then keep your head forward and tucked into chest. It is *not* bad for your neck to let your head fall back. It is only bad if it causes you pain. Pain, serious misalignment,

Figure 5.13

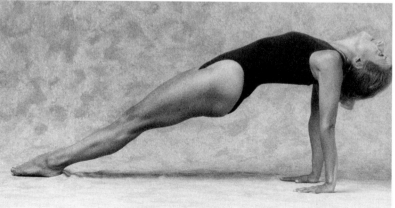

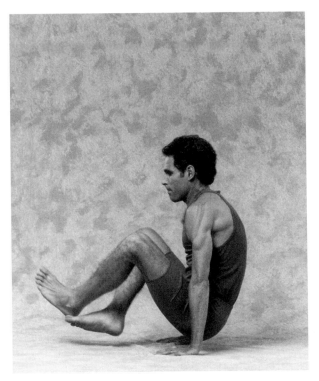

Figure 5.12c

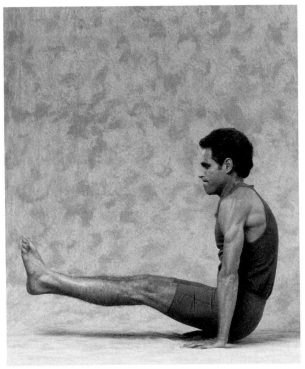

Figure 5.12d

or injury would cause this move to be contraindicated. If it causes you pain, don't do it. Do not hold your head halfway between forward and back. This is stressful. Let it go all the way back, resting on the ledge created by the shoulder muscles (trapezius), or keep it all the way forward.

THIS IS INTENSE EAST STRETCH POSTURE—HOLD FOR FIVE BREATHS (FIGURE 5.13).

Inhale, to prepare for release.
Exhale, release posture, come down.
Exhale, take it up into Quaky Posture (repeat the *vinyasa* or connecting movement sequence that we just learned).
Exhale, walk or jump back.
Inhale, Face Up Dog.
Exhale, Face Down Dog.
Inhale, jump through back to seated position, with legs extended straight out, as in Stick Posture, or hop

feet back to hands, sit down, and straighten legs. *Exhale,* as you land and prepare for next posture.

3

BOUND HALF LOTUS INTENSE WEST STRETCH POSTURE: *ARDHA BADDHA PADMA PASCHIMOTTANASANA*

Ardha means "half." *Baddha,* like the word *bandha,* comes from the root word *bandh,* which means "bond" or "lock." The adjective *baddha,* then means "bound," "caught," or "restrained." *Padma* means "lotus." *Paschima* means "west." *Uttana* means "intense stretch." The long detailed name for this posture simply means that this is another intense Forward Bending Stretch with one foot in bound half lotus position.

Note of caution: This is the seated version of Standing Bound Half Lotus Posture. Follow all the precautions given in the preceding chapter for the standing posture. *Anytime there is tightness in one area of the body, another area is often forced to compensate in a stressful or inappropriate way.* In this particular posture, as in the standing version, the knee will be the first area to feel compensation for tight hips. So be sure to keep the breath flowing smoothly, and pay attention to the correct method.

Remember that "binding," or catching, the toe with the hand coming from behind *must* happen before you attempt to bend forward. Forward bending without binding can put too much downward pressure on the knee in an incorrectly aligned position and cause injury to the knee.

TECHNIQUE

Inhale, bring the right leg up into half lotus position, and press the right heel into the lower left abdominal wall toward the navel (Figure 5.14).

Beginners' Modification: Pull the right foot up toward the little valley formed where the top of the left thigh meets the pelvis. Keep the ankle on top of the thigh, trying to press the heel into the abdominal wall. If tight hips restrict your mobility in this posture, then bring the foot all the way across the left thigh so that one knee is above the other and move the foot in as close to the thigh as possible. Lift the chest, extend out through the right heel, and keep the right thigh contracted. Sit up straight and take your five breaths in this position. Gaze straight out in front of you.

Exhale, reach right arm around back, and bind with foot (Figure 5.15). Take the outside of the left foot with the left hand.

Beginners' Modification: If you are unable to "bind" with the foot, hold right foot with left hand, reach right arm around back, and "bind" on left forearm. This becomes your "posture." *Do not attempt forward bending until you bind with foot!* Take your five breaths in this position (Figure 5.16).

Figure 5.14

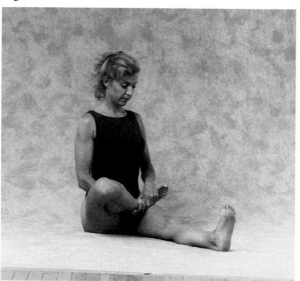

Figure 5.15

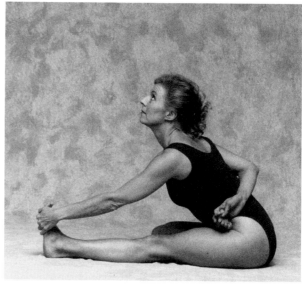

Inhale, lift chest, and extend back with left arm straight. The head is up and the gaze is up.

Exhale, bend forward using left arm to pull torso toward hips. Press right shoulder toward right knee. Shoulders should be equidistant from the floor (Figure 5.17). Left thigh is working. Gaze out toward toes.

THIS IS BOUND HALF LOTUS INTENSE WEST STRETCH POSTURE—HOLD FOR FIVE BREATHS (FIGURE 5.17).

Inhale, lift the head and look up, extend arms and back.

Exhale, release posture.

Note: What follows is the connecting *vinyasa,* or movement between the two sides of the posture, which is the same as what you just did between Intense West Stretch and Intense East Stretch. Correctly, this connecting movement is done between every half posture. However, it takes time and regular practice to build up the arm muscles and overall endurance to do repeated *vinyasas.* For the rest of this chapter, beginners may wish simply to change from right to left, leaving out the *vinyasa* between sides and putting only the connecting movement between successive postures or groupings of postures. Slowly you will become strong enough to do all the *vinyasas.*

Inhale, take it up.

> *Beginners:* Put hands down, cross legs, roll over feet.

Exhale, jump back.

Inhale, Face Up Dog.

Exhale, Face Down Dog.

Inhale, jump through.

> Repeat instructions for left side.

Figure 5.16

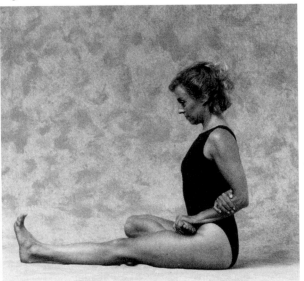

Figure 5.17

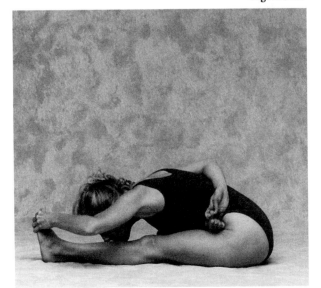

4

HORIZONTAL FACING ONE LEG INTENSE WEST STRETCH POSTURE: *TIRYAN MUKHAIKAPADA PASCHIMOTTANASANA*

Tiryan means "going or lying crosswise," "horizontal," or "transverse." *Muka* means "face." *Eka-pada* means "one leg." *Paschima* means "west" or "hinder" and refers to the back side of the body. *Uttana* means "intense stretch." This posture is another forward bending pose with one leg folded back alongside the thigh.

Note of caution: For some body types this posture carries a risk of injury if it is done *incorrectly.* In general, but particularly in this posture, incorrect form tends to be much more hazardous for people who are tight with limited range of motion than for those who are loose as a goose. Often in class, when I first teach this posture to beginners, a few folks will jump into what they anticipate the posture will be and do everything wrong. I go flying across the room like a shot out of a cannon to correct their form.

Many athletes have been injured doing the "hurdle" stretch, which has been *incorrectly* adapted from this yoga posture, and unfortunately, this is the reason they get injured doing it. Generally those who tweak themselves with this stretch are extremely tight. This, along with ignorance of the correct form and method, causes their alignment to be frightful. As they push the stretch, all of a sudden *"boi-oi-oi-oing, kersnap!"* something pops! Consequently, this stretch is contraindicated in the field of sports medicine. The irony is that, like the Half Lotus Posture in the last chapter, there is *nothing* wrong with the posture when it is practiced correctly. The following preliminary work will teach you the correct form and the safe way to practice.

PRELIMINARY WORK

Before Horizontal Facing One Leg Posture can be

Figure 5.18

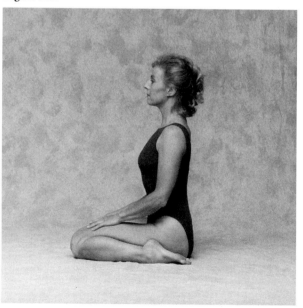

Figure 5.19

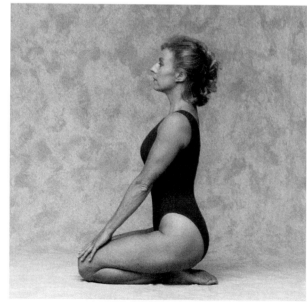

practiced safely, you must be able to sit in the position shown in Figure 5.18. This is actually a posture called *Virasana,* or Hero Posture. While it is not actually part of the form at this point, it is prerequisite to Horizontal Facing One Leg Intense West Stretch. Once this position is achieved, only then are the hips, legs, and ankles open enough to allow both buttock bones and all five toes on each turned-back foot to be flat on the floor.

This means that there is sufficient flexibility in the hip joint and in the ligaments on the medial (inner) side of the knee, and also in the rotational range of the ankle, to allow the posture to be safely done on one side only.

Kneel on the floor. First, bring the knees and feet together and then sit on your feet. This is Phase A (Figure 5.19). If this is difficult or immediately hurts your knees or ankles or feet, skip to the modifications given below for knee or foot resistance or tightness. If this is only moderately difficult, keep going, and try to sit here for a few breaths until it gets easier and/or more comfortable.

Once this becomes comfortable and uncomplicat-

Figure 5.20

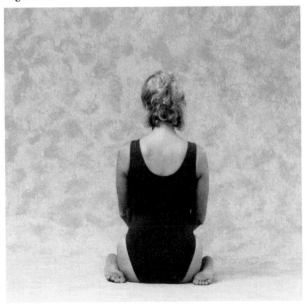

ed, continue to Phase B. Spread the feet about eighteen inches apart. Sit between the feet with the buttocks resting on the floor as shown in *Virasana,* Figure 5.20. Keep the knees together and *the feet parallel to the thighs.*

Note: Do not let the feet turn out to the sides. This is incorrect form—extremely stressful and potentially injurious to the knee. If this posture, done correctly, is painful, difficult, or impossible, follow the subsequent steps. Sit here and let gravity do a little work for you, but keep the breathing and *bandhas* going.

MODIFICATIONS—KNEES AND FEET

If this hurts your knees—you have two options: Don't do it at all or ease into it progressively!

Note of caution: If you are just coming back from arthroscopic surgery or are merely tight, or have knee pain or knee injuries, then this position can be very therapeutic for your knees. However, you will need to be extremely careful when beginning. This is simply a part of the work done in this whole sequence of postures that restores the range of motion and biomechanical balance to the knees. However, *you must ease into it.* One way of easing into it, as I explained earlier, is to sit on top of your feet, with your feet together as shown in Figure 5.19. If this is still too much for the knees, another way to ease into the posture and relieve stress on the knee joints is to place a pillow under your butt (Figure 5.21), between your thighs and your calves. Try to hold this for five breaths and do this as your fourth posture in this series. *If it still hurts your knees, then you may need to leave out this posture altogether.*

If this hurts your feet—you have only *one* option: Do it!

Note: If this position hurts the tops of your feet, it means you have limited (either mild or severe) plantar flexion and stiff ankles, which makes you a prime candidate for heel (cancaneal) spurs, Achilles tendinitis, plantar fascia tendinitis, or chronic sprained

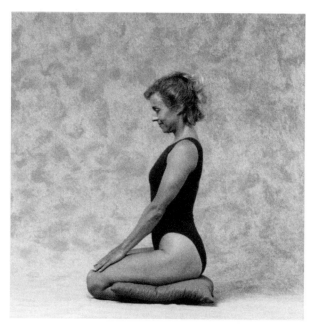

Figure 5.21

ankles. It also means you must practice this *religiously.* Since the objective of this practice is not to cause pain but to eliminate it, you should also ease into it using pillows as above, but the work must be done. If the posture as described above is difficult (Figures 5.18, 5.19, or 5.21), try placing one foot on top of the other in the sitting position. Then, gradually over the weeks, work your way into the successive positions, eventually with the feet outside the thighs, and with

Figure 5.22

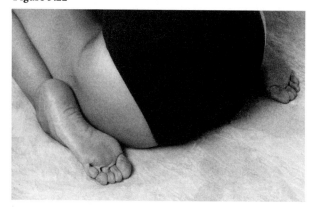

all five toes of each foot resting flat on the floor (Figure 22). At this point, *and only at this point,* can you proceed to the posture itself, Horizontal Facing One Leg Intense West Stretch.

This posture is excellent for flat feet. Because of the stretching of the tops of the feet and ankles, plantar flexion is restored, and it is possible that the arches will eventually be developed or restored. However, as Patanjali says in the *Yoga Sutras* with reference to progress in yoga, this takes a *durga kala,* or a very long time, and requires *nairantarya,* which literally means "without break"—that is, daily practice of the pose for at least two to three minutes over a period of many months. For those with heel pain or bone spurs on the heels, eventually the pain *and* the spurs can disappear.

If this hurts your thighs—you have only one option: Do it!

Note: If this position hurts your thighs, it is probably because they are very tight from skiing, cycling, skating, sprinting, or running hills. You *need* to do this! Follow the directions as given above for tight feet and ankles. Once Hero Posture is attained, then you can begin to work on directions for Horizontal Facing One Leg Posture at this point in the sequence.

TECHNIQUE

Inhale, fold the right leg back to the side, with right calf and foot parallel to the right thigh (Figure 5.23). Keeping buttocks bones firmly grounded to the floor, take the left foot with both hands, straighten the arms, contract thigh, extend the back, and look up.

Exhale, fold forward, using arm and shoulder muscles to pull torso towards leg (Figure 5.24). Do not round back. Keep heart "open" (which means don't hunch the shoulders, close down the chest, and crush the inner organs). Elbows up. Gaze out toward toes.

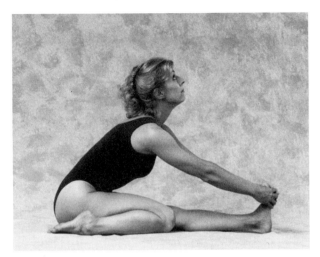

Figure 5.23

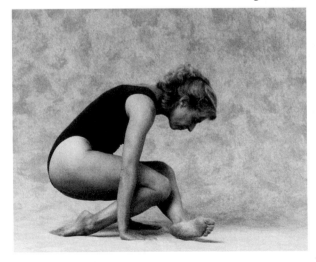

Figure 5.24

THIS IS HORIZONTAL FACING ONE LEG INTENSE WEST STRETCH POSTURE—HOLD FOR FIVE BREATHS (FIGURE 5.24).

Inhale, lift head, look up, straighten arms.
Exhale, release.

   Beginners: Remember you may leave out the *vinyasa* here and simply change sides, repeating the instructions for the left side.

Inhale, take it up. Try to take it up in horizontal facing one leg position (Figure 5.25 sequence), swing left leg under and
Exhale, jump back.
Inhale, Face Up Dog.
Exhale, Face Down Dog.
Inhale, jump through.
   Repeat instructions for left side.

Figure 5.25a

Figure 5.25b

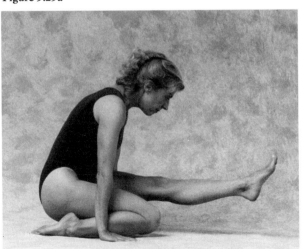

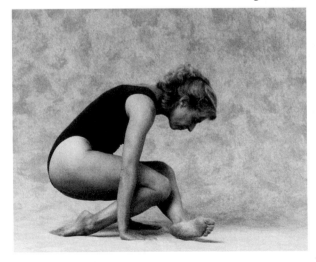

5

SINGLE LEG FORWARD BENDING (HEAD OF THE KNEE) POSTURES A AND B: *JANU SIRASANA A AND B*

Janu means "knee." *Sirsa* means "head."

Note: When using the English expression for this posture, I most frequently refer to it as Single Leg Forward Bending Posture, because it is easy and self-explanatory (like calling Intense West Stretch, *Full Forward Bending*). This posture is sometimes incorrectly called Head to Knee Pose, which is misleading because it encourages people to round their backs in the posture and struggle to get their heads to their knees. The Sanskrit translation I am most happy with is Head-of-the-Knee Posture, which refers to the "head," or kneecap, of the bent leg.

SINGLE LEG FORWARD BENDING A

TECHNIQUE

Inhale, bring right heel into groin, and open bent leg ninety degrees out to the side (Figure 5.26). Take left foot with both hands, center torso over extended leg, lift chest, extend back, and look up. If hamstrings are tight, take shin or ankle instead of foot with both hands. Press back with the "head" of the bent knee.

Exhale, fold at hips, using arm and shoulder muscles to bring torso to thigh (Figure 5.27). As you stretch out, lead with your chin. This helps to extend and stretch out the spine. Place the chin on the shin *below* the knee. Gaze out to toes.

Beginners' Modification: If you are holding the shin or ankle, hold high enough up on leg to leave some "slack" (extra length) in the arms so you can bend elbows and pull with arms and shoulders. Do not round back. Hold the chest lifted, head up, and spine in *extension* (Figure 5.28).

Note: This is a twisting as well as a forward bending posture. Attempt to twist torso out over extended leg, centering chest over thigh bone (femur). Shoulders, torso, and arms should be kept level. Keep heart open and elbows up. Do not struggle to touch the head to the knee. Forget about your head. The head is the last part of the torso to touch the leg, after

Figure 5.26

Figure 5.27

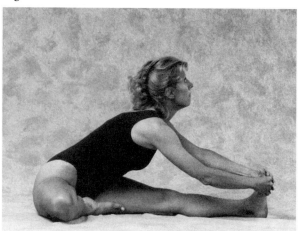

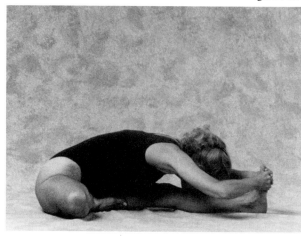

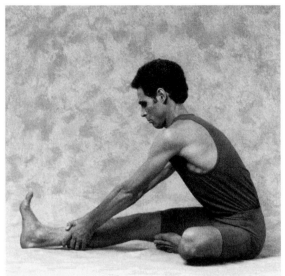

Figure 5.28

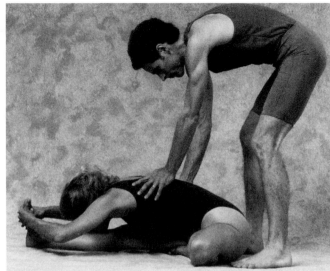

Figure 5.29

the belly, the rib cage, and the chest. The spine is kept lengthened and the back is not allowed to round. In the completed posture the crown of the head extends out beyond the knee of the extended leg, as in Figure 5.27.

Once you have been practicing for some time on a *regular* (read: daily) basis, you might wish to get some help in the posture from a training partner who can give you a push and help to lengthen the stretch. You must be hot and sweaty to do this, and very familiar with your limitations and capabilities. Start with very easy pushing and then slowly increase the intensity. It should feel good, not painful! (Figure 5.29).

THIS IS SINGLE LEG FORWARD BENDING A POSTURE—HOLD FOR FIVE BREATHS (FIGURE 5.27 OR 5.28).

Inhale, look up and lift the chest, going back into the preparatory position, as in Figure 5.26.

Exhale, release.

> *Beginners:* Leave out the *vinyasa* and simply change sides, repeating the instructions for the left side.

Inhale, Take it up.

Exhale, jump back.

Inhale, Face Up Dog.

Exhale, Face Down Dog.

Inhale, jump through.

> Repeat instructions for left side.

SINGLE LEG FORWARD BENDING B

Inhale bring right heel into groin as in Single Leg Forward Bending A, then lift up the pelvis and move the hips forward so the buttocks are resting on the foot (Figure 5.30). The heel of the foot should be placed into the perineum (the small muscle between the anus and genitals). Open the bent leg eighty-five degrees out to the side. Take the left foot with both hands. Head up, arms straight, extend the back, tighten left thigh, look up.

Exhale, bend forward using arms and shoulders to pull torso toward thigh and crown of head toward foot, as in Single Leg Forward Bending A. Do not round the back. Gaze out toward the toes (Figure 5.31). Placement of the foot should remind you to hold *mula bandha!*

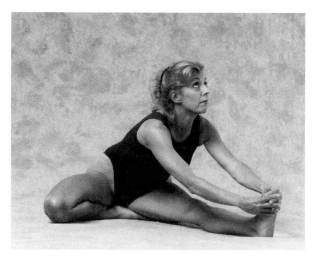

Figure 5.30

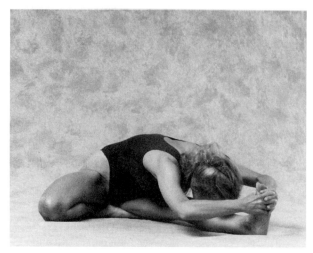

Figure 5.31

Beginners' Modification: Grab foot or ankle, pull as far forward as possible, keeping chest lifted, head up and back straight, as in Position A. If weight on foot is uncomfortable, work with a double-thickness mat, or use hands to support some of weight, or practice Hero Pose (previous posture modification) until the foot becomes more flexible and can tolerate the position. Continue to hold the "pull," using strength, or muscular contraction, throughout the posture.

THIS IS SINGLE LEG FORWARD BENDING B POS-TURE—HOLD FOR FIVE BREATHS (FIGURE 5.31).

Inhale, lift chest, extend back, look up.
Exhale, release.
   Beginners: Leave out the *vinyasa* and change sides.
   Go to "Repeat instructions for left side."
Inhale, take it up.
Exhale, jump back.
Inhale, Face Up Dog.
Exhale, Face Down Dog.
Inhale, jump through.
   Repeat instructions for left side.

6

MARICHYASANA POSTURES A–C: *MARICHYASANA A–C*

The posture Marichyasana is named after the sage Marichi, son of the Creator, Brahma. Marichi, Beam of Celestial Light, was begotten, according to Hindu mythology, of the god Brahma's pure spirit, and his only wealth and glory were his sanctity and devotion. Marichi was also the grandfather of Surya, the Sun God. (Remember, we refer to Surya in the Sun Salutation warm-ups, called *Surya Namaskar* in Sanskrit.)

This is a wonderful but somewhat complicated series of postures. I don't think there is anyone new to yoga who will be able to just whip through all three of them. I love this grouping of postures, even though I still struggle a bit with C. Often, in beginning classes, we do only Marichyasana A and C. Marichyasana B requires the half lotus position, which is not easy for anyone who does sports. (There is actually a Marichyasana D posture in the Primary Series, which we do only in advanced classes and is not included in this book.)

Shoulder sprains, injuries to the rotator cuff, or

dislocations of the shoulder joint are all relieved by the practice of the Marichyasana series. Also lower- and middle-back pain from compression through running, swimming, or biking are also relieved by these postures. Hips are realigned, often alleviating hip pain. The internal benefits include toning and rejuvenation of the liver, pancreas, spleen, intestines, and lungs.

Marichyasana B, although it takes some time for many of us to master the elusive half lotus position, is wonderfully therapeutic for the abdominal organs. On the right side, the left heel presses into the ascending colon. On the left side, the right heel presses the descending colon. This can help to stimulate the colon, prevent stagnation or constipation in the large intestine, and thus reduce the risk of colitis or cancer of the colon. In women, the heels press into the ovaries and uterus, which stimulates circulation and health. With regular practice, in many cases this can help to relieve menstrual cramps.

MARICHYASANA A

TECHNIQUE

Inhale, bend the right knee, and place the sole of the right foot flat on the floor. Bring the heel as close to the right buttock bone as possible. The right calf should press against the right thigh. Separate the inner side of the right foot from the inner side of the left thigh by at least a palm's width. The outside of the right foot should line up with the side of the right hip and function as an outrigger to help give stability to the form (Figure 5.32). This is the prep position.

Exhale, reach forward with the right arm, and drop the right shoulder inside the right knee until the armpit touches the right knee and shin. Continue *exhaling* and wrap the right arm back around the right shin and thigh (Figure 5.33). Keep the right palm facing away from the body and then bring the left arm back, grabbing the left wrist with the right hand (Figure 5.34, close-up). If that is not possible, grab the palms or fingers together.

Beginners' Modification: If the hamstrings (back of the legs) or hip joints are very tight, it may be

Figure 5.32

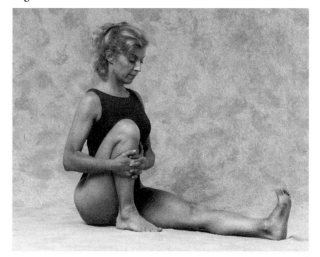

Figure 5.33

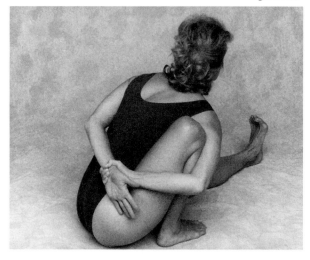

difficult at first to get the shoulder forward enough to wrap the arm. In this case simply take hold of the right shin with both hands and use the arms to extend the back and sit up straight (Figure 5.35). Once you are able to keep the right foot in place without "hanging on" to the shin, release the hands, clasp the left shin, and work on forward bending (Figure 5.36). Don't attempt to wrap the arms if you can't get your shoulder and armpit in front of the kneecap, as you see in Figure 5.37. Eventually, after many months of practicing the preceding three *asanas,* the back of the legs and the hips will develop enough suppleness to allow the correct practice of Marichyasana A.

Inhale, extend spine, lift head (Figure 5.37).
Exhale, bend forward, resting forehead, then the

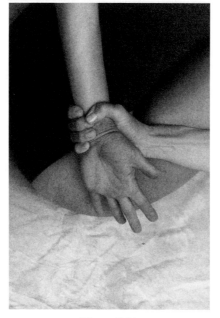

Figure 5.34

nose, and finally the chin on the shin (Figure 5.38). Gaze out toward toes. Extend out through left heel. Keep left thigh working. Use arms and abs to pull into stretch.

Beginners' Modification: Hold left shin with both hands and work on forward bending, as in Figure 5.36. Lift the back and sit up straight.

THIS IS MARICHYASANA A POSTURE—HOLD FOR FIVE BREATHS (FIGURES 5.35, 5.36, OR 5.38).

Inhale, lift head, look up, extend back and lift chest.
Exhale, release the posture.
Beginners: Go to "Repeat instructions for left side."
Inhale, take it up.
Optional Advanced: Take the right leg up over the right arm, pushing the leg back and trying to "hang" the right leg over the shoulder (Figure

Figure 5.35

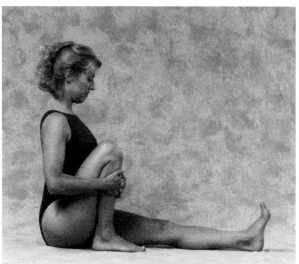

Figure 5.36

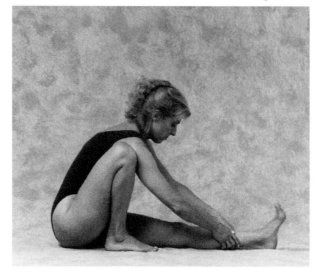

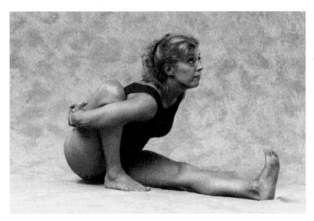

▲ Figure 5.37

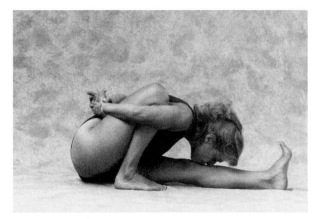

Figure 5.38 ▲

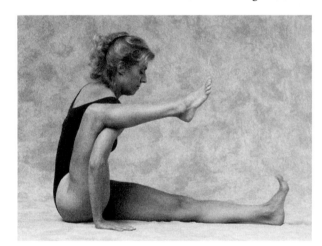

Figure 5.39 ▲

5.39). Try to lift up the left leg and straighten the right leg (Figure 5.40), then bend the left knee and bring the left leg through and under. Bend the right leg back and rest on the back of the right upper arm (Figure 5.41). Then, from that position,

Exhale, jump back.
Inhale, Face Up Dog.
Exhale, Face Down Dog
Inhale, jump through.

Repeat instructions for left side.

▼ Figure 5.40

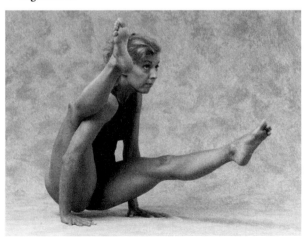

Figure 5.41 ▼

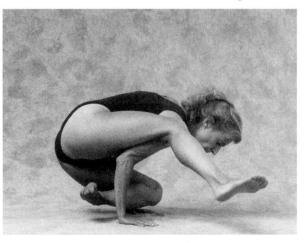

MARICHYASANA B

TECHNIQUE

Note for beginners: Depending on the frequency of your practice, a considerable amount of time will be spent just working on the first segment of this posture, which is half lotus position. Intermediate students who take our classes in New York City generally agree that attaining correct half lotus position can often take as long as one to two years, especially if one continues to aerobically train (i.e., run, skate, bike, swim). As in the fourth posture in this chapter, where Hero Posture must be achieved before attempting Horizontal Facing One Leg Posture, so here, half lotus must be completed before continuing with Marichyasana B (see Modification for Hips that follows).

Inhale, bend left knee, and bring left leg into half lotus position. The left heel should press into the lower right half of the abdominal area.

Exhale, bend the right knee, and pull the foot in toward the buttock bone (Figure 5.42). The right foot is flat on the floor.

> *Beginners' Modification:* Once half lotus position is achieved, then you can begin to bring up the right leg. It may be helpful to sit up straight, using the arms and shoulders to pull the right thigh into the chest, and working in this position to open the hips (as in Figure 5.42), before continuing with the binding of the arms.

Inhale, sit up straight, stretching the spine into extension. Look up.

Exhale, reach forward with the right arm, holding the right shin with the left hand and trying to get the right armpit in front of the right kneecap. Then roll the shoulder inward and try to wrap the right arm around behind the back. Keep the right palm facing away from the body. Reach around behind the body with the left arm and grab the left wrist with the right hand. If this is not possible, grab the palms or fingers together.

Inhale, using back extensor muscles, lift the chest up. Look up.

Exhale, extend the spine, and bend forward, resting the head on the floor between the right knee and the left foot (Figure 5.43). Keep the line of the shoulders parallel to the floor. Gaze out past the end of the nose.

> *Modification for Hips:* If your hips are very tight, half lotus position will be tough. This is a modification that helps to open the hips and is a good way to loosen up for deeper practice in Marichyasana B.
>
> Lie down, lift the legs, and place the left ankle on the right thigh, as close to the hip as possible. Keep the buttocks on the floor and reach through the space between the thighs with the left hand. Hook the hands together around the right shin. Pull the right leg in toward the chest. You will feel the stretch deep in the left buttock and hip (Figure 5.44).

THIS IS MARICHYASANA B POSTURE—HOLD FOR FIVE BREATHS (FIGURE 5.42 OR 5.43).

Figure 5.42

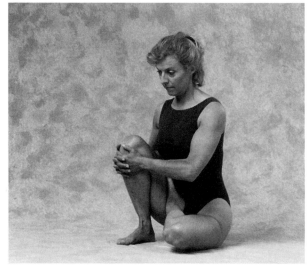

Inhale, lift torso, look up.

Exhale, release the posture.

> *Beginners:* Leave out the *vinyasa* and change sides. Go to "Repeat instructions for left side."

Inhale, take it up.

> *Optional Advanced* (Figure 5.45 sequence): Put hands down in front of you, stand on one leg, jump up, unhook leg in half lotus and,

Exhale, jump back.

Inhale, Face Up Dog.

Exhale, Face Down Dog.

Inhale, jump through.

> Repeat instructions for left side.

MARICHYASANA C

Note: It may take you several breaths to get yourself fully twisted and into this posture. That's okay. Take as many as you need. The important thing is to keep breathing and to always do the move described on the recommended breath. For example, if it says "Exhale, take the arm around behind the back," then make sure to exhale as you work on this movement.

Figure 5.43

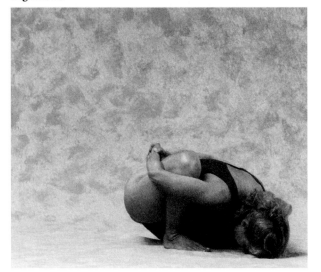

TECHNIQUE

Inhale, bend the right knee, and bring the right heel up to the right buttock bone. The right foot is flat on the floor and the outside of the right foot should be lined up with the outside of the upper thigh, as in Marichyasana A prep position.

Exhale, twist out to the right. Turn the chest ninety degrees, if possible, and try to clear the chest past the right thigh (Figure 5.46). Take the left arm over the right thigh so that the back of the upper arm muscle (tricep) is pushing against the outside of the right leg (thigh, knee, or shin). Extend out through left leg.

Beginners' Modification: At first it is very difficult to make this ninety-degree twist with the torso. If your back is tight and your torso rotation is limited, it may result in your left shoulder hunching up around your neck and ear when you try to take your arm around your thigh. If this is the case for you, then wrap your left arm around your right leg from behind the leg, as shown (Figure 5.47). Look back over the right shoulder toward the right corner of your eyes. *Do not attempt to go further than this. Hold this*

Figure 5.44

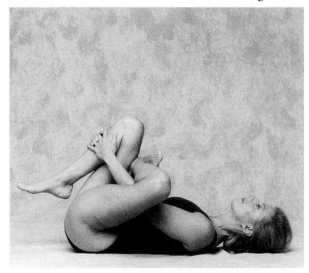

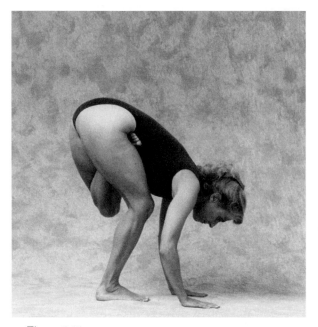

▲ **Figure 5.45a**

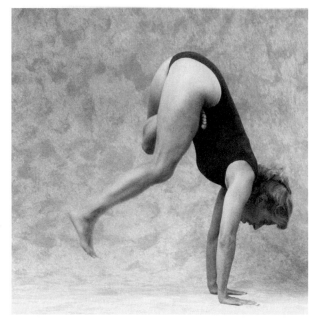

Figure 5.45b ▲

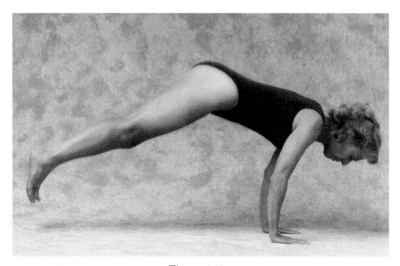

Figure 5.45c

position as your posture until, through regular practice, your torso rotation increases and you are able to proceed to the next phase of the posture. Skip to "This is Marichyasana C—hold for five breaths."

Inhale, rotate the left shoulder forward, twist the arm inward (pronation) and back, and take the left hand behind the back at the waist.

Exhale, take the right arm behind the back, and attempt to clasp the right wrist with the left hand. (At first you will probably just manage to hook the fingers together, then the palms, and finally to

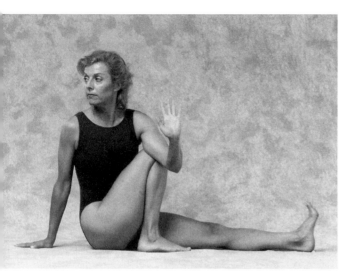

Figure 5.46

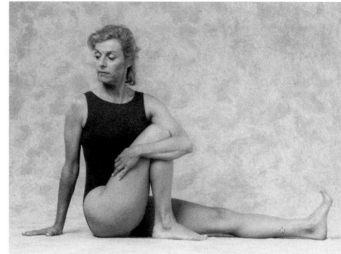

Figure 5.47

hold the wrist.) Look back over the right shoulder, out of right corner of your eyes (Figures 5.48 and 5.49).

Note (includes comments on difficulties and limitations): Take as many breaths as necessary to get yourself into this posture, or the modification of it you are

doing. The important thing, though, is to keep *ujjayi* breathing going while struggling! Hold root and abdominal lock and keep your gaze steady. The left arm should lock tightly around the bent right leg. Work to eliminate any space or gap between the left armpit and the right knee.

Pull with the arms to continue the rotation. This

Figure 5.48

Figure 5.49

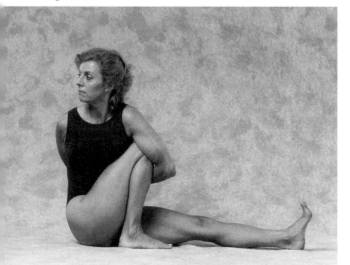

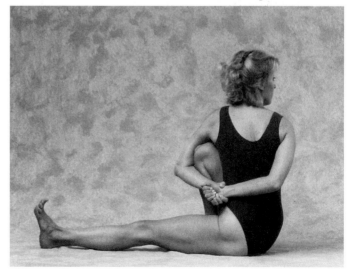

posture may take a long time to master, particularly if your back and shoulder muscles are very tight from training. Swimmers, for example, who maintain good range of motion and rotation in the shoulders (particularly butterflyers!) have a far easier time with this posture than do cyclists, baton twirlers, or golfers, for example, who can have tremendous rigidity and tightness in the shoulders.

If you can make the rotation with the torso, but cannot make the shoulder rotation and take the arm behind the back, then you probably are limited by tightness in the shoulder joint (rotator cuff muscles), or in the front of the shoulders (anterior deltoid muscles). Many athletes at this point ask, "Well, what can I do to loosen this tightness?"

This! This is what you can do for the tightness. Work at this posture repeatedly, slowly working the hand up the back, until the hands connect behind the back.

THIS IS MARICHYASANA C POSTURE—HOLD FOR FIVE BREATHS (FIGURES 5.46, 5.47 OR 5.48, AND 5.49).

Inhale.
Exhale, release the posture.
   Beginners: Leave out the *vinyasa* and change sides.
     Go to "Repeat instructions for left side."
   Inhale, take it up.
   Optional Advanced: Put right leg behind and up over right shoulder, as shown for the exit from Marichyasana A in Figure 5.39, then lift up, swing through, and
Exhale, jump back.
Inhale, Face Up Dog.
Exhale, Face Down Dog.
Inhale, jump through.
Repeat instructions for the left side.

If you are continuing, go directly to the first posture in chapter 6, *Navasana,* or Boat Posture. If you are just beginning to work with this chapter, you should stop here and skip to chapter 7 for the Modified Closing Sequence. Postures 15, 17, 18, and 19 in the next chapter are an especially critical part of the sequence to safely prepare for the Amended or Complete Closing Sequence. *Thus, do not begin work on the Amended or Complete Closing Sequence until you have completed practice through the end of chapter 6.*

Practice the sequence thus far—chapters 3 through 5, plus your modified closing from chapter 7—until you are familiar with alignment, the order of the postures, and special directions. Work with this chapter until you "get" it. After a few days of working with the book, try a few days working without the book, going from one posture to the next from sense memory. Then, when you feel ready, both physically and mentally, go on!

6
fine-tuning

THE PRIMARY SERIES—SEATED POSTURES II

*Anyone who practices can acquire the yoga siddhis (powers), but not one who is lazy.
Yoga siddhis are not obtained by merely reading textbooks. Nor are they reached
by wearing yoga garments or by conversation about yoga, but only
through tireless practice. This is the secret of success.
There is no doubt about it.*

Hatha Yoga Pradipika (Chapter 4, Verses 65–66)

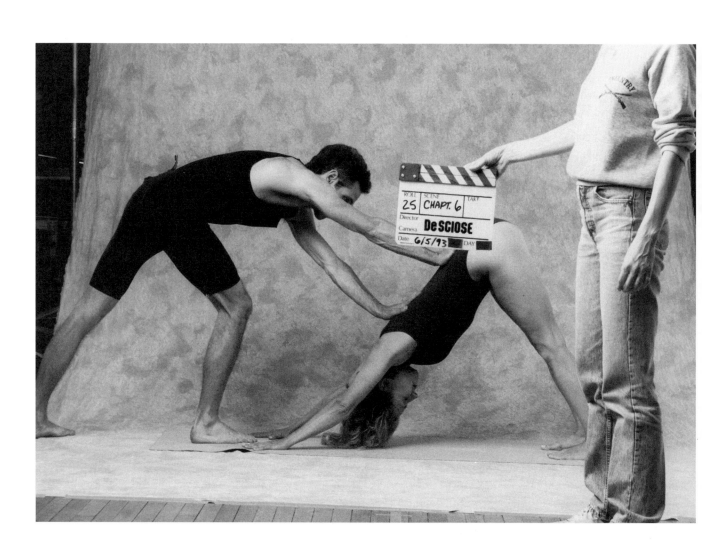

The Primary Series

SEATED POSTURES II

The Peak of the Heat

The secret to "getting" the postures in this chapter, if there is any secret, is something I have mentioned numerous times—heat! The postures that you will now be working on come at the peak of your heat in the Primary Series. You have been practicing the Sun Salutations for weeks and months now. You have learned the standing postures pretty much by heart. After Sun Salutations and standing postures, you are about thirty minutes into the practice and sweating pretty good. The first six postures in the Primary Series, which we learned in chapter 5, should take another fifteen minutes, once you have learned them and are able to flow through them and the *vinyasa* without stopping.

So now you are forty-five minutes into the practice. If anything is going to enable you to begin to make progress in these poses, it is the heat. Work hard, focus on the *bandhas* and the breathing, even as you are learning new postures. This will help keep the heat up. Be prepared to continue at least through seven more postures, as once you begin work on this chapter, that is the first place you may stop. Beginners will only do five postures, as there are two that they will omit in the early stages of practice. Most important, please remember that this chapter is a continuation of the preceding one. You may only practice the postures in this chapter if you have first done everything that precedes it. And this means every time you practice. It doesn't mean that if you did the postures in chapter 5 last week or last month,

it is okay today to skip to the postures in this chapter. This is a sequence. You are learning a dance.

Playing the Edge

One of the key elements to finding your way into the practice is to learn a technique called *edge playing.* The expression has been around in yoga circles since the early seventies, and I'm not sure who used it first—maybe a yogi by the name of Joel Kramer. In any case, it really helps you to pay attention to where you are in a pose.

You move as deeply as you can into the posture, using your breath and the *bandhas*, as we have been practicing. You go to your "edge," where discomfort starts to intensify and, perhaps, becomes pain, and at that point you back off slightly and breathe and relax, still holding the *bandhas* and doing *ujjayi* breathing. You take your five breaths. Then you go to the "edge" again, and see if it has moved. Take another five breaths. And again. Each time, you are trying to move the edge further and further away from you. It's a very effective way to trick the mind into going further into a posture than you might think you can, and also an effective way of allowing the body to "surrender" into a posture, rather than attempting to force the body into a posture. This process of riding out to explore your boundaries and then repositioning them in ever-widening circles is an effective way to learn to confront your limitations and go beyond them.

You will find that if you really wish to do this, you will. If you don't, you won't. I have seen the most incredibly tight men and women begin to "get" some of these postures after anywhere from six to twenty-four months of regular practice. I have also seen students who have been coming to class one time per week for three or four years make no progress. Why is that? Because that is all they do—come to class once a week! And that's not nearly enough to make any change in an extremely tight body, or in any body, for that matter. This is a discipline. This is about learning to do a little training every day and building on that. Increasing mindfulness, strength, endurance, and, oh yes, flexibility.

Keep in mind that these postures are given in sequence and in series for a reason, which is an integral part of the therapy. There are places that lend themselves anatomically and biomechanically to an exit, and others that don't. All the postures serve as coun-terpostures to others in some way. They don't always follow one another immediately. Sometimes there might be two or three poses between a posture and its counterpose. In certain cases, if you do one posture and not the counterposture, the spine could be left off-balance. So it is always important to do the minimum number of postures recommended in each grouping and be conscious of returning the spine to "neutral."

As in chapter 5, there are a couple of points within this cycle where it is possible to end your practice and move to closing. These will be pointed out as you go along. It is at this point in your practice that you begin to end with either the *Amended* or the *Complete Closing Sequence.* (The only reason you might still be doing *Modified Closing Sequence* is if any of the postures in *Amended* or *Complete Closing Sequence* are contraindicated for you. In that case it is perfectly acceptable to do *Modified Closing Sequence* to end your practice.)

7

BOAT POSTURE: *NAVASANA*

Nava means "boat."

TECHNIQUE

Inhale, jump through.

Exhale, from the jump through, lift the legs straight into the air, making a ninety-degree angle between the extended legs and the torso (Figure 6.1). Keep the back *straight,* arms parallel to the floor. Head is up. Gaze is at the big toes.

Beginners' Modification:

Exhale, bend the knees, pull the feet up, and place them flat on the floor (Figure 6.2). Hold the knees with the hands and sit with the back erect.

Inhale, lean back until the feet come off the floor, balancing *between* the buttock bones and the coccyx (base of the spine). If you are resting on the coccyx bone, you are leaning back too far!

Exhale, let go of the legs with the hands (Figure 6.3). Don't collapse! If you disintegrate (i.e., the back rounds) when you let go, you have to back up and continue to hold the

Figure 6.2

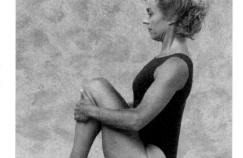

Figure 6.1

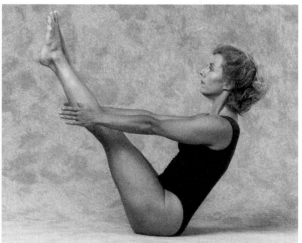

Figure 6.3

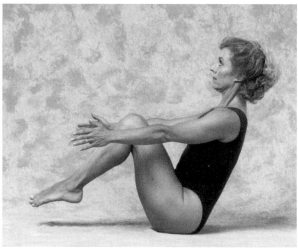

knees with the hands, becoming less and less dependent on support from the hands to keep the back straight.

Note: Do this modification as the posture, until the abdominals become strong enough to hold the legs extended without "caving." Attempting to straighten the legs and do the posture prematurely, before the abdominals are strong enough, results in sloppy practice and puts an enormous strain on the psoas muscle, which can strain the lower back. Make sure you have ninety-degree angle or slightly less between the torso and the extended legs. Also, the chest should be lifted and back lengthened before you try to hold the legs extended.

THIS IS BOAT POSTURE—HOLD FOR FIVE BREATHS (FIGURE 6.1, 6.2, OR 6.3).

Inhale, take it up.
> *Beginners:* Cross legs, put hands at sides, push down with hands, lifting buttocks off the floor.
> *Intermediate/Advanced:* Cross legs, put hands at sides, take it up, and tip slightly forward, holding the tucked legs off the ground (as in the *vinyasa* move for previous postures).
Exhale, come back into Boat Posture, or the modification you are doing.

THIS IS BOAT POSTURE—HOLD FOR FIVE BREATHS. REPEAT THIS SEQUENCE FOUR MORE TIMES FOR A TOTAL OF SIX REPETITIONS.

(Remember to hold root and abdominal locks, *mula* and *uddiyana bandha,* to protect the back, maintain heat, keep energy "up" for this work, and focus concentration!)

Inhale, take it up.
Exhale, jump back.
Inhale, Face Up Dog.
Exhale, Face Down Dog.
Inhale, jump around (to the outside of) the arms to prepare for the next posture (Figure 6.4).
Exhale, work shoulders under and behind knees.

8

PRESSURE ON THE SHOULDERS POSTURE: *BHUJAPIDASANA*

Bhuja means "shoulder" or "arm." *Pida* means "pressure" or "to squeeze." Thus, the name of the posture implies pressure against or the squeezing of the shoulders. This posture simultaneously works (contracts) the adductors (the muscles in the inner thigh that move the legs together), and stretches the abductors (the muscles that work opposite to the adductors and open the thighs). We will see in a subsequent counterposture how these two muscles are worked in exactly the opposite way.

TECHNIQUE

Inhale, instead of jumping through the arms on the inhale, in this *vinyasa* you jump around the arms, with the back of the thighs landing on top of the back of the upper arms, as in Figure 6.4. With the palms flat on the floor, lift the feet, balance on the hands (Figure 6.5).
Exhale, cross and interlock the ankles (Figure 6.6), and tip forward, placing the head on the floor (Figure 6.7). Gaze is at or past the tip of the nose. Attempt to lift feet so they clear the floor.

Beginners' Modification (somewhat easier):
> *Inhale,* jump the feet to the outside of the hands so that the palms are flat on the floor about shoulder width apart, between the legs. If you are tight in the back of the legs (hamstrings) or the hips (hip flexors), this position might not be possible, in which case you will need to

work one side at a time (see following *Beginners' Modification: most easy*). Continue to breathe. Realistically, it will take some struggling and quite a few breaths to work yourself into this posture.

Exhale, work the shoulders and elbows in behind the knees, pressing against the shoulders with the inner thighs and trying to wedge the shoulders in back of the knees. The hands should be placed on the floor between and slightly behind the feet, as in Figure 6.4.

Inhale, lift the feet up, balancing on the hands with the back of the knees resting over the back of the upper arms, as in Figure 6.5. Try to interlock the feet at the ankles, as in Figure 6.6.

Difficulties: In the beginning, the legs will slip down the arms, and you may repeatedly tip over backward as you try to pick the feet up and place the

▼ **Figure 6.4**

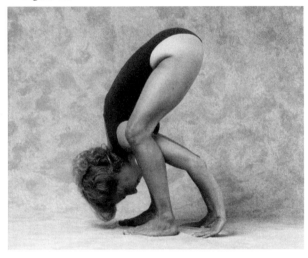

Figure 6.5 ▼

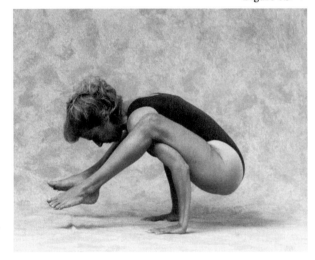

▼ **Figure 6.6**

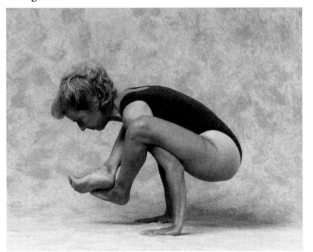

Figure 6.7 ▼

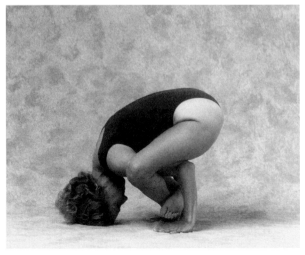

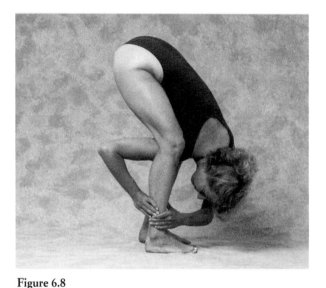

Figure 6.8

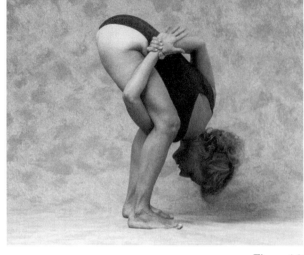

Figure 6.9

weight on the arms and hands, finding balance difficult. This work is dependent on progress in forward bending, and as the back of the legs get opened up, the legs will go up higher on the arms. Eventually you will be able to place the palms flat and balance on the hands.

Note of caution: Resist the temptation to put the thumbs back to help prop you up. This is a common tendency if you are tight in the hips and back of the legs. (The legs are low down on the arms and you are trying not to tip over backward, so you stick your thumbs back.) However, you *want* to be free to roll backward without any risk of straining, or putting too much weight on the thumbs, so keep your thumbs pointing forward.

Beginners' Modification (most easy):

If you are too tight in the hips to manage the "rest the back of the knees over the tops of the shoulders" position, then begin working one side at a time. Instead of attempting to jump the feet to the outside of the hands, from the last posture on the connecting movement, simply jump the feet *to* the hands.

Separate the feet about two feet apart. Bend the knees slightly and lean forward, keeping the shoulders down and the buttocks up. Don't squat.

Phase 1: Work to take the right shoulder toward and eventually *under*, the right knee, using the hands holding the ankle to help pull the shoulder behind the knee (Figure 6.8). Push the right knee in toward the right shoulder, using the inner thigh (adductor) muscles. Using the inner thigh muscles is an important aspect of this posture.

Keep pressing the buttocks toward the ceiling or sky. Take five breaths in this position, then change sides. This will continue the opening process in the hips and, with practice, slowly the shoulders and knees will come closer together.

Phase 2: Once you can start to work the shoulder behind the knee, you can begin to take the arm back, then up and over the buttocks. Keep the right palm facing away from you. Reach around with the left hand and grab the right wrist, pulling the right hand up and in toward the spine (Figure 6.9). Take five breaths, then change sides. This not only provides introductory work for Pressure on the Shoulders Posture, but it prepares you for the following posture as well.

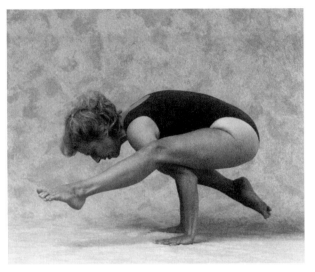

Figure 6.10a

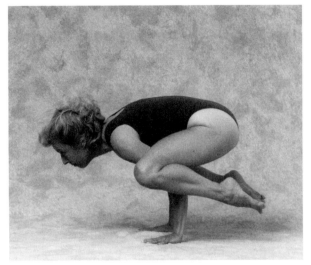

Figure 6.10b

THIS IS PRESSURE ON THE SHOULDERS POSTURE
—HOLD FOR FIVE BREATHS (MAKE SURE TO RE-
PEAT THE MODIFIED POSTURE ON BOTH SIDES)
(FIGURE 6.6, 6.7, 6.8, OR 6.9).

Inhale, lift the head up, bring the feet through the
arms and uncross the ankles. Unwind the legs one
at a time and take them back to balance on the upper arms (Figure 6.10 sequence).

Exhale, either jump back from this balanced position, or if unable to jump back, rest the feet on the
floor first and jump back from there.

Inhale, Face Up Dog.

Exhale, Face Down Dog.

Inhale, jump around the arms again, as for last posture.

> *Beginners' Modification:* Jump through and come
> into Stick Posture (*Dandasana*).

Figure 6.11

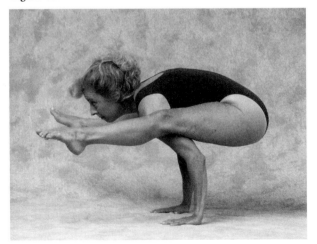

9

TORTOISE POSTURE: *KURMASANA*

Kurma means "turtle" or "tortoise."

TECHNIQUE

Inhale, jump the feet around the hands again, with
the back of the knees landing on the back of the
upper arms, near the shoulders. Press up, lift the
feet, straighten the legs (Figure 6.11), and

Exhale, bend the arms, and lower the buttocks to the

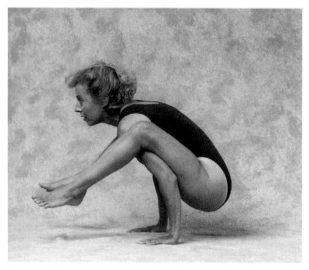

Figure 6.12

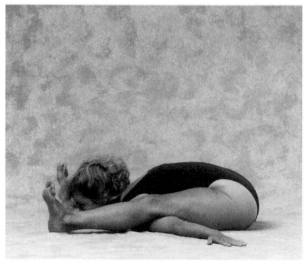

Figure 6.13

floor (Figure 6.12). Reach the hands under the knees and point the hands slightly back, then stretch the arms straight out to the sides. By pushing down with the thigh muscles and straightening the legs, you will stretch the middle-back muscles and push the shoulders and chest toward the floor. By also pressing down with the chest and back, the shoulders will eventually come to rest on the floor. At this point, reach out with the torso, extending the back, and bring the forehead, then chin, and finally the chest to the floor. Gaze is straight—at or past the end of the nose (Figure 6.13).

Beginners' Modification (somewhat easier):

From Stick Posture (*Dandasana*), spread the legs, bend the knees a little, and slide the feet back slightly toward the shoulders.

Exhale, bend forward, and push the hands one by one under the knees. Notice that this work feels similar to the preceding pose, Pressure on the Shoulders Posture. Continue to breathe! As much as possible, stretch the arms straight out to the sides and slightly back. Reach out with the torso, lifting the chest and extending the back. Push forward with the legs and thighs, as in Figure 6.13.

Beginners' Modification (most easy):

Many of you will start out looking something like Figure 6.14. As you make progress in all of the preceding postures, you will find that Tortoise Posture becomes easier.

Bring the soles of the feet toward one another, but don't pull the heels in toward the groin. Keep the feet out, about an arm's length away from you. Grab the ankles with the hands, and pull the chest toward the calves. Keep attempting to lift the chest and extend the spine (Figure 6.15). As the hips and the back of the legs open, and the shoulders get closer to the knees, you will slowly begin to be able to slide the arms under the knees.

Note: Whatever modification you choose, find your posture and hold that position.

This is Tortoise Posture—hold for five breaths (Figure 6.13 or 6.15).

Go directly into next posture, Sleeping Tortoise.

Beginners' Modification: If you did the *Beginners' Modification* in this posture, hold for five more

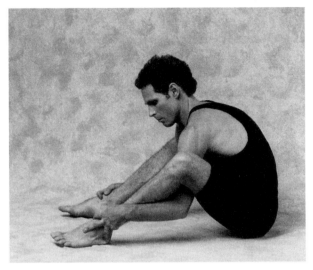

Figure 6.14

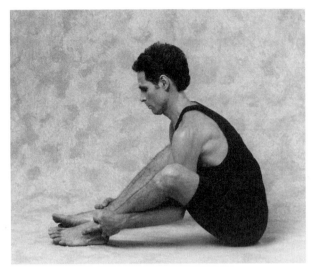

Figure 6.15

breaths, then skip this next posture (Posture 10, Sleeping Tortoise Posture), and continue with the *vinyasa* that follows Posture 10. Follow that with the *Beginners' Modification* for Posture 11, or Embryo-in-the-Womb Posture.

TECHNIQUE: INTERMEDIATE AND ADVANCED ONLY

Inhale, turn the palms face up, bend and lift the knees slightly, lift the chest slightly, coming up out of Tortoise Posture, bend the elbows, internally rotate the shoulders, and move the arms back alongside the hips (Figure 6.16).

10

SLEEPING TORTOISE POSTURE: *SUPTA KURMASANA*

Supta means "reclining" or "sleeping." *Kurma* means "tortoise" or "turtle."

Caution: This pose is a continuation of Tortoise Posture, and should be attempted only when you have begun to make some progress getting the shoulders down under the knees in the preceding posture. There really is no modification for this posture, other than what I have described for the previous pose, Tortoise Posture, which beginners may repeat here.

Figure 6.16

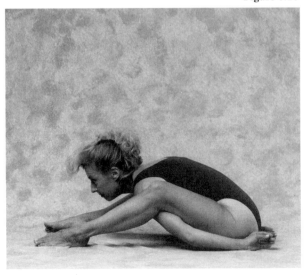

Exhale, move the hands up and over the hips, and clasp them behind the back at the waist, if possible. Now move the feet in toward one another, eventually crossing one foot over the other and interlocking them at the ankles. Last, tuck the head in between the feet and take the forehead to the ground (Figure 6.17). Gaze is straight past the end of the nose.

Note: Using an extension device (in this case a towel), to connect the hands can facilitate the work in the pose (Figure 6.18).

THIS IS SLEEPING TORTOISE POSTURE—HOLD FOR FIVE BREATHS.

Inhale, lift the head.

Exhale, release the hands and feet, but keep the legs in position.

Inhale, sit up with the knees still hanging over the back of the upper arms, and place hands in front of groin (Figure 6.19), then press forward and up, lifting up on to the hands, legs extended (Figure 6.20) out over the shoulders or top of arms.

Exhale, lean forward slightly, and fold first one leg back, then the other leg back, resting the knees on the back of the arms as you did in the exit *vinyasa* move for Tortoise Posture above. Jump back.

Inhale, Face Up Dog.

Exhale, Face Down Dog.

Inhale, jump through.

▼ **Figure 6.17**

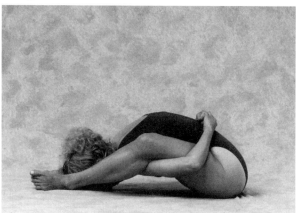

Figure 6.18 ▼

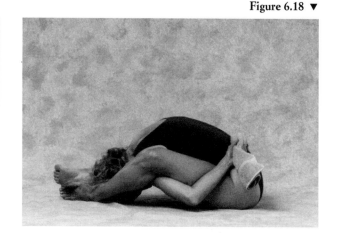

▼ **Figure 6.19**

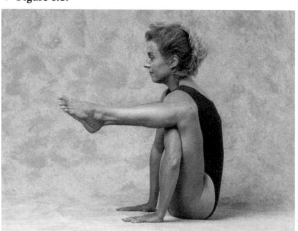

Figure 6.20 ▼

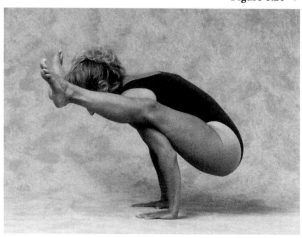

11

EMBRYO-IN-THE-WOMB POSTURE:
GARBA PINDASANA

Garba means "womb." *Pinda* means "embryo." This posture resembles the position of an embryo in the womb, except, of course, that in this case, the legs are folded in a full lotus position.

This is an interesting posture and generally causes a bit of commotion when we first introduce it into a beginners' class—mostly because it is not easy, and partially because it brings comic relief! Correctly practiced, this posture requires the Full Lotus Posture. But since this is difficult for many of us, I have designated the posture "Advanced Only." There is a *Beginners' Modification* that follows, and it accomplishes much of the same benefit as the true posture itself.

TECHNIQUE: ADVANCED ONLY

(Beginners should see the following Modification.)
Exhale, sit in Full Lotus Posture (*Padmasana*), with the right leg folded in first (Figure 6.21).

Inhale.
Exhale, push the right hand through the space between the thighs and calves (Figure 6.22), and then the left hand (Figure 6.23), one on each side.

Note: At this point you are probably saying, "She must be joking! What space between the thighs and the calves?" I know, there isn't much. And some of us have less space than others. Slathering the forearms with a little water does wonders to assist in sliding the arms through what may be virtually a nonexistent space. However, *don't* use oil. It will totally screw up the rest of your practice.

Keep breathing. Push the arms through until you can bend the elbows. Then lift the thighs and catch the sides of the head or face with the hands, holding the ears, if possible. Press the spine forward and the shoulders back to straighten the torso and help with balance.

(Make sure that you push the hands through at the section where the calves are pressing into the thighs, between the ankles and knees—*not* between the ankles and the groin. Work the hand through as close in to the ankle as possible; there is more space at this point than there is closer to the knee, where the calf muscle is fleshier.)

Inhale. First, make certain you are centered on your

Figure 6.21

Figure 6.22

Figure 6.23

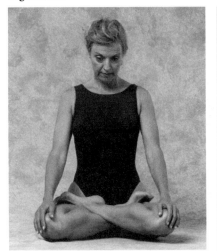

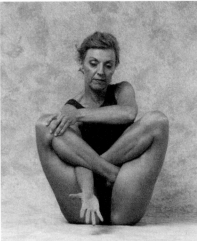

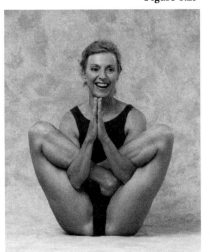

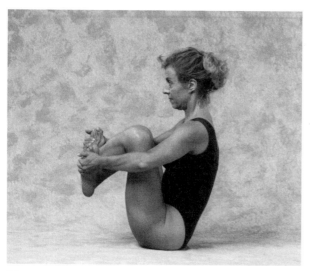

Figure 6.24

yoga mat or carpet. While maintaining your posture, with either the hands holding the head (more difficult), or simply clasped together in front of you, roll backward on the inhale and forward on the exhale, while turning a complete circle of 360 degrees. Try to complete the circle in nine rolls.

Beginners' Modification:

Inhale, if you are unable to sit in Full Lotus Posture, bend the knees and cross the ankles.

Exhale, gather the legs into the chest (Figure 6.24), then grasp the left foot with the right hand and the right foot with the left hand.

Inhale, rock back on the inhale, rolling all the way back onto the shoulders, with the feet coming to the floor behind you, and then.

Exhale, roll forward again on the exhale, continuing to rock back and forth on the inhales and exhales. You may feel a little silly doing this, but it feels wonderful and massages the middle-back muscles, which really need some attention after the Tortoise and Sleeping Tortoise series.

THIS IS EMBRYO-IN-THE-WOMB POSTURE—ROLL FOR AS MANY BREATHS AS NECESSARY TO COMPLETE CIRCLE. (FIGURE 6.23 OR 6.24).

When you have completed the circle and are back to where you started, you roll all the way upright and *go directly into the next posture* (Figure 6.25). Beginners who are practicing the modification, skip the next posture (Posture 12, Rooster Posture) and go on to Posture 13, Bound Angle Posture.

Note: In the Tortoise Postures, the erector spinae muscles (the muscles that go up the middle of the back on either side of the spine and extend the lower back, and are also called lumbar extensors) are constantly being contracted by the lifting of the chest action, then stretched intensely by the downward pressure of the legs over the shoulders. They really get worked over in these two postures. In *Garba Pindasana,* these muscles are massaged and relieved by the rolling-around action on the back.

12

ROOSTER POSTURE: *KUKKUTASANA*

Kukku means "rooster," which is sort of what this posture looks like.

TECHNIQUE: ADVANCED ONLY

(There are no modifications.)

Inhale, coming directly from Embryo-in-the-Womb Posture (*Garba Pindasana*), roll up, place the hands flat on the floor, and lift up to balance on the palms (Figure 6.25). Keep the head up and be sure to hold *mula bandha* while balancing. Look straight ahead. Focus on a point on the wall to help maintain the balance.

THIS IS ROOSTER POSTURE—HOLD FOR FIVE BREATHS (FIGURE 6.25).

Exhale, release posture, sit back down, pull hands out from between legs. Disengage legs.

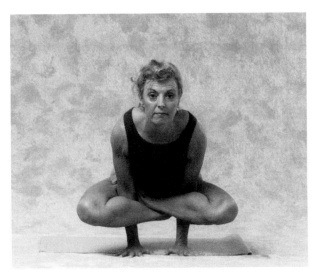

Figure 6.25

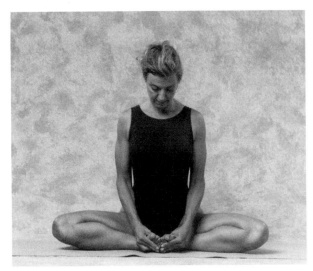

Figure 6.26

Inhale, take it up. Don't get lazy with the "take it ups." Remember to place hands at sides, cross feet and push down with hands, lifting buttocks, torso, and legs up off the floor! Try to "dangle" back and forth and swing back.

Exhale, jump back.

Inhale, Face Up Dog.

Exhale, Face Down Dog.

Inhale, jump through.

Exhale, sit down, extend legs.

13

BOUND ANGLE POSTURE: *BADDHA KONASANA*

Baddha means "fixed, restrained, or bound." *Kona* means "angle."

Note: This posture is the counterposture for Posture 8, Pressure on the Shoulders Posture. In this case, you are pressing the thighs out and down, thus stretching the adductors, and working or contracting the abductors, just the opposite of what you did in Pressure on the Shoulders Posture.

TECHNIQUE

Inhale, bring the soles of the feet together, pulling the heels in as close to the perineum as possible. Take hold of the feet and try to open the feet out, like the pages of a new book (Figure 6.26).

Exhale, fold at the hips, moving the torso toward the floor. Do not round the back or collapse the front of the body. Lead with the chest and follow through with strength from the back muscles, eventually taking the chest and chin to the floor. Keep the buttocks on the floor (Figure 6.27). The gaze is straight ahead.

Beginners' Modification and Helpful Hints:

For many of you, especially men and most runners, the adductors will be extremely tight, and when you bring the feet together, you will look something like Figure 6.28. This posture is one of the many that dramatically illustrate how tight we can get and how far away from normal anatomical range of motion it is possible for us to go as a result of training. "How," you may ask, "if I look like Figure 6.28, will I ever progress to look like Figure 6.27?" Good question.

The most common mistake made by beginners in this posture is to hunch the shoulders and round the back in an attempt to get the head down and "look"

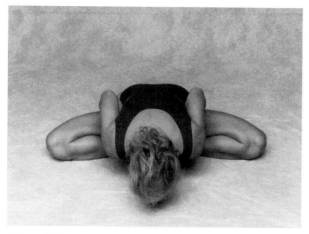

Figure 6.27

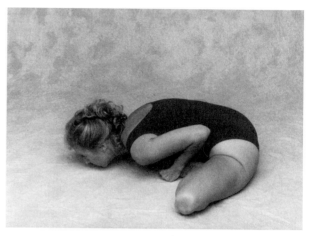

Figure 6.27, side view

flexible. *Absolutely, do not let the back round or the shoulders hunch.* Instead, think of stiffening the back and "leading" with the chest as the torso moves forward. To help keep the back straight, hold on to the ankles with the hands and use the arm and shoulder muscles (Figure 6.29) to hold the back erect. Press out and down with the inner thighs, eventually taking the knees to the floor. However, before you can push down on the knees, the heels must be in tight to the groin. Do not push down on the knees if you cannot pull the feet in close to the groin.

If necessary, to help straighten the back, place a pillow under the hips. This will help to tip the pelvis forward and straighten the lower back. Once you've been practicing this regularly on your own, you might wish to have a friend sit behind you and place her feet against the lower back "plate" and press forward, giving a lift to the back (Figure 6.30). Try to hold this position after your friend releases the support.

Once you are able to hold your back straight by yourself, you may wish to have your friend sit behind you and place her legs over your inner thighs (Figure 6.31). This weight on the thighs will help the inner thighs to release and open. Do this only when you have been doing regular practice for some time on your own. Then, using your arm and shoulder mus-

cles, pull forward, keeping the back straight, into the hip stretch.

Remember to breathe and hold the *bandhas* while you are working in this posture, whatever modification you are doing.

THIS IS BOUND ANGLE POSTURE—HOLD FOR FIVE BREATHS (FIGURE 6.27, 6.28, 6.29, 6.30, OR 6.31).

Inhale, lift the head, extend the back, and come to a sitting position using the lumbar extensor muscles.
Exhale.
Inhale, cross the feet, take it up or roll over the feet.
Exhale, jump back.
Inhale, Face Up Dog.
Exhale, Face Down Dog.
Inhale, jump though.
Exhale, extend legs.

This is a possible closing point within the Primary Series. For those of you who wish to stop at this point, the next step is to go to chapter 7 and begin "closing," or ending your practice. You must do at least the Modified Closing and, once you complete the rest of this chapter, do the Amended or Complete Closing, if possible, in order to release and relieve the

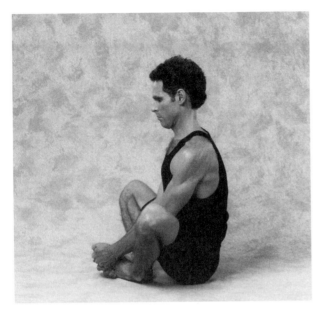

Figure 6.28

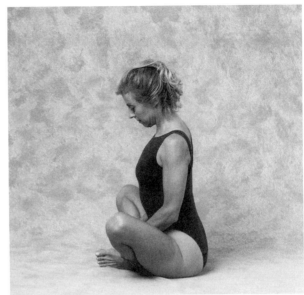

Figure 6.29

spine of any tautness that may remain from any of the preceding postures. Remember, this is therapy! That is why you must do the appropriate postures in the given order. That way, the poses and counterposes work with and against one another to return the spine to neutral when you finish practice and come to rest. Don't do Amended or Closing Sequence until you complete all postures in chapter 6.

Figure 6.30

Figure 6.31

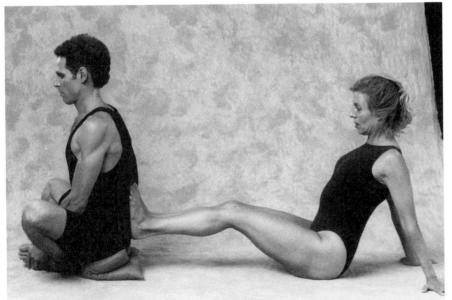

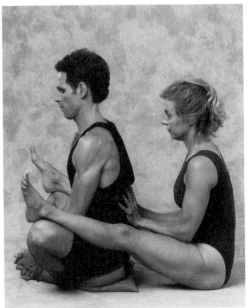

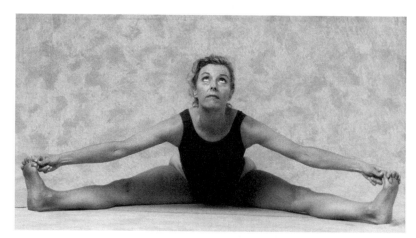

▲ Figure 6.32

Figure 6.33 ▼

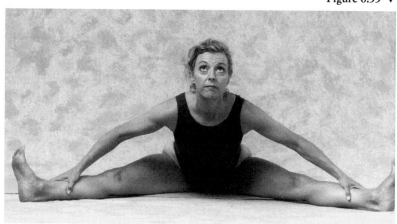

▼ Figure 6.34, side view

Figure 6.34 ▼

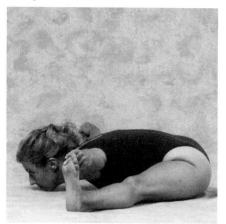

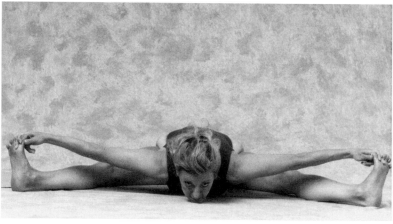

14

SEATED ANGLE POSTURE: *UPAVISHTA KONASANA*

Upavishta means "seated." *Kona* means "angle."

TECHNIQUE

Inhale, separate the legs as wide apart as possible. Take the big toes with the thumbs and index and middle fingers. Lift the chest, keep the spine straight, extend the rib cage, look up (Figure 6.32). If you cannot catch the toes, take the ankles or shins. Do not bend the knees (Figure 6.33).

Exhale, bend forward as far as possible. Do not round the back. Keep the thighs contracted, pushing the back of the knees into the floor. Keep the kneecaps pointing straight up. Focus on holding the contraction of the thighs. Forget about achieving flexibility. Hold *mula bandha* (contract the perineum!) to *prevent overstretching* the hamstrings. Beginners especially: Do not drop the head forward in order to seem more flexible. As you bend forward, remember to keep the head up and the back *straight!* The gaze is straight ahead.

Eventually, as you develop flexibility, you will bend all the way forward and take the head to the floor. Then extend the back and place the chest and chin on the floor. Gaze up and out (Figure 6.34).

THIS IS SEATED ANGLE POSTURE—HOLD FOR FIVE BREATHS (FIGURE 6.33 OR 6.34).

Inhale, bend the knees slightly while maintaining the hold on the toes, and lift the legs into the air to a balanced position. Extend the legs. Bend the elbows slightly, if possible, to pull the legs upward and out. This uses the arms more effectively and helps with balance. Head is up and the gaze up just past the level of the big toes (Figure 6.35).

Beginners' Modification: If it is not possible for you to extend the legs all the way, then keep the knees slightly bent and just focus on finding balance.

THIS IS (BALANCED) SEATED ANGLE POSTURE— HOLD FOR FIVE BREATHS (FIGURE 6.35).

Figure 6.35

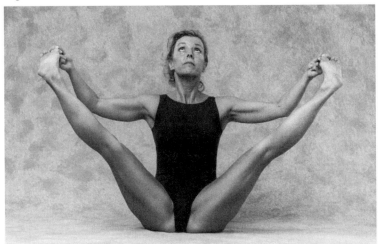

Figure 6.35, side view

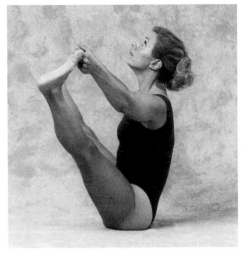

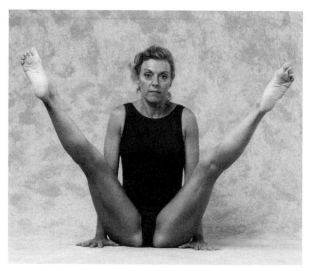

Figure 6.36

Inhale, put your hands down at your sides, holding the legs up in the air (Figure 6.36). Take it up.
Exhale, jump back.
Inhale, Face Up Dog.
Exhale, Face Down Dog.
Inhale, jump through, lie down.

Important note: Once you go on to the next posture (Posture 15, Lying Down Angle Posture), you must complete the remainder of this chapter, plus the Amended Closing Sequence (six postures) or Complete Closing Sequence (eleven postures) in chapter 7.

▼

15

LYING-DOWN ANGLE POSTURE: *SUPTA KONASANA*

Supta means "reclining" or "lying down." *Kona* means "angle."

Note of caution: Contraindications for inverted postures: This is the first of the inverted postures. What is meant by inverted posture is one in which the body is upside down. There will be slightly different cau-

tionary advice for each of these postures, but in general, the inverted postures should not be practiced by the following groups: (1) persons with hypertension (high blood pressure), (2) women in the first few days of their menstrual cycle (when flow is heavy), (3) anyone with eye disorders that create pressure in the eyes (such as detached retina), (4) persons with neck pain or irregular configuration of the vertebrae in the neck (such as a reverse cervical curve), and (5) persons with lower-back pain or injury. See following Modification for Injury or Pain.

TECHNIQUE

Preparation: To begin this posture, you should be lying down with the legs and feet together, and arms at your sides. This is where you left off at the end of the preceding *vinyasa,* and it is like *sama-sthiti,* or attention position, lying down.
Exhale, lift legs over head to floor, separating the legs and taking same angle between legs, as in previous posture, Seated Angle Posture. Take the big toes with the first two fingers and thumb. The head is centered with chin pressing into notch in collarbone. Do not move the head once you come into this posture (Figure 6.37). Gaze is at the heart *chakra,* or the center of the chest. If you cannot take the toes, grab the calves (Figure 6.38).

Figure 6.37

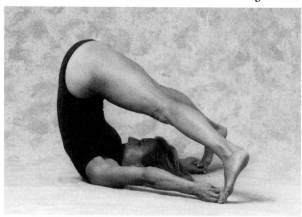

Modification for Injury or Pain: Let's examine the neck and lower-back contraindications in a little more detail.

First the lower back: If you have lower-back pain, compressed vertebrae, or disk problems, or are very tight in the lower back and back of the legs, this posture might aggravate your back if done incorrectly. If your problem is tightness, when you do this posture the limited flexibility in the back of the legs will cause the buttocks to come too far over the head, rounding and straining the lower back. What you might do as an alternative is to rest your legs against a wall, which will prevent the strain and compression in the lower back (Figure 6.39).

In order to do this posture safely in the presence of any lower-back irregularities, the rules are the same as in forward bending, because this is actually just a forward bending posture turned over 180 degrees. The spine must be kept in extension, with no rounding and no compression. If done correctly, this is a very therapeutic posture for the entire spine. However, if you have back pain or injury and are uncertain whether to do this posture, I would recommend that you *leave it out.*

Second, the neck: If you have neck injury from whiplash, a reverse cervical curve, misaligned vertebrae in the neck causing pain or numbness in the shoulders or arms, compressed or inflamed cervical disks, or simply general misalignment of the cervical vertebrae that may or may not be causing you pain, this posture may aggravate your neck problems. If you can only do infrequent or short practice, then leave it out! *You certainly cannot do this occasionally, out of sequence, or half-seriously and expect any benefit whatsoever.*

However, it *might* also eliminate your neck problems when done in sequence as part of the *full* Primary Series. But in order to work, the complete Primary Series must be done, every day, roughly six days a week; this will take approximately seventy to eighty minutes per day, for anywhere from three weeks to three months. Since this is a major commitment, requiring a lot of time and dedication, it is much safer to simply omit the posture if you are uncertain whether you can find the time.

The rest of the practice will sufficiently strengthen and align the spine to alleviate most tension and pain in the neck and lower back.

Important Note: If you omit this posture for any of the above contraindications, then you will also leave out the inverted postures in Closing Sequence. This means that you will *only* practice the Modified Closing Sequence.

THIS IS LYING-DOWN ANGLE POSTURE—HOLD FOR FIVE BREATHS (FIGURE 6.37, 6.38, OR 6.39).

Inhale, hold on to toes, and roll through up to a bal-

Figure 6.38

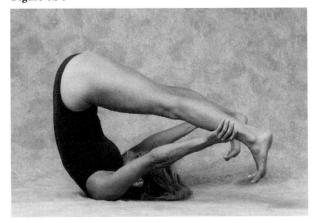

Figure 6.39

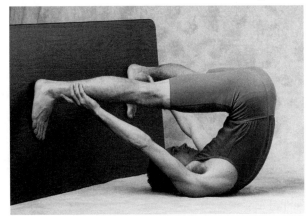

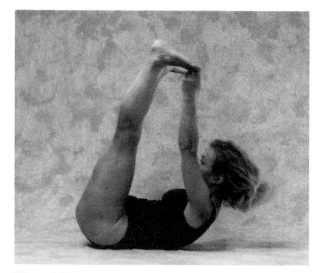

Figure 6.40a

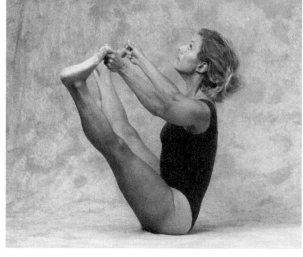

Figure 6.40b

anced position, without bending the knees (Figure 6.40 sequence). This takes a little practice until you get the hang of the roll-up and balance routine. Balancing at the top of the roll means sort of "catching" yourself between the abdominal and back muscles. At first you won't be able to hang on to the toes. Then you won't be able to roll without bending the knees. Then you'll figure out

how to keep your legs straight but won't be able to hit the balance point. Once you get the hang of it, hold at the "top" for a beat and then

Exhale, lean forward, release the balance, and slowly roll down to touch the calf muscles on the floor while still holding on to the toes. *Land on the calves with the feet dorsiflexed, or pulled back* (Figure 6.41 sequence).

Figure 6.41a   **Figure 6.41b**   **Figure 6.41c**

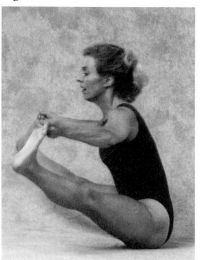

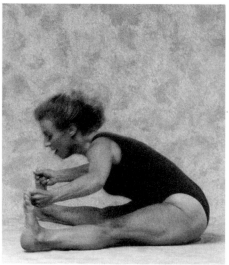

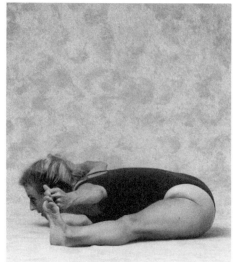

Important note of caution: Be careful to flex the feet far enough so that when you land, you do so on the calf muscles and not the heel bones. Landing on the heels can bruise the heel bones and is definitely not recommended! Be very careful if you try this and be sure to practice first on thick padding or carpeting!

Inhale, cross legs, take it up.

Exhale, jump back.

Inhale, Face Up Dog.

Exhale, Face Down Dog.

Inhale, jump through.

Exhale, lie down, feet together, arms at sides.

Very important note: This posture begins the stretching and opening of the back of the neck, and prepares the spine for the postures in Complete Closing Sequence that continue the therapeutic alignment of the vertebrae. In order for this posture to be effective, it must be done in sequence (as I have mentioned more than a few times already) *and as part of the complete practice. If you do this posture, you must be prepared to do either the Amended or Complete Closing Sequence.* If you have omitted this posture, continue with the next posture.

16

Lying-Down Big Toe Posture: *Supta Padangustasana*

Supta means "reclining" or "sleeping." *Pada* means "foot." *Angustha* means "big toe." This posture is the same as the standing posture, Extended Hand–to–Big Toe Posture, catching the big toe with the hand.

Technique

Preparation: This posture begins from a lying-down position, like supine *sama-sthiti.*

Inhale, bring the right leg straight up in the air and grab the big toe with the first two fingers and thumbs of the right hand (Figure 6.42). If you cannot reach the big toe, take the ankle or back of the calf. Do not bend your knee. Keep the left leg straight, with the thigh contracted and the foot flexed. Place the left palm on the left thigh.

Exhale, lift the torso up using the right arm and abdominals. Pull the head toward the knee. The gaze is up at the right big toe. The back should be off the ground, so work the arm and abdominal muscles strongly enough to lift the torso (Figure 6.43).

This is Lying-Down Big Toe Posture Part A—take five breaths (Figure 6.43).

Exhale, open right leg out to side. Turn head and gaze to your left out of the left corner of your eyes. Use the left hand to press down on the left hip and thigh (Figure 6.44). Keep both thighs working (contracted!) and both legs straight. Work to keep the left leg pressing down into the floor.

> *Beginners' Modification:* Do not bend the knees. You may need to back off or readjust your hand position in order to open the leg to the side (Figure 6.45). You may also need to back off the angle of the leg slightly.

This is Lying-Down Big Toe Posture Part B—take five breaths (Figure 6.44 or 6.45).

Inhale, bring the leg straight back up to where you started, as in Figure 6.42 (changing your hand position again if necessary) using the inner thigh muscles to lift the leg. Do not bend the knees of either leg. Both thighs should remain contracted throughout the entire sequence.

Exhale, lift torso again and, if possible, touch head to knee, as in Figure 6.43.

Inhale, head down as in Figure 6.42.

Exhale, release leg, return to lying-down position.

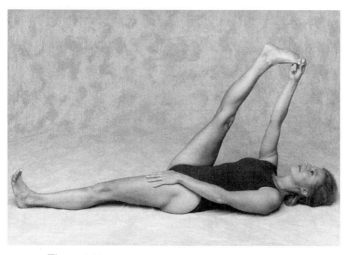

Figure 6.42

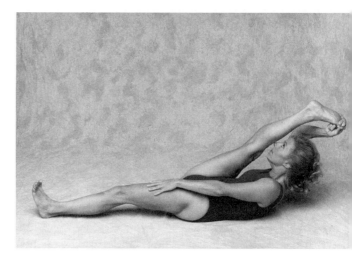

Figure 6.43

Repeat instructions for left side, then follow with a *vinyasa:*

Inhale, sit up, cross legs, take it up.
Exhale, jump back.
Inhale, Face Up Dog.
Exhale, Face Down Dog.
Inhale, jump through, lie down.

Important note: This is another possible closing point in the Primary Series. For those of you who wish to stop at this point and skip to Closing Sequence, there are two options. If you omitted the previous pose, Lying-Down Angle Posture, do Modified Closing Sequence next and then take rest. If, however, you did the previous posture and wish to end at this point, you must close with Amended or Complete Closing Sequence.

Figure 6.44

Figure 6.45

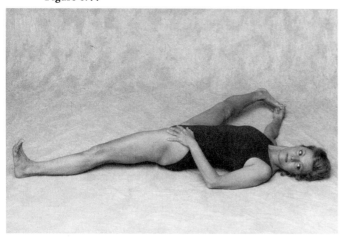

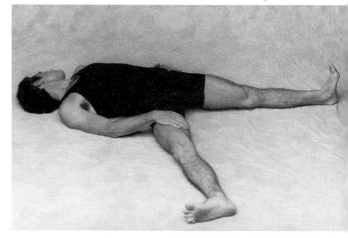

17

BOTH BIG TOES POSTURE:
UBHAYA PADANGUSTHASANA

Ubhaya means "both." *Pada* means "foot." *Angustha* means "big toe." In this posture, you take both big toes with the hands.

Important note of caution: Contraindications for inverted postures: This is the second of the inverted postures. All of the same contraindications apply as for Lying-Down Angle Posture (Posture 15). If you did not do Posture 15, do not do this (or the following) posture either.

TECHNIQUE

Preparation: Begin posture from lying-down position.
Exhale, bring both legs over the head, toes to the
floor. Reach back with the arms and grab both big
toes with the thumb and the first two fingers of
both hands (Figure 6.46). Keep the head centered.
If you cannot reach the toes, grab the ankles or
back of the calves. Don't bend your knees. Hold
on tight!

Beginners' Modification: If the feet do not reach
the floor, go only as far as feels comfortable
without creating strain (see lower-back contraindications in Posture 15).

Inhale, roll up to balance while *holding on to your
toes or whatever you are holding.* Don't bend the
knees (Figure 6.47).
Exhale, hold the arms straight, legs extended, head
back. Look up (Figure 6.48). Do the best you can
with this. If you need to bend the knees slightly,
it's okay. Remember to hold *mula* and *uddiyana
bandha.*

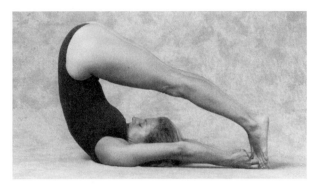

▲ **Figure 6.46**

Figure 6.47 ▼

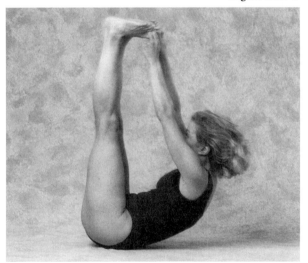

Figure 6.48 ▼

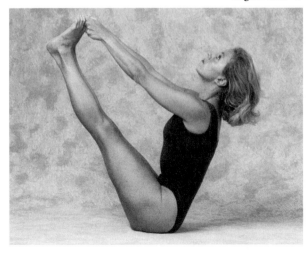

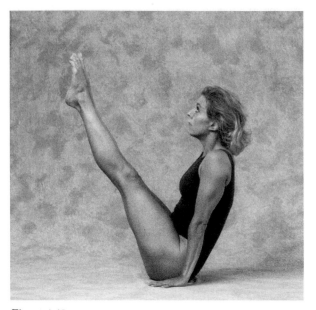

Figure 6.49

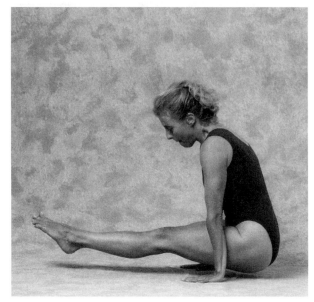

Figure 6.50

Note: Like the "roll up to balance" move out of Lying-Down Angle Posture (*Supta Konasana*)—this will be tricky for a while. You might not get enough steam going and only get halfway and then roll backward. On the other hand, you might use too much steam and come flying though the point of balance and continue to the floor. If this happens, be careful to bend your knees and catch yourself on your feet. Don't crash.

THIS IS BOTH BIG TOES POSTURE—HOLD FOR FIVE BREATHS (FIGURE 6.48).

Inhale, put your hands down, take it up, keeping the legs in the air, if possible (works the abs!) (Figures 6.49 and 6.50).
Exhale, jump back.
Inhale, Face Up Dog.
Exhale, Face Down Dog.
Inhale, jump through, lie down again.

18

UPWARD-FACING INTENSE WEST STRETCH POSTURE (FULL FORWARD BENDING): *URDHVA MUKHA PASCHIMOTTANASANA*

Urdhva means "upward." *Mukha* means "face." *Paschimo* means "west" or "posterior." This is the same posture as Intense West Stretch (forward bending), except the posture is rotated ninety degrees and the face is tipped upward.

Important note of caution: This is the third of the inverted postures. All the same contraindications apply as for Posture 15, Lying-Down Angle Posture. If you did not do Posture 15 or Posture 17, omit this one also.

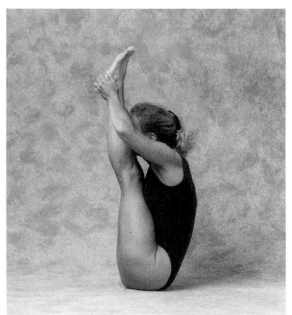

Figure 6.51

TECHNIQUE

Preparation: Begin this posture from a lying-down position, like supine *sama-sthiti.*

Exhale, bring both legs over the head again, as in the last posture, with toes to the floor. Same modifications and adjustments apply as for last posture. Reach back and this time grab the outside edges of the feet near the heels with the hands.

Inhale, roll up to balance, as in last posture.

Exhale, pull torso into thighs using abs and arms (Figure 6.51). Lift chest, extend the spine, do not round the back. Balance is tricky here. Concentrate on the interplay between the back muscles and the abdominal muscles. Gaze is up at toes. Don't bury head and round shoulders.

THIS IS UPWARD-FACING INTENSE WEST STRETCH —HOLD FOR FIVE BREATHS (FIGURE 6.51).

Inhale, take it up (release hands, place hands at sides, keep legs in air, and lift yourself off the ground, as you did in last posture).

Exhale, jump back.
Inhale, Face Up Dog.
Exhale, Face Down Dog.
Inhale, jump through.
Exhale, lie down.

19

BRIDGE POSTURE: *SETU BANDHASANA*

Setu can mean "ridge of earth," "bank," "causeway," "dam" or "bridge." When used in conjunction with *bandha,* it means "the forming of a causeway or bridge."

Important note of caution: The true Bridge Posture is an advanced posture and not easy to learn on one's own. If your balance is not secure, it is possible to tip over and fall out of this posture, which is generally not pleasant and *could* result in injury. Therefore, it is not recommended for beginners and, also, is contraindicated for persons with neck injuries, or for those who have already decided to omit the three inverted postures that preceded this.

However, the modification given here is excellent for those with neck injuries, and is a wonderful counterpose for much of the preceding work. Consequently, I recommend that *everyone* except advanced Power Yoga and *astanga yoga* students, do the Modification.

TECHNIQUE: ADVANCED ONLY

(Beginners and Intermediates, do the Modification.)

Note: Other than Face Up Dog Posture, this is the only backward bending posture in the Primary Series. It strengthens the neck and tones all aspects of the spine. The extensor muscles of the back, which many of you have been attempting to stretch out in the forward bending postures (and develop as well

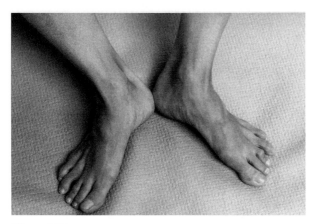

Figure 6.52

by reaching out with the chest and extending the back), become very powerful through the practice of this pose.

Preparation: Lie down with feet and legs together. This is lying-down attention position.

Inhale, bend the knees and bring the heels in toward the buttocks. Place the heels together and open the feet out, with the sides of the feet pressed firmly into the floor (Figure 6.52). Bring the elbows up alongside the body, push the chest up off the floor, and arch the back of the neck, resting the top of the head on the floor. Pull the head back as far as possible by lifting the lower and middle back. Fold the arms across the chest and hold the shoulder blades with the hands (Figure 6.53).

Note: Eventually, this will all be done in one move on one breath. While learning, however, keep breathing and take as many breaths as necessary to reach the lift-off position.

Exhale, lift the hips up, roll up and back over the head to the forehead. If the placement of your feet has been the correct distance from your buttocks, the legs will be able to extend all the way. Keep the heels together and outside edges of the feet pressed strongly into the ground. Gaze is up and back at the point between the eyebrows (Figure 6.54).

Eventually, with a little practice, you will get the feet the correct distance from the hips when you start the posture. Thus, you can fully extend the legs and will not have to readjust the feet once you lift up off the ground. Also, with practice, you will be able to fully roll back on the head almost to the forehead. Very scary, yes! But a wonderful posture and easy to learn if you can find a professional *astanga yoga* or Power Yoga teacher to spot you in this. However, until you can find someone to help, practice the Modification.

Beginners' Modification:

Inhale, bend knees, bring heels up to buttocks. Separate feet hip-width apart. Keep feet parallel.

Exhale, raise buttocks in the air and interlock fingers underneath hips (Figure 6.55). Squeeze shoulder blades together, working to open the chest and heart *chakra* and stretching the pectoral muscles at the front of the shoulders. Keep chin tucked into throat with the head on the floor and the back of the neck relaxed. Do not move head. Lift buttocks as high as possible, using thigh muscles.

THIS IS BRIDGE POSTURE—TAKE FIVE BREATHS (FIGURE 6.54 OR 6.55).

Inhale.

Exhale, release arms, place hands on the floor (Figure 6.56), bend knees and lower legs and buttocks to the floor, release head and slide head out along the floor, straightening neck as you go. Lie flat. Or, if you did the modified pose, simply release the hands and lower the buttocks to the floor.

Inhale, sit up, cross legs and take it up.

Exhale, jump back.

Inhale, Face Up Dog.

Exhale, Face Down Dog.

Inhale, jump through, lie down.

This is the end of the Primary Series. From here you continue to the Closing Sequence. However,

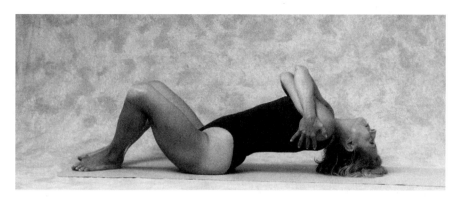

▲ Figure 6.53

Figure 6.54 ▼

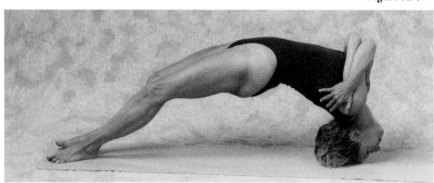

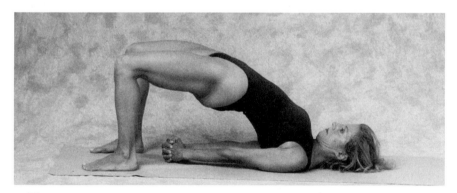

▲ Figure 6.55

Figure 6.56 ▼

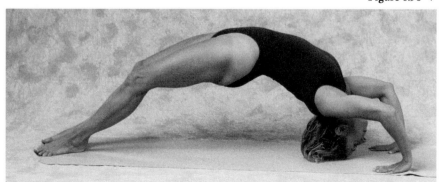

there is one posture which, though technically a Second Series posture, is frequently practiced at the end of the Primary Series. Upward Bow (*Urdhva Dhanurasana*) is generally done (with full forward bending, or *Paschimottanasana,* as a counterpose) at the end of Second Series. You may practice it here with forward bending to prepare for Second Series. I would recommend at least twelve to sixteen weeks of regular, earnest practice with the basic Primary Series postures before adding this optional posture.

20

UPWARD BOW POSTURE: *URDHVA DHANURASANA* (OPTIONAL)

Urdhva means "upward," as we remember from *Urdhva Mukha Svanasana,* or Face Up Dog Posture. *Dhanu* means "bow," as in an archer's bow and arrow, and *dhanur* means "bow-shaped," "curved," or "bent."

Important note of caution: Face Up Dog Posture, and the preceding posture, Bridge Posture, are the only backward bending postures in the Primary Series. If, because of back problems, you have modified Face Up Dog and Bridge Postures, it is advisable to leave out this posture, as it is also a backward bending pose. If your shoulders are tight or limited in their range of motion, the lower back and sacroiliac joint (the place in the lower back where the lower backbone, sacrum, and hip bone, or ilium, come together) will compensate for the limited movement in the shoulders. This is not great for the lower back. I know, because I went through it for six months, using root and abdominal lock ferociously to take the compression out of the lower back and work more into opening the shoulders. The posture, misleadingly, looks as though it requires a lot of strength. It doesn't. It requires a lot of flexibility in the back and shoulders. Occasionally someone will try this for the first time and go right into

it with full extension in the arms and legs. It took *me* ages just to get my head off the floor! When I started really focusing on getting my shoulders, breastbone, and heart opened up, things started to move. But the point is, you can put lots of strength into this, struggle like crazy, and go *nowhere* because of limited range of motion in the shoulders. I have seen weight lifters who can press hundreds of pounds, but who can't lift themselves off the floor! You have to master this posture with intelligence, planning, patience, and perseverance, *not* strength!

Like the back-bending postures in the Second Series of *astanga yoga* (see Introduction to Second Series, chapter 8), this pose really works to open the chest and shoulders. This may sound a little corny, but not only does it open the chest, it opens the heart as well. And I mean that in the full psychological sense of the word. If you have been carrying around a lot of sorrow in your heart, whether very old or very recent, there is something about doing this work that breaks it loose and frees you up. Again, this may sound a little too far out there for some of you and might cause a few sidelong glances and raised eyebrows: "Uh-oh, here she goes again." Just wait till you do the work.

TECHNIQUE

Preparation: Begin from a lying-down position.

Inhale, bring the feet up toward the buttocks bones, keeping them flat on the floor and about hip-width apart. Turn the toes in slightly (to help keep the feet parallel once you come into the posture) and place the hands, palms down, alongside the ears (Figure 6.57).

Exhale, press up into the air (that's it!). Keep feet flat on the floor and parallel. Then try to straighten arms and legs. Be sure to let your head relax or hang back. Don't try to hold the head up. Gaze back toward the point between the eyebrows and down toward the floor (Figure 6.58). If you feel any pain or serious discomfort in the lower back, work with one of the following modifications, or wait until the end of the Second Series to begin practicing this posture.

(Even though I have been training very hard for many years, you can still see the tightness in my shoulders. The vestige of some kind of repetitive training with the arms and shoulders is evident, in spite of the fact that it was thirty years ago.)

Modifications and Helpful Hints

There are a number of things you can do to begin the opening process required in the back and shoulders for this posture. All of them require the use of a chair or bench, blocks, training partner, or wall. There really are no modifications comparable to those of previous postures that just involve altering body position.

Modification No. 1

If you are tight in the shoulders, as I am, it might be helpful to use a training partner's ankles as the prop. If you don't have a training partner, you can use two small (five-by-nine-by-six-inch) wooden blocks propped against a wall. Your partner stands behind you with his feet about as far apart as your shoulders. If you are using blocks, place them snugly up against the wall, also shoulder-width apart. Lie down with your head just in front of, and centered between, your partner's feet or the blocks.

Inhale, place hands on partners ankles or the

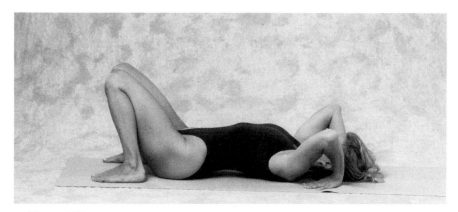

▲ **Figure 6.57**

Figure 6.58 ▼

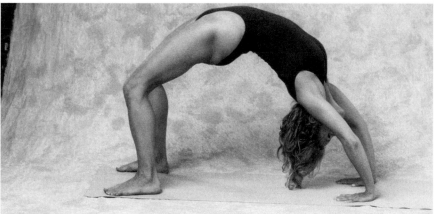

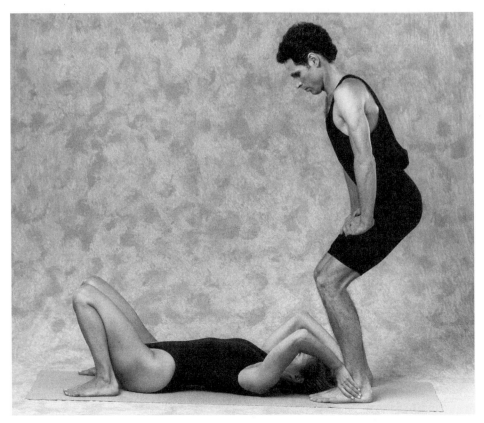

▲ Figure 6.59

Figure 6.60 ▼

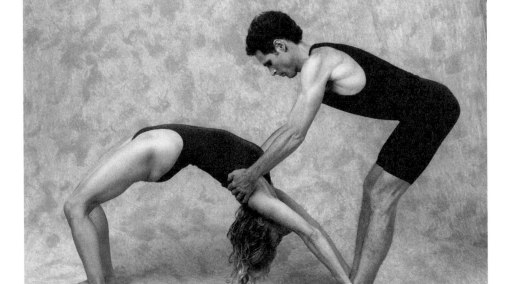

blocks, with the insides of your wrists facing away from you (Figure 6.59).

Exhale, press up into the posture. If you have difficulty, your partner might reach under your *shoulder blades* and help to lift you up. This will give you some leverage and help you to open the chest and straighten the arms (Figure 6.60).

Modification No. 2

In this case, instead of raising up the hands to reduce the backward curve of the body and lessen the distance of the arch, we will raise up the feet. Take a sturdy bench or chair and place it firmly against your wall. Place your feet about hip-width apart on the bench. As you raise up, your feet will flatten on the bench.

Inhale, place your hands alongside your ears (Figure 6.61).

Exhale, press up. Pressing up here requires a bit more arm strength, because more of the weight of the torso is angled into the arms, but once you get up, it's easier. You might want to come up to the top of the head first (Figure 6.62). Working with the feet elevated takes a lot of compression out of the lower back (Figure 6.63) and really lets you stretch out. I feel like King Kong when I do this modification. You can also have your training partner help you in this version (Figure 6.64).

THIS IS UPWARD BOW POSTURE—TAKE FIVE BREATHS (FIGURE 6.58, 6.60, 6.63, OR 6.64).

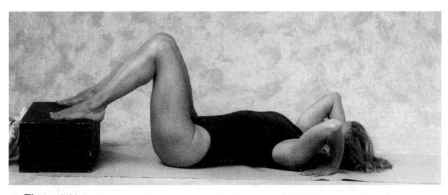

▲ **Figure 6.61**

Figure 6.62 ▼

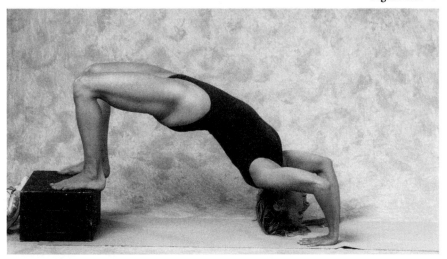

Inhale.

Exhale, release, come down, take a recovery breath or two, then do again. Repeat three times (at least) and hold each repetition for five breaths.

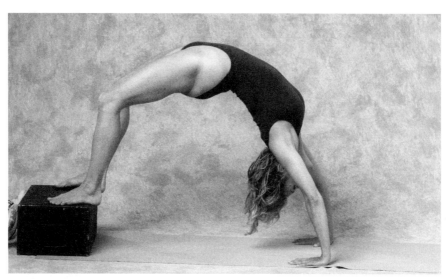

▲ **Figure 6.63**

Figure 6.64 ▼

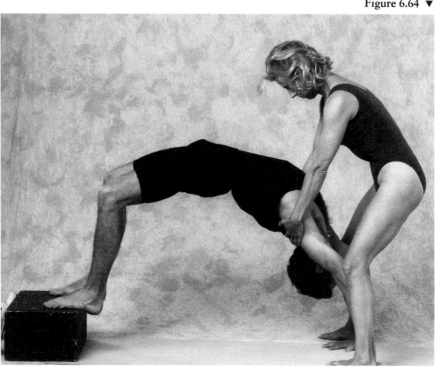

21

INTENSE WEST STRETCH POSTURE (FULL FORWARD BENDING): *PASCHIMOTTANASANA*

Important note: This posture is a counterpose to Upward Bow and *must* be done if you have completed the preceding posture. It is the first posture of the seated Primary Series postures and is fully described at the beginning of chapter 5.

TECHNIQUE

Preparation: Sit up, come into Stick Posture, *Dandasana.*

Inhale, with legs extended straight out, take sides of feet or ankles, straighten arms, look up, lengthen spine.

Note: If you have modified this posture somewhat to compensate for tightness or injury, use the same adjustment here. The purpose of this posture as a counterpose at this point is to get into the lower back and remove any compression that may have occurred (although it's not supposed to happen, it can and does) in the preceding posture. So if you have to bend the knees to get out of the hamstrings and into the lower back, do it.

Exhale, fold at hips, bend elbows, pull with arms, don't round the back. Extend the back. Create space between the vertebrae!

You may wish to have your training partner give you a push here. Only do this after you have been following regular practice for at least six to eight weeks. Make sure your partner pushes low enough down on the back so that it helps the rib cage to move forward and extend out, as opposed to contributing to the rounding of the back. When the back of the legs open enough so that the rib cage can rest on the thigh bones, then the push can come from higher up (Figure 6.65).

Figure 6.65

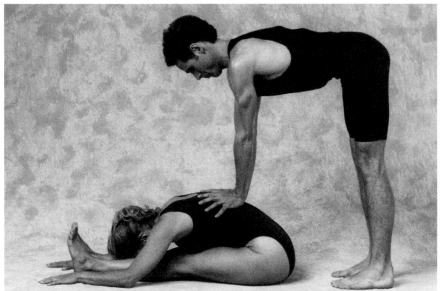

THIS IS INTENSE WEST STRETCH POSTURE—TAKE FIVE BREATHS (FIGURE 6.65).

Inhale, head up, straighten arms.
Exhale, lie down.

THIS IS THE END OF THE PRIMARY SERIES.

▼

VERY IMPORTANT NOTE: *OPTIONS FOR PRACTICE*

What happens after this? Once you have worked through the complete Primary Series (chapters 5 and 6), and have developed minimal strength in the arms and shoulders (can hold yourself in Four Limbed Stick Posture (*Chaturanga Dandasana*), or push-up position), you can begin to work on the Closing Sequence. The Amended Closing Sequence is offered as an alternative to the Complete Closing Sequence and is to be used *only* as preliminary work when first learning chapter 7, or when time is limited. Correctly performed, the practice always ends with the Complete Closing Sequence.

So at this point, you continue to chapter 7 and begin learning the Closing Sequence, starting with the postures that comprise the Amended Sequence. I would recommend working with chapters 3 through 6, plus chapter 7, for anywhere from several months to one year, depending on your prior experience and your progress, until you pretty much know the form by heart.

So, no matter what your practice will be or how long it will take, it *always* begins with Sun Salutations and ends with some version of Closing Sequence. There are a number of ways that you can put the practice together to make a workout that suits your time schedule and fitness level.

Full Practice = Sun Salutations, Primary Series, Complete Closing Sequence, and rest. Ideally, this is what you would like to get in four or five days a week.

Shorter Options = (1) Sun Salutations (five or six of each or more), plus Modified Closing and rest; (2) Sun Salutations (three to five of each), Standing Postures, a Closing Sequence, and rest; or (3) Sun Salutations only (as many as you like).

This last option of only Sun Salutations is a great warm-up for any sporting activity, whether going out for a run or a game of tennis.

Once you know the sequence, your practice will be dictated by the needs of your body and mind and the limitations of your time. The truly liberating aspect of the practice, once you learn the form, is the ease with which the mind flows from one posture to the next. You don't have to stop and ask yourself, Well, gee, what should I do now? The form takes care of that question and the body automatically goes from one posture to the next without thought. That is ultimately the point: practice without thought. Patanjali, in the Yoga Sutras, defines yoga in the second sutra of Book One as *yogas citta vrtti narodahah,* or "yoga is the cessation of the fluctuations of the mind." This is truly mind control, control of our *own* minds. If you can control your mind, you have controlled everything, according to Yoga philosophy. There is nothing in this world that can bind or limit you.

7

protection in the unprotected state

THE CLOSING SEQUENCE

Faith is the bird that feels the light and sings when the dawn is still dark.

RABINDRANATH TAGORE, "Fireflies"

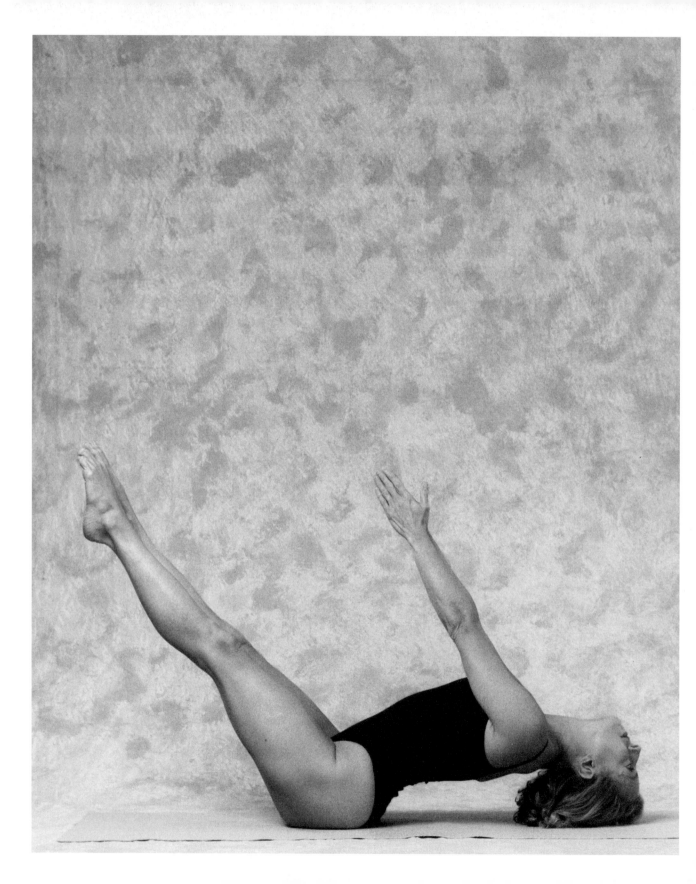

THE CLOSING SEQUENCE

EXTENDING POSSIBILITY

From the very first day I discovered this practice, I had an intuitive feeling that it was some form of protection—protection against not only sports injury, but disease, depression, debility, and generally being in the wrong place at the wrong time. When I run through my practice in the morning, I usually feel that it's about the toughest thing I will encounter for the day. It gives me a psychological feeling of strength and centeredness.

This doesn't mean I think I'm invincible. It means the practice makes me feel alive, conscious. It doesn't presuppose that I can be asleep and still have the protection; I feel that I have to do my part. I try to pay attention. But the work with the breathing, the struggle in the postures, the effort to "consciously evolve" makes me feel humble. I think of all the persons who have come before me, who have been struggling with the postures just as I am here today, and I feel grateful for their effort to keep the practice alive. I sense I have done my work on myself. I have dematerialized toxins, both physical and mental. I have zapped negative thoughts and feelings. I have tried to make myself a better person for that day. Doing the yoga practice, I am maintaining youth, health, and fitness on a physical level, as well as establishing a clear and balanced mental outlook.

One of the things my husband, Thom, says the practice does for him is to eliminate the fear of injury during speed work and high-intensity training. We might not all be elite athletes, but we can all relate to wanting to do a little better, or go a little further, or work a little more effectively at our training or our lives in general.

Thom explains: "The minute an elite athlete starts doing high-quality ballistic training, like sprinting (speed work) for a distance runner—say, running between twenty-five to twenty-nine seconds for two hundred meters, the fear of injury becomes a measurable reality. Each motion is like a full thrust effort, as opposed to distance running, where each step might be effort, but it isn't nearly the same intensity as all-out sprinting."

Every one of us comes to the point in our higher level type of training, whether we are kayakers, hikers, golfers, climbers, or cyclists, where we are face-to-face with some constraint. Part of this inhibiting factor is sheer physiological limitation—tightness or weakness. The rest is fear. The fear is that you will literally extend yourself past the range of possibility, that if you go one nanosecond faster—or higher or longer—something will tear or rip or collapse or blow up completely. This holds you back. And it's a legitimate fear. Thom continues: "But because of the range of motion you go through and develop in this yoga practice, you know that the muscles will take this extension."

So first of all, you are more in touch with what the muscles are capable of and where they are at in terms of range of motion. Second, this makes you more secure mentally, and the fear of injury falls away. With the calm, quiet confidence you build with the breathing, you know your limitations have changed and the realm of your personal possibility has extended, both mentally and physically.

Coming face-to-face with limitations in our practice helps us to recognize inhibiting factors in other areas of our lives, not necessarily physical ones. The fear that we will extend ourselves past the range of possibility is one that permeates all aspects of life. Whether it is swimming in the ocean or walking on the moon, isn't it some form or another of this fear that holds us back from achieving many of the things we dream of?

But in our practice, we get to know a particular restraint very well. We work with it every day. And eventually, although we could never have imagined it when we started, we watch it change form and slowly disappear into the distance. We learn that through the regular practice of confronting our restrictions, we can loosen their ability to obstruct our range of "motion." This helps us to realize that not only our muscles, but ourselves, as whole persons, can extend further than we ever thought possible.

THREE OPTIONS FOR ENDING PRACTICE

The sequence of postures in this chapter is the now-famous Closing Sequence that I have referred to frequently throughout the book. This is the sequence that puts you back into "neutral," so to speak, after the Primary or Second Series. As I always tell my classes, "This is a sequence. Each posture is a counterpose or supplement to one that precedes it. If you do any, you must do all of either the full or abbreviated progression of postures, and you must do them in order." These are the postures that chill you out, establish the metabolic rate for the day, return the system to cruise control, and bring all the body's systems into balance. Most important, the Closing Sequence postures also work out any physical hitch or twinge that might be hanging around from the practice. There are three variations of the Closing Sequence:

1. The first is the *Modified Closing Sequence.*
2. The second is the *Amended Closing Sequence.*
3. The third is the *Complete Closing Sequence.*

At a number of points in the early chapters of this book, I have recommended ending your practice with the *Modified Closing Sequence.* For those of you just starting out and working only with chapters 3 and 4, using this routine is an excellent way to finish off your practice. It is also a possible ending to use when you are limited in time. However, it is not recommended as a general rule once you progress to full practice. This method is not part of the "form," and the movements are not technically yoga postures. However, they do provide a sense of closure, both physically and mentally, and allow you to come into the final relaxation Posture, *savasana,* with comfort and balance.

For those of you just beginning to work with this chapter, it is recommended that you begin with the practice of the *Amended Closing Sequence.* This is a shortened sequence of six postures that will give you most of the benefits of the *Complete Closing Sequence,* as well as the three basic counterpose functions of the full progression.

A specific example of what I mean by counterpose function can be found in the relationship between Shoulder Stand and Fish Posture. In Shoulder Stand the chin is pressed forward into the neck, contracting the front of the neck and stretching out the back of the neck. In Fish Posture, then, the back of the head is pressed into the back of the neck, contracting the back of the neck and stretching out the front of the neck. These postures, in sequence, work as all the counterposes in the practice to balance and support one another, both strengthening and stretching the associated muscles, tendons, and ligaments.

The six postures that comprise the *Amended Closing Sequence* are (1) Shoulder Stand, (2) Plow Posture, (3) Press the Ear Posture, (6) Fish Posture, (9) Bound Lotus Posture, and (12) Relaxation Posture. These postures are designated with an asterisk (*) following the title of the posture.

The *Complete Closing Sequence* consists of all twelve postures in this chapter, including Relaxation Posture. This is the correct form, and once you progress past beginning level, provided none of the contraindications for inverted postures apply to you, you should always end your practice with the *Complete Closing Sequence.*

Note: Eventually, in the *Closing Sequence,* whether *Amended* or *Complete,* you go from one posture to the next with only a breath for transition. However, when you are first learning the postures, it will take several breaths for you to make the shift from one pose to the next.

MODIFIED CLOSING SEQUENCE

TECHNIQUE

Begin by lying down and bringing both knees to your chest. Wrap the arms around the knees and hug the thighs to your torso. Roll around a bit, back and forth or side to side, over the lower back and the sacroiliac joints (the flat part of the lower back), as if massaging the back muscles with the pressure of the floor. If there are any protruding vertebrae, and this is not comfortable, make sure you are lying on a mat or carpet. This will give some padding to the spine.

Then open the arms straight out to the sides of the body, and keeping the knees bent and together, lower the knees to the right, trying to touch the right elbow with the knees. Keep the shoulders on the ground as best you can. Look in the opposite direction. Let the knees touch down, even if the shoulder comes up. Relax and breathe into the stretch. Allow the back to let go and open up. Hold for five or ten breaths. Then reverse it and work the other side. Come back to center, give yourself one more hug. Then put the feet down on the floor, with the knees still bent. Separate the feet about hip-width apart. Then extend the legs out into relaxation pose (see Posture 12 in this chapter). If the back still feels any discomfort, do Modified Bridge Posture (Posture 19, chapter 6) and then repeat above.

THE POSTURES

AMENDED* AND COMPLETE CLOSING SEQUENCE

1

SHOULDER STAND POSTURE:
SALAMBA SARVANGASANA *

Alamba means "support" or "prop." The prefix *sa* means "accompanied by." *Salamba,* then, means "supported or propped up by." *Sarva* means "complete" or "all." *Anga,* as we already know, means "limb" or can mean "body." So *sarvanga* means "all the limbs, the whole body." The literal translation might therefore be, "all the limbs, or the whole body, accompanied by support." The posture has come to be known in yoga circles as Shoulder Stand, since all the weight is borne on the shoulders.

Note of caution: This posture, as all inverted postures, including Plow and Head Stand Posture (later in this chapter)—should *not* be practiced by

1. menstruating women
2. pregnant women (unless they have been practicing since the first month and are working with a professional specializing in prenatal yoga)
3. persons who are obese
4. persons with high blood pressure, high cholesterol levels, or any other high-risk factors for heart attack or stroke
5. persons with detached retina or who are recovering from eye or cosmetic surgery or are under the care of an eye doctor (consult with doctor first!)

6. persons with any cervical (upper-spine) or lumbar (lower spine) misalignment or injury, without the prior consultation of a trained *astanga yoga* therapist or Power Yoga professional.

Note: An Illuminating Story
Back in 1986 I was suffering what is called "referred" shoulder and arm pain, meaning that the cause of the pain is somewhere else. In my case it resulted from a reverse cervical curve (the spinal curve at the back of the neck). A misaligned vertebra was pressing against a nerve running to the shoulder and arm. The misalignment originally resulted from an old accident in college in which I was thrown off a horse and landed on my head. It was then aggravated twenty-five years later by a bang on the head in a very minor auto accident in which I was a passenger and did not wear a seat belt.

The chiropractor I was seeing told me not to do this posture or the Plow Posture. Indeed, anytime I did do it for demonstration purposes, it seemed to provoke the pain again. However, once I began doing it daily (as I mentioned in chapter 4), as part of the entire *astanga* Primary Series, with all the poses and counterposes, it was extremely therapeutic for the neck. After three weeks of practice, the pain was gone. After three months of practice, the reverse cervical curve had begun to reverse itself.

So whether this is helpful or injurious *can* depend on how you approach it. If you have any specific questions about your own situation, it is always best

* Postures in *Amended Closing Sequence* are designated with an asterisk.

to consult your orthopedic physician, preferably one who is also a yoga therapist and practices yoga!

TECHNIQUE

Preparation: Lie down, bring legs and feet together, arms touching sides. This is the equivalent of attention position, lying down. Take five breaths.

Inhale, lift legs about thirty degrees.

Exhale, continue to raise legs all the way over the head into "plow" position. Clasp the hands together and straighten the arms. Press the hands toward the floor. This will stretch open the front of the shoulders. Work the upper arms in toward one another so that they are parallel, then release the hands and place them on the back, as far down the back toward the floor as possible as in Figure 7.2. Center the head and keep the neck relaxed. Take as many breaths as necessary to get the hands, arms, and shoulders in position. *Once you become more familiar with the alignment necessary for Shoulder Stand Posture, it is not necessary to go into Plow Posture first, and you should come directly up on this* exhale *into Shoulder Stand.*

Note of caution: Do not press the chin into the throat. This will tend to "flatten" the natural upward curve of the cervical spine. Rather, relax the neck and allow the notch in the chest between the collarbones to come up toward the chin, so that the head is centered. When Shoulder Stand is done correctly, the weight should be on the shoulders. The spine does not touch the floor at all. That is why it is important to squeeze the arms together and pull the shoulder blades together. This creates a shoulder ledge for the

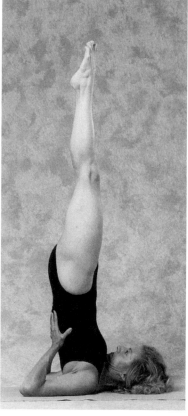

Figure 7.1

weight of the body to rest on. The body weight does not rest on the neck or spine.

Inhale, raise the legs up into Shoulder Stand position (Figure 7.1).

Exhale, support the back with the hands and arms. Toes are lined up directly over the forehead. Gaze at the toes. Breathing is slow and relaxed. Lift and extend the spine in order to make the torso perpendicular to the floor.

Note of caution: Once you are up in position, do not move the head to look around. Keep the head still and centered. Moving the head more than a fraction of an inch or so for adjustment can strain the neck while in Shoulder Stand.

THIS IS SHOULDER STAND POSTURE—TAKE FIVE BREATHS (slowly work up to 20 to 25 breaths) (Figure 7.1)

Inhale, prepare to change position to next posture.

2

PLOW POSTURE: *HALASANA* *

Hala means "plow."

Important: See contraindications in preceding posture.

TECHNIQUE

Exhale, lower legs over head to the floor (Figure 7.2).

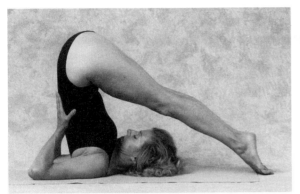

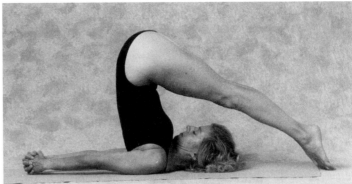

Figure 7.2

Figure 7.3

Keep feet together, toes pointed. Release hands from back, extend arms along the floor, and interlace fingers (Figure 7.3). Keep working shoulder blades together, taking the shoulders back and under. Press the arms together. Do not press chin into chest. Keep neck relaxed. Gaze (past the end of the nose) at the heart *chakra* or the center of the chest.

THIS IS PLOW POSTURE—TAKE FIVE BREATHS (FIGURE 7.3).

Inhale, prepare to change position to next posture.

3

PRESS THE EAR POSTURE: *KARNAPIDASANA**

Karna means "ear." *Pida* can mean "pressure," "pain," or "discomfort." In this usage, *pida* means "to press the ears gently with the knees," or "bring the knees to the ears." This is sometimes called Knee-to-Ear Posture.

TECHNIQUE

Exhale, lower knees to the floor alongside the ears (Figure 7.4). Arms remain in same position as in

Plow Posture. Gaze at the heart *chakra,* or the center of the chest.

Beginners' Modification: If this posture is difficult or the knees do not come all the way to the floor, just relax and do the best you can. Rest knees on the forehead if necessary.

THIS IS PRESS THE EAR POSTURE—TAKE FIVE BREATHS (FIGURE 7.4).

Go directly to next posture unless you are doing the *Amended Closing Sequence,* in which case you place the hands flat on the floor and roll out of Press the Ear Posture back down toward the floor (Figure 7.5). Skip to Posture 6, Fish Posture.

4

UPWARD LOTUS POSTURE: *URDHVA PADMASANA*

Urdhva means "upward." *Padma* means "lotus." Remember *urdhva* from *Urdhva Muka Svanasana,* Face Up (or upward facing) Dog Posture, and *padma* from *Ardha Baddha Padma Paschimotanasana* Bound Half Lotus, in the first part of Primary Series?

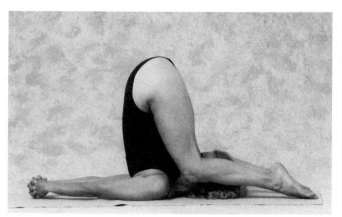

Figure 7.4

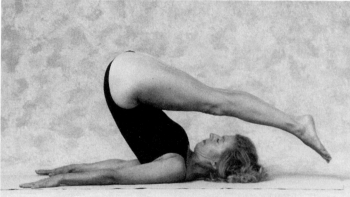

Figure 7.5

TECHNIQUE

Inhale, raise the legs into the air, back into Shoulder Stand Position. Support the back again with the hands.

Exhale now, using the hands if necessary, and put your legs into full lotus position. Fold the right leg in first (Figure 7.6), and then bring the left leg in over the right. This is a little tricky and will take some practice. If you cannot do lotus, simply cross the legs. Keep breathing. At first this is going to take several breaths to get into.

Reach up with the arms and support the knees with the hands (Figure 7.7). If your knees are crossed, you can also reach up and rest the knees on the hands. Gaze is up toward the ceiling.

Note: Correctly, the weight of the torso should be back far enough so that there is a downward pressure of the knees onto the hands. The hands are actually pushing up on the knees, supporting them and keeping the weight from rolling backward. If, however, the weight is not far back enough over the head, there will be a tendency to roll back down from the posture. This will often happen when there is tightness in the back of the neck, or fear of rolling over backward. As the neck and shoulders open, the pose will become easier.

THIS IS UPWARD LOTUS POSTURE—TAKE FIVE BREATHS (FIGURE 7.7).

Inhale, prepare to change position to next posture.

Figure 7.6

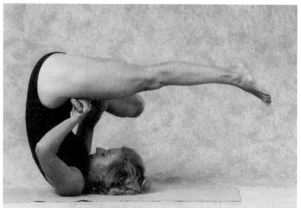

Figure 7.7

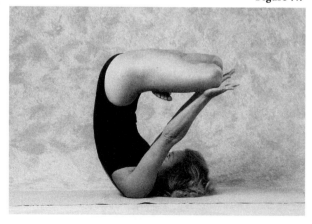

5

EMBRYO POSTURE: *PINDASANA*

Pinda means "embryo." This posture resembles the fetal position of an embryo in the womb.

TECHNIQUE

Exhale, lower the legs, still in full lotus position or folded to the chest. Wrap the arms around the folded legs (Figure 7.8). Gaze is same as preceding pose.

Note: As in the posture before this one, for people with tightness or restriction in the back of the neck, it will be difficult to keep from rolling back down out of this posture. If you don't really get stretched out in the back and back of the neck in the inverted postures which precede this, then you won't get up high enough on the shoulders to hold the posture.

THIS IS EMBRYO POSTURE—HOLD FOR FIVE BREATHS (FIGURE 7.8).

Inhale, prepare to change position to next posture.

6

FISH POSTURE: *MATSYASANA**

Matsya means "fish." Whether you are doing the *Amended* or *Complete Sequence,* this is a key posture as a counterpose for Shoulder Stand, Plow Posture, and Press the Ear Posture. This posture must be done to balance the work of the earlier poses in this sequence!

TECHNIQUE

Exhale, release arms, and place the palms down on the floor along your side. Then, keeping the legs the same, either in full lotus position or folded and crossed, roll down out of the posture (Figure 7.9).

Inhale, place elbows alongside, and using the arms, arch the chest up and press up onto the crown of the head.

Exhale, press the knees to the floor and if the legs are in full lotus position, grasp the big toes with the hands (Figure 7.10). If the legs are folded and crossed, rest the hands on the inner thighs. Gaze is up and back past the point between the eyebrows.

Note: Do not support the weight of the body with the arms. The elbows should be off the ground. The

Figures 7.8

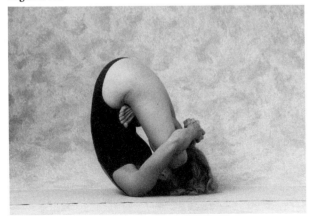

Figures 7.9

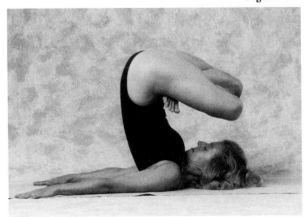

chest should be lifted with the back muscles. The neck muscles are also working to lift the chest. This is excellent strengthening and stress-relieving work for the muscles of the neck and shoulders.

THIS IS FISH POSTURE—HOLD FOR FIVE BREATHS (FIGURE 7.10).

Inhale, prepare to change position to next posture.

7

EXTENDED LEG POSTURE: *UTTANA PADASANA*

Uttana means "stretched out" or "lying on the back with the face up." It has been used as a root in a number of previous postures, such as *Parsvottanasana,* in the standing postures, where *uttana* (ottana) is an interior part of the word (literally *ut* means "intense" and *tan* means "extend or lengthen"). *Pada* means "leg."

TECHNIQUE

Exhale, unwrap the legs, and extend straight out in the air at about a forty-five-degree angle to the floor. At the same time, extend the arms, with palms together (Figure 7.11). Gaze is the same as for Fish Posture.

Note: This may feel as if it is stressful for the lower back, but actually it is very strengthening for the lumbar extensors, which maintain posture and height. Of course, if there is any acute pain, this should be omitted, as should any movement that causes sharp pain. A counterpose follows, as I have explained earlier, and it will balance this work and stretch the lower back in the opposite direction.

THIS IS EXTENDED LEG POSTURE—HOLD FOR FIVE BREATHS (FIGURE 7.11).

Inhale.
Exhale, release posture, then sit up.
Inhale, take it up.
Exhale, jump back.
Inhale, Face Up Dog.
Exhale, Face Down Dog.
Inhale, jump to knees.

Figure 7.10

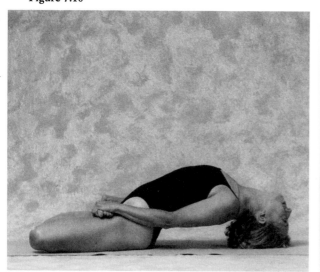

Figure 7.11

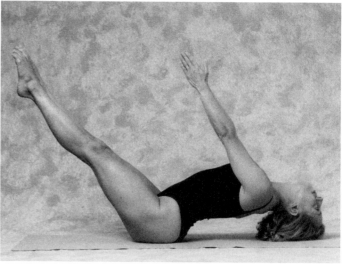

8

HEADSTAND POSTURE: *SIRASANA*

Sirsa means "head." In the ancient *hatha yoga* texts, Headstand has been called the king of *asanas*. It is an extremely important posture, as it brings vitality and clarity to the brain and the mind. It is a very strong healing and regulatory posture in that it conveys an abundant blood supply to the pituitary and pineal glands in the brain. Studies have actually shown that regular practice of Headstand can increase the hemoglobin content of the blood.

Weight Placement

When I begin teaching Headstand in our intermediate/advanced classes, I always instruct students to support the weight equally with the wrists, forearms, and elbows only, not with the head. This develops strength in the arms and shoulders, keeps the body centered, keeps the weight *off* the head, and avoids injury in the neck and spine.

As practitioners become more advanced, generally after three to four years of practice only, slowly they begin to take more and more weight on the head, with the forearms and hands only used for balance. In this way, the neck muscles that support Headstand, build strength gradually and are able to keep the spine lengthened. The vertebrae in the neck should not compress in Headstand, but maintain their normal range from one to another. The neck, back, and shoulder muscles are responsible for preserving this spacing.

Another factor to be considered in determining how much of the body weight can safely be supported by the head is the size of the person doing Headstand. Obviously, a person weighing 200 pounds would want to keep most of the weight *off* the head, while a person weighing only 105 pounds might be able to take a bit more weight.

Duration

In the beginning you will find holding the pose for ten breaths (approximately one minute) to be extremely difficult. Eventually, the posture can be held comfortably by more advanced practitioners from fifty to sixty breaths, which will be about ten minutes! If you have been working regularly with the practice for some time now and are fairly familiar with the Primary Series, I would recommend you always end practice with Complete Closing Sequence and attempt to hold Headstand for at least ten breaths before coming down. Then, perhaps, you can shorten some other aspect of the practice in order to spend a little more time in Headstand.

Alignment

Once you are in headstand position, keep the shoulders lifting up away from the floor and stretching "sideways" as much as possible. Maximize the distance between the ears and shoulders. Be careful to keep the elbows in line with the shoulders and maintain an equilateral triangle between the elbows and hands. This "base" is the foundation of the Headstand and must be kept stable and aligned. The wrists should be held perpendicular to the floor. Don't let the hands collapse out.

When viewed from the side, the heels through the buttocks to the ears should be in a straight perpendicular line with the floor. Also, the midline of the body should be in a straight perpendicular line with the floor. You might wish to have a friend observe whether or not you are leaning to one side or another, or forward or backward.

Often there is a tendency to collapse in the middle of the trunk with the back arched and the belly protruding. This can be caused by tight shoulders, weak back or abdominal muscles, tight hip flexors (especially the psoas muscle), or by too much weight forward on the elbows. If there is too much arch in your back, holding *mula* and *uddiyana bandha* will help to bring the spine into alignment.

Falling

Everyone is afraid of falling when they begin work on this posture. The best way to face the fear of falling is the best way to face any fear—look it straight in the face. You might as well accept the fact that at some point or another, you will fall. Everyone falls. It is not so awful as you might imagine, and can be done safely.

If you overbalance, simply remember to relax, release the finger grip, tuck the chin, round the back, and bend the knees and roll out. The other way to fall out is to release the hands, arch the back, and go over landing one leg at a time on the feet. One of these methods will probably come more instinctively than the other. I had to teach myself to roll out, but arching over came naturally. Practice both ways a couple of times on a very thick mat until falling isn't so scary anymore. If you don't have a thick mat, use a mattress or pillows.

Correct Technique

The correct form for raising up into—and down out of—the Headstand is with the legs together and completely firm and straight, pressing off the toes for the ascent and touching down on the toes on the descent. This will seem difficult at first, but it is the correct method and should be learned. My teacher would *never* allow me to bend my knees going into Headstand, or use a wall, although he did spot for me. In the beginning I had to practice walking the toes toward the head from the preparatory position, as you will do (see Figures 7.14 and 7.15), until I could finally lift them an inch off the floor. Then I had to hold them there for as long as I could hold the position. Finally, I began to raise the legs in the air, of course falling over the first few times.

Note of Caution: This is not an easy posture. I never teach this pose in beginners' or intermediate classes, and only introduce it to students once they have been doing practice for some time. A good way to prepare for Headstand is by developing strength in

the arms and shoulders with the Sun Salutations and the repeated practice of the *vinyasa.*

If you have questions as to whether or not the condition of your health allows for the practice of Headstand, ask your consulting physician. See contraindications for Inverted Postures at the beginning of this chapter.

TECHNIQUE

Preparation: Come to a kneeling position.

Inhale, place your forearms on the center of your mat, folding the arms so that the hands wrap around the elbows (Figure 7.12). Maintaining this distance between the elbows, release the folded arms and interlace the fingers so that the hands are folded (Figure 7.13), and with the forearms, form an equilateral triangle.

Exhale, place the head inside the hands so that only the crown of the head is on the mat and only the pads of the thumbs touch the back of the head (Figure 7.14).

Inhale, walk the feet up toward the elbows (Figure 7.15), tuck the toes and

Exhale, try to raise the toes off the floor (Figure 7.16). Although, correctly, the knees do not bend, you will probably find your knees will bend a little in order to get your hips high enough to raise the feet off the ground. Hold this position for a few breaths when you are first learning this method. At first, balance is difficult, even for a few breaths. But as the orientation of being upside down becomes less confusing and more comfortable, balance will come with practice.

Inhale, lean backward slightly with the buttocks, and raise the legs off the floor. Counterbalancing with the hips will help bring the legs off the floor.

Exhale, raise both legs together, pressing with arms and abdominals to the halfway point (Figure 7.17). There will be a lot of pressure on the neck and shoulders in this position. At first you will only be

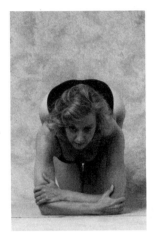

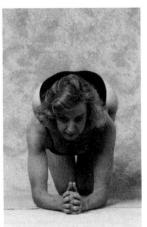

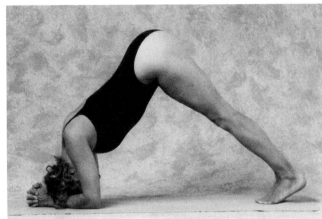

Figure 7.12   **Figure 7.13**   **Figure 7.14**

able to hold this "half-bend" (or literally, Upward Stick Posture, *Urdhva Dandasana*) for a few seconds. As you become stronger, you will be able to stay in this position for a longer period of time.

Inhale, continue to raise the legs all the way up to perpendicular.

Exhale, slowly raise the legs past the halfway point and press the buttocks slightly forward, returning them to a perpendicular line with the floor (Figure 7.18). If you don't adjust the position of the hips as you raise the legs, you will find the weight of the

torso is too far back and you will go right over. Gaze is steady and out at one stationary point along the floor or a point in your view.

Note: Practice raising up and down, finding balance, and developing strength. Be sure to use arms and shoulders for support, keeping weight off the head. Once you have the feeling of balance, try to maintain for five breaths. After practicing this for some time, begin to work with the "half-bend" position that follows Headstand.

Figure 7.15   **Figure 7.16**

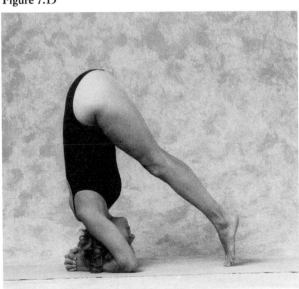

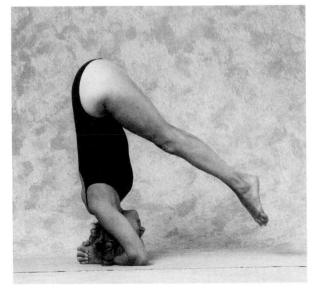

THIS IS HEADSTAND POSTURE—HOLD FOR FIVE BREATHS (gradually work up to ten breaths, and eventually in advanced practice, twenty-five to fifty breaths) (Figure 7.18).

Inhale, begin to
Exhale.

> *Beginners:* Lower down to floor.
> *More Advanced:* Lower down to half-bend position (see Figure 7.17). Hold, if possible, for five breaths.
> *Inhale,* raise legs back into Headstand. Hold for one breath.
> *Exhale,* come down slowly on one exhale, keeping the legs together and straight, slowly folding at the hips as you descend. Come down in control.

Inhale, bend the knees, rest the buttocks on the heels, and

Exhale, lower the forehead to the floor. Rest in this position for the same amount of time you held Headstand, or for at least ten breaths.

Inhale, place the hands on the floor, under the shoulders.

Exhale, jump back.

Inhale, Face Up Dog.

Exhale, Face Down Dog.

Inhale, jump through.

Exhale, sit down.

Figure 7.17

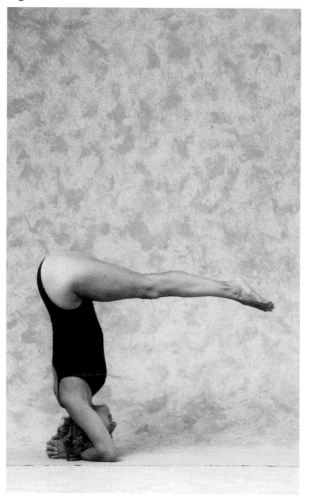

Figure 7.18

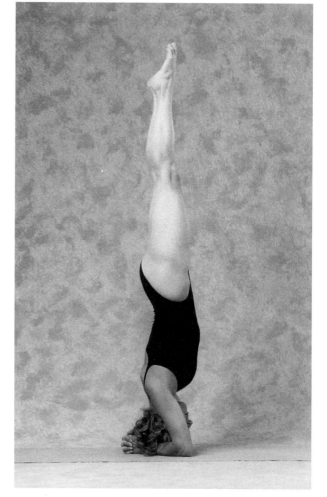

9

BOUND LOTUS POSTURE: *BADDHA PADMASANA* *

Padma means "lotus." *Baddha* means "bound, tied, or fixed." Remember Bound Angle Posture, *Baddha Konasana,* and Bound Half Lotus Intense West Stretch (whew!), *Ardha Baddha Padma Paschimottanasana* in Primary Series?

TECHNIQUE

Inhale, bring the right leg into half lotus position.

Exhale, bring the left leg over the right, into full lotus position. This might take several breaths to accomplish. Keep breathing as you work into the pose.

Inhale, reach up and around with the left arm, and grasp (or bind) the left foot with the left hand.

Exhale, reach up and around with the right arm, going over the left arm, and grasp the right foot with the right hand. You might have to lean forward slightly to make the connection (Figure 7.19). If you are in full lotus position but cannot reach your feet, or if you are not in full-lotus position and simply have your legs crossed, then just cross or fold your arms behind you.

Inhale, look up. Gaze is up and back. Hold this position for one breath, then

Exhale, fold forward, bringing first the forehead, then the nose, and then the chin to the floor (Figure 7.20).

Note: This posture, when bending forward, is actually called *Yoga Mudrasana,* which means Sealed Yoga Posture. *Mudra* in yoga refers to a position, generally of the hands, that seals or closes off a *nadi,* or energy channel.

Beginners' Modification: Since this posture is an important counterpose to Fish Posture, specifi-

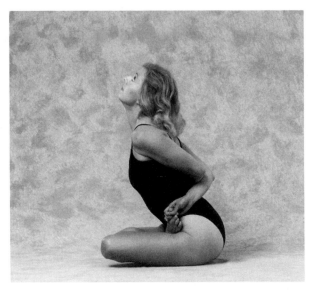

Figure 7.19

cally for the lower back, you must do some modification. So even if you are not able to sit in full lotus, bind, or reach the floor with your head, you could simply sit with your legs crossed and bend forward from the hips, bringing your head toward the floor. Gaze out at a stationary point in line with the end of the nose.

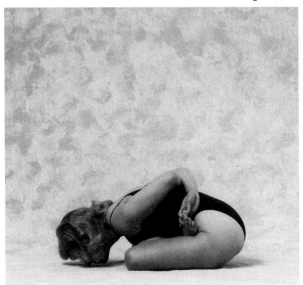

Figure 7.20

THIS IS BOUND LOTUS POSTURE (OR MODIFICATION)—HOLD FOR TEN BREATHS (FIGURE 7.20).

Inhale, look up while bending forward, lift the chest.
Exhale, sit up.
Inhale, look up again, extend the back.
Exhale, release.

10

LOTUS POSTURE: *PADMASANA*

Padma means "lotus flower."

TECHNIQUE

Inhale, bring hands to knees, forefinger and thumb touching, back of palm resting on knee (Figure 7.21).
Exhale, lift the lower back and chest. Tuck the chin slightly in toward the notch between the collarbones. Relax shoulders but hold the *bandhas* strongly. Gaze is straight out in line with the end of the nose, which is pointing slightly down toward the floor.

You will take ten breaths in this posture. This should be very slow, long, controlled breathing, with each inhalation and exhalation reaching to ten or fifteen seconds in duration. If you cannot sit in full lotus position, simply sit with legs crossed in front of you.

THIS IS LOTUS POSTURE—HOLD FOR TEN BREATHS (FIGURE 7.21).

Go directly into next posture.

11

SCALE POSTURE: *TOLASANA*

Tola means "pair of scales." Notice how this posture looks like one of the pans in a set of balance scales.

TECHNIQUE

Inhale, place the hands at the sides.
Exhale, lift up off the ground, holding the knees up as high as possible (Figure 7.22). This is much easier if you are in full lotus position. If you are not in full lotus, just press up and hold as strongly as possible. Gaze is up between or past the eyebrows.

THIS IS SCALE POSTURE—HOLD FOR FIVE BREATHS (work up to twenty-five breaths) (Figure 7.22).

Inhale lower down.
Exhale, release posture.

Figure 7.21

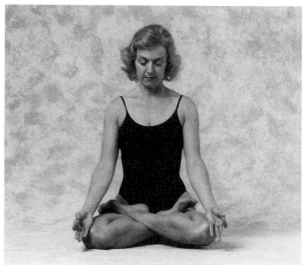

Inhale, put the hands down and take it up (still in full lotus, if possible!).

Exhale, jump back.

Inhale, Face Up Dog.

Exhale, Face Down Dog.

Inhale, jump through.

Exhale, lie down.

TAKE REST!!

12

CORPSE OR RELAXATION POSTURE: *SAVASANA*

Sava means "corpse or dead body." This does not mean that we are trying to be dead in this posture, only "still" *like* a corpse.

Figure 7.22

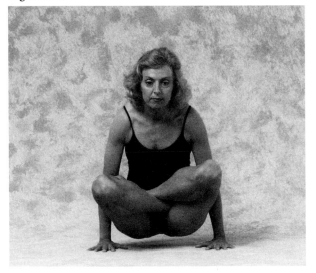

TECHNIQUE

From a lying down position, separate the feet twelve to eighteen inches and allow them to fall out to the sides. Move the arms out away from the sides one to two feet and turn the palms up. In order to be still in this pose, you must first be comfortable. The following adjustments will help you to iron out any remaining glitches or points of discomfort that may be taking your attention from relaxation:

1. Dorsiflex the feet (pull toes toward shins), stretching out the back of the legs.
2. Then relax and let the feet fall open again.
3. Squeeze the shoulder blades together slightly underneath you, which will fan open the chest, then release.
4. Allow the chest to sink back down toward the floor, "pinning" the shoulder blades underneath. Relax.
5. Press the lower back into the floor.
6. Then let go and relax, allowing the natural upward curve of the lower back to return.
7. Press the chin into the chest.
8. Relax and let go, allowing the natural upward curve of the back of the neck to return.

Note: Many of you will find that the chin juts upward toward the ceiling in this position, compressing the muscles at the back of the neck. This is incorrect alignment and corresponds to the imbalanced postural stance referred to in chapter 3 as "forward" head. The chin should be level with the forehead in Relaxation Posture. Work to pull the chin "in" and extend the back of the neck. It may be necessary to place a small pillow under the back of the head in order to elevate the head and bring it into correct alignment.

Also, the above sequence of adjustments should alleviate any discomfort you might be feeling in the lower back. If you still feel a little tension in your back, doing the knee-to-chest position and cross-stretch as given in the *Modified Closing Sequence* will help.

This is Relaxation Posture—hold for ten to thirty minutes (always remain in this posture for at least five minutes when completing practice).

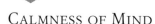

Calmness of Mind

The purpose of Relaxation Posture is to give the body an opportunity to rest and cool down after the practice, and to allow the tension, tightness, and toxins dislodged by the practice to be carried off by the various organs and systems of elimination. Going further, the objective is to be motionless and without thought. By keeping the body still, you are training the mind to be still and relax. You cannot relax while the mind is jumping around like a monkey from one stressful or stimulating thought form to another.

Practice should always end with *savasana,* for anywhere from five to thirty minutes. No matter what your time limit, you always need to allow *at least* five minutes just to cool down and reset the body's baseline metabolism. However, I try to encourage people to take longer rest periods and make this a time for meditation and restoration as well.

When I first introduce this posture in classes, people often think, Oh boy, this is great, I get to sleep. And beginners often do fall asleep, especially after evening classes. But this is not sleep. It is conscious relaxation. It doesn't take long to realize just how difficult this posture actually is, because unlike the rest of the practice, there isn't all this activity, like breathing, *bandhas*, postures, and so forth to keep our attention. Suddenly we are still. There is nothing to "do." For *karma* (action) yogis, this can be difficult. The mind jumps around thinking about how soon this will be over, or what to eat for dinner, or the phone calls that didn't get made today, or the list of things to do tomorrow, and so on. And when the mind is busy, usually the body will fidget. It's always

easy to spot the "thinkers" in class because they can't keep still—either the fingers are busy working, or the toes or the face.

But through the practice of watching yourself, you begin to become aware of this mental activity and subsequent physical tension, and eventually, you start to settle down. With practice, the mind learns to follow the breath and stay focused, and fall into light meditation. The posture is then extremely restorative and refreshing. Verse 32 of Book One in the classic *Hatha Yoga Pradipika* says, "Lying full-length on the back like a corpse is called *savasana.* With this *asana* tiredness caused by other *asanas* is eliminated; it also promotes calmness of mind."

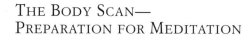

The Body Scan— Preparation for Meditation

An excellent way to prepare both your mind and body for Relaxation Posture is with a procedure I call the *body scan.* This is a technique I've been using for dozens of years that basically lets you skim over the various systems of the physical body and take a look at what is going on.

You begin by getting comfortable, as recommended above. You then try to visualize or imagine or feel (whatever works best for you) the body's physical structure—the bones and muscles. How do they "feel," or look? Are the bones spaced evenly, correctly? Are they balanced? Is the right hipbone pressing into the floor in a similar way to the left one, for example? How about the right heel bone and left heel bone? Are they fairly symmetrical?

Sometimes I just scan the structure, other times I scrutinize. It depends on how I'm feeling and what is going on. If there is a tightness or bruise or a "holding," I'll take a little time to inspect that. Visualizing sometimes comes easily. Sometimes I can climb over my hip bones or shoulder blades as I might ascend mesas in Arizona. Other times it doesn't go so well and I just have a quick "flyover."

After arranging the superficial structure of the bones and muscles, you sink a bit deeper into the circulatory and respiratory systems. You can start by entering through the nose and traveling along on the breath to the lungs. You might imagine you are bumping around inside the lungs like a helium balloon inside the Astrodome. From there the scope of the journey is up to you. (This is one of my favorites: I like to squeeze through the walls of the lungs with the oxygen molecules and travel to the heart.) You might try to "see" or imagine the passages into and out of the heart. See them as clear and smooth and free of debris and obstacles. See all the little trapdoors swinging easily and functioning without resistance or stress.

From there you might be pumped out of the heart and sent tumbling into the vast network of rivers, streams, and creeks that make up the circulatory system. At this point you might wish to construct a little boat or raft for yourself and set out down the main artery leading from the heart. As you travel downstream, you might notice the condition of the "banks" of the river. Look for debris or litter. If you see any, then imagine a big trash-collecting "boat" (a white blood cell) traveling down the river, sucking up the debris and transporting it to the recycling station. Imagine that all the walls of the blood vessels are plaque-free—pink and smooth. Or the banks of the river are pristine and untrampled. See a beautiful and healthy environment, however it may appear to you. Go along as far as you like. Notice the branches and tributaries of the main river that go off to the various manufacturing stations (organs) and how well organized the delivery of supplies and the removal of waste are along these passageways.

When you are ready, sink deeper still—into the nervous system. The scenery changes. Now, perhaps, you will see great networks of tracks and trails and pathways. Observe how well maintained they are. Polished, shiny stainless steel, perhaps. No rust. No broken tracks. Check the connections, the intersec-tions, and the switching stations of the countless *nadis* (channels). Look around for static or interference, especially if you have had a stressful day. If you find any impediment that is creating poor reception, do some rewiring and breathe in a little *prana* to that stretch of track.

When you are finished with the nervous system, settle deeper still into the digestive and elimination systems. Now you get to roam around in the stomach and get a look at that last meal up close. This can be frightening or rewarding. It depends on how you have been treating yourself for the past few days. If you've been eating lots of nutrient-dense high-fiber foods like oatmeal, atole (blue-corn porridge—my favorite breakfast), rice, barley, any whole grain or whole grain bread, fruit, fresh seasonal vegetables with tempeh or tofu, things should look pretty good. Plenty of vitamins and minerals. Matter that is easy to digest and move along the system. No problems. But let's suppose you had a bagel or hard roll for breakfast, a cheese sandwich for lunch, and pizza or a hunk of beef for dinner. You'll be lucky if you can make it through from one end of the stomach to the other, and you'll have a hard time squeezing through the intestines. The intestines will be clogged up like the local expressway at rush hour. All that white flour! It's like glue. Remember the papier-mâché stuff you made in grade school and what you used for glue—flour and water! Plus cheese is extremely congestive for most people and meat is not nearly as easy for the balanced body to digest as vegetables, for example.

So see if you are clogged up or flowing smoothly and easily. This is an important aspect of your health to have awareness of. Some people just gulp antacids or laxatives, not connecting what goes in the mouth with what goes on in the stomach and intestines. This always amazes me. There was a popular TV commercial for an antacid that showed the daughter of a middle-aged man worrying about her father having an ulcer. She is then relieved to find out from his doctor that all he needs, of course, is a little of this antacid stuff.

What amazes me is that there isn't a health consultant on every corner to tell this guy to lay off coffee, white flour, dairy, and meat for a while and eat oatmeal and rice and steamed veggies instead. Also, fresh vegetable juices are extremely healing, and since an irritated stomach can't take the high-fiber content of raw vegetables, putting the veggies through a juicer brings all the healing qualities, but none of the irritating ones. Anyway, pay attention to your intestines. They can bring you years of joy or misery—it's up to your mouth!

LETTING MEDITATION HAPPEN

At this point, your body scan is finished. The whole process may have taken five or twenty-five minutes. Now you are ready to settle into beginning meditation. I have found over the years that it is somewhat easier for most people to experience a glimpse of the meditative state after their *asana* practice than it is without the preceding physical work. The reason for this I always attribute to Newton's third law of motion: "For every action there is an equal and opposite reaction." Which means that the degree to which you work "hard" at the practice is the degree to which you can let go "soft" for relaxation. What seems to happen is that after the body works out at the postures, it is easier to let go for relaxation. And if the body is letting go and relaxing, than the mind can follow along after the example set by the body, and spontaneously fall into moments of the elusive state of meditation. Which, by the way, is the only way meditation happens—spontaneously. You cannot make meditation happen. You have to *let* it happen by letting go of tension, thought, desire, effort. And the only way you can find it is through practice. You practice one-pointed concentration and, with luck, meditation comes. That's all.

When I was a biofeedback researcher, I taught meditation with the aid of electroencephalographic biofeedback devices. These instruments measured brain waves and gave people audio feedback when they were going in the right direction—that is, slowing the brain waves and moving toward the state of meditation. I did lots of preliminary autosuggestive work with subjects, such as having them repeat phrases like "I am relaxed," or "I am letting go of all tension," or "My muscles are relaxed and melting into the floor," etc. But that was as much as I could do. As far as getting people into meditation, all I could suggest was that they stop "trying" to meditate and allow it to happen. Not very tangible help. But that is the most any guide can do for you.

No one can teach you to meditate. All you can be taught is a technique for learning to concentrate. After that, it takes tons of practice. And what you need to practice is the sixth *anga,* or limb, *dharana,* or concentration—staying focused on one thing, which is what you have been training yourself to do for the past months and years with the Power Yoga practice.

During this practice you have been using the techniques of listening to and counting your breath and continually gazing at one point, so those might be the most effective and familiar procedures to continue to use for Relaxation Posture. However, there are many, many methods for learning meditation, from the Tibetan technique of listening to the surrounding environment to the Zen technique of counting your breath. It doesn't matter too much what technique you use—whether you concentrate on a prayer, a picture, a flame, a flower, a sound, your breath, or a *mantra*—as long as you pick one that suits you and stick with it. Here are two different techniques that you might use for your own *savasana,* or Relaxation Posture.

REPETITION OF *MANTRA*

A popular yoga technique used to prepare for meditation is the recitation of *mantra*, or sound. The word *mantra* comes from the Sanskrit root *man,* which means "to think, imagine, or believe," and a *mantra* is a thought or intention expressed as a sound. It can be a single sound or a string of sounds with no meaning. It can also be a string of sounds comprising a mystical verse, incantation, or sacred prayer, or hymn. The root *mantras* are the single sounds, and are made up from the primary sounds of the Sanskrit alphabet, and repetition of any of these *mantras* is an excellent technique for beginners.

The "om" sound is the oldest and most venerated of all the yogic *mantras*. This sacred monosyllable symbolizes divine universal energy in both the Hindu and Buddhist traditions. A Hindu sage in India whom I had spent many weeks tracking down once told me that the "om" sound represented the sound of the universe—all it parts and inhabitants working together. I always liked that explanation. It was generic and nondenominational, and yet spiritual enough to be worthy of my concentration.

I recommend that you start this practice while still sitting in *Padmasana,* or Lotus Posture. Practice humming (chanting!) the sound out loud. Don't be shy about the sound of your voice. If you feel silly, simply imagine that this is an exercise for your diaphragm—which it is! And that this is also an excellent way to clear out any remaining cobwebs hanging around in your head. Break the sound into four parts. First hum an "ah" sound. Then an "oo" sound. Then an "mm" sound. And last, a nasal humming sound that ends the chant. Practice each sound individually at first. Take a deep inhale through the nose, and then let the sound run out the mouth first and then the nose for the duration of the exhale. After you have practiced them each separately, put them all together in one breath. Take a deep, full (top to bottom, which you should be fairly adept at by now) breath, and this time start with the "ah-h-h" and end

with the "mm-m-m," giving 25 percent of your exhale to each sound. Use your diaphragm and the *bandhas* to support the sound.

Imagine that you are throwing out a very clear, focused, steady sound and trying to "thread" it through the eye of a needle a few feet in front of your face. Don't be feeble or tentative. Create a strong sound—not necessarily loud, just powerful. Get some resonance. Feel the nasal humming part buzzing around in your head. After you have practiced this a bit, you will be able to hear it continue even after you have stopped reciting it. Then move into Relaxation Posture and continue the repetition mentally.

You might wish to leave out the body scan, if and when you start to use *mantra* repetition, so that you can go right into it from the last sitting posture. Try to keep the sound going around in your head, like a tape loop. Every time the mind strays, which it will a million times, bring the attention back to "om." Eventually, the concentration will get stronger and longer.

At some point, the sound may drop off, there will be no thought, and you might just feel joyful or as if you are floating, sinking, or just being. This, as best as anyone is able to communicate in words, is the beginning of the state of meditation.

WATCHING THE BREATH

The second technique is to simply listen to your breath, which should be a fairly familiar pastime by now. Listen to it come in and listen to it go out. That's all. Every time you lose concentration, refocus your attention on the breath, as you might refocus a camera. When the breath object has become fuzzy and fades off into background, simply bring it back into sharp focus in the foreground and keep your attention on it as long as possible. There are no tricks to make this easier. Don't waste your time hunting around for an easier method. There are no easier methods. But if the mind does get bored with following the breath, here is an exercise to do that will reawaken your interest in your breathing. Close your mouth. Hold the nostrils tightly closed with your fingers and see how long it takes before you become vitally interested in your breath again.

MISSION ACCOMPLISHED

Around the time I was putting the final touches on this chapter, a major "awakening" hit me one day during my practice. That particular morning, because of a lot of distractions and excitement in my brain, I was really *using* the practice (and all its built-in techniques for *dharana,* or concentration) to discipline my mind. I was watching very carefully, noting every time my mind was distracted by the clock, the birds outside, the bank account, thoughts of writing, thoughts of going to the beach and running, thoughts of eating, and on and on. Each time I was distracted, I would refocus on the *bandhas*, the breath, and the gaze. Slowly it dawned on me in a completely new way that if you *aren't* using the practice to train your mind, you aren't doing yoga! You might be stretching, you might be breathing, you might be sweating and gaining some fitness and strength, but if you are letting the mind run wild, you aren't *doing* yoga!

Duh! Now this might sound fairly obvious to you, and it has always been fairly obvious to me, too. But this time it was as if the elevator had gone up a few floors, and instead of stepping out on the fourteenth floor as I had always done in the past, l was now on the twenty-second. All of a sudden I saw things that I knew were there but hadn't actually "seen" before. It's hard to explain, but it goes back to what I mentioned in chapter 1 about plateaus, and also about not being able to explain to people who call on the phone asking about Power Yoga what the practice will be like for them in two years or even two weeks. This practice reveals things to you about yourself and your world as you go along that a week earlier you wouldn't have been capable of getting.

Really *doing* yoga means *using* the act of listening to the breath, *using* the act of directing the eyes, *using* the control of *prana* through the *bandhas* and *ujjayi* breathing, and *using* the postures to stop the mind from running wild each and every time it gets up to go and rebels from the monotony of one-pointed concentration.

We cannot listen and think simultaneously. Either we are transmitting and processing or we are receiving, but we can't do both at the same time. It has long been clear to me, in trying to become a better listener, that the secret of good listeners is that they simply suspend their thinking process. Poor listeners cannot turn off their minds. You can see their impatience and watch them thinking while you are talking to them. They are simply waiting for you to stop talking before they begin to fill the space with their own stored-up thoughts.

Yoga is a difficult discipline. The mind basically resents it. The mind does not like to be restrained. The mind would rather go to the movies and be entertained than do yoga. I said that in class once and one of my regular students, who had brought a boyfriend to class for the first time that night, started to laugh. She looked at me, then at him, then back at me. "How did you know?" she asked. "We almost skipped class and went to the movies."

Remember that I said back in chapter 1 that one of the meanings of *hatha* was "force." When we practice the *astanga* form, this very ancient and classical form of *hatha,* what we are doing in one sense is "forcing" the postures onto a misaligned or imbalanced body. Not forcing in an aggressive way, like shoving a size 8 foot into a size 7 shoe, but in an encouraging way, to create health and balance. More important, though, we are forcing focus on the fluctuations of the mind. It is so easy to say, "Oh, I'll practice tomorrow," and allow the whimsical imaginings of the mind to excuse us from practice. But tomorrow never comes.

By applying force to the mind and directing it into a narrow field of focus, we limit the fluctuations, and become better receivers. The mind is less noisy. We are less distracted. Each time we lay on the potency of the practice, we get stronger in our commitment to continue. The mind begins to gain power as it learns to surrender to the practice of *dharana*.

Based on this dynamite revelation—that we can't think and listen at the same time—the ancient *astanga* yogis very cleverly devised these methods that force you to be a receiver. Every time you try to transmit, there is a red flag there saying, "Hey, you there! You are supposed to be receiving! You are missing some important data here—receive! receive!" And back you go to mindful listening. This whole practice never ceases to dazzle me in new ways!

This completes the Power Yoga practice (Figure 7.23). Now your true yoga "practice" begins.

Figure 7.23

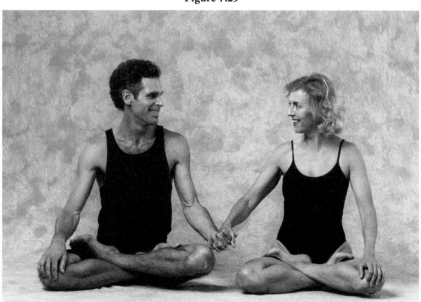

leap into nothingness

INTRODUCTION TO THE SECOND SERIES

Reaching for the stars,
I stumbled on a sack of wool,
and inside found the Golden Fleece!

MARY CROVATT HAMBIDGE, "Apprentice in Creation"

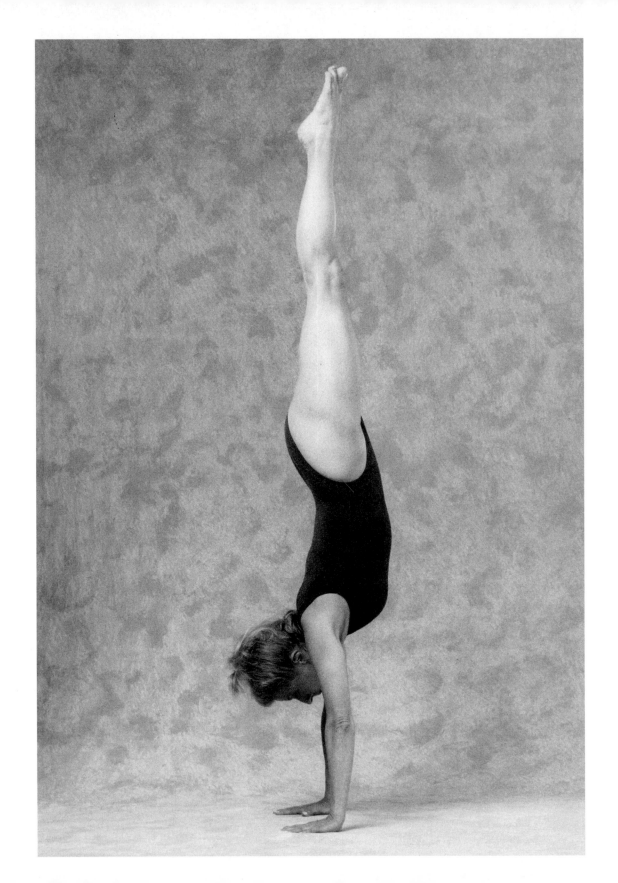

Introduction to the Second Series

Back-Strengthening and Back-Bending Postures

A Different Adventure

The forward bending postures (Primary Series), which essentially are everything we have done so far, have a certain groundedness and security about them. They may not always be easy, but they feel safe. Six months of grunt work on "opening" the back of the body; not always "fun," but rewarding.

The Second Series of *astanga yoga* begins the work of the backward bending postures. Backward bending is a very different kind of adventure. For me, beginning the Second Series was like taking off in an airplane. You are leaving the relative (and illusory) safety of the ground, where you have been practicing for many months, and soaring into space. Now, for some people, this will be a more comfortable place; for others, less comfortable. I can't say that it was more or less comfortable for me, just different. Looking out at the clouds from the window of an airplane many miles in the air is a very different perspective than looking at those same clouds from the ground.

Traditionally, back-bending has always been said to conquer fear, whereas forward bending conquers ego. The back-bending postures create a feeling of vitality and energy that is different from the revitalization of the Primary Series. I have always felt that this was a result of opening and stretching out the front of the body, a place much more protected and psychologically vulnerable than the back of the body.

Let me use one of the postures from this chapter as a sample to explain just what is different about back-bending. In *Laghu Vajrasana,* which translates as "Beautiful Thunderbolt," you start out by kneeling, and then, while leaning backward and looking back over your head, you reach behind you, clasp your calves, and lower your head all the way to the floor. It's challenging and a little scary.

We are used to and comfortable with what is in front of us. We are not so used to and comfortable with what is behind us. If we turn around to see what is behind us, then it isn't behind us anymore—it's in front of us, and becomes familiar. Doing backward bending is like confronting the world upside down and backward. It's not exactly what we are used to, so it isn't exactly reassuring.

Your mind, at first, is not cooperating. It's a trifle worried about falling on your head, straining your back, or tearing loose your thigh muscles. Even though you have done all the preliminary work and it is a perfectly safe and logical next step, doing a backbend still takes a little courage in a way that none of the Primary Series postures do. It takes determination. You sort of come face-to-face with the challenge, then turn around, take a few breaths, and dive in—backward. I frequently say in class that Second Series develops your "intentionality," or your design to do something. By that I mean it helps to crystallize your mental picture and fortify your focus. You have to take a deep breath, visualize where you are going, see it happen, and then jump in. It takes *nerve.*

Nerve Purification and Fortification

"Nerve" is an interesting choice of words, because the Second Series of *astanga yoga* is called *nadi shodana,* which means "nerve purification." *Nadi,* as we know, literally means "channel," referring specifically to the passageways that channel the *prana; shodana* means "purification." This series of postures continues the work of the first series, but undertakes a more direct action on the nervous system. It sands, polishes, and streamlines the wiring.

Now you might be reading this and say that "nerve" is jumping out of a plane or hang gliding or kayaking or mountain climbing, but yoga? You might be thinking, *Aren't you exaggerating a bit when you say yoga takes nerve?* Well, yes and no. Yes, in that compared to hang gliding, I guess Beautiful Thunderbolt Posture is pretty mellow. No, in that they are also similar in many ways. You are exploring previously unexplored territory and a new way of accessing that territory.

If you think of the analogy of the construction of a house as corresponding to the yoga practice, then the Primary Series deals with the basic understructure and framing. In order for the completed house to be a solid, durable structure, a proper foundation must be laid and everything framed out evenly, with all the angles and board lengths correct, so that when it is all put together, the corners all correspond and line up properly. In this way, the house will be evenly balanced, with equal weight distribution and all parts of the foundation taking equal stress.

The Second Series works on the wiring. In order for the electric current (*prana*) to flow safely and efficiently along the appropriate channels, all wires, switches, connections, etc., must be in sequence and correctly insulated, switched, cleaned, matched, and maintained. Then there is no fear of overloading the system.

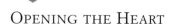

OPENING THE HEART

Anyone who participates in endurance sports like cross-country skiing, cycling, skating, running, or swimming needs *maximum* space within the thoracic cavity for full lung capacity. Ironically, many people who pursue these sports actually have *reduced* space as a result of a "collapsed" demeanor of the chest. You may remember that I first discussed this condition back in chapter 3. The chest appears caved in slightly, the shoulders round forward, the upper back is bowed and the shoulders are tight. This closed condition in the front of the chest can indicate anything from an abusive upbringing and consequent lack of self-esteem to simple overtraining of the muscles in the front of the shoulders, like the pectorals (the "pecs") and the anterior deltoid muscles (front of the shoulders), as well as overdeveloped latissimus dorsi muscles (the "lats"), the back muscles that flex or round the spine forward.

The back-bending and back-strengthening postures are extremely therapeutic for this situation. They stretch out the front of the body, strengthen the back of the body, and free the lungs from the downward pressure of the chest. This is especially important training for all of us (runners, cyclists, swimmers, climbers, skiers, kayakers, skaters, rowers, golfers, etc.) whose sport brings tightness to the shoulders and chest.

This tightness in the front of the shoulders and chest can be a strong, protective psychological mechanism against feeling, or exploring feeling. In yoga therapy, tightness in this area indicates a closed emotional condition and a closed heart *chakra,* or storage center for love and compassion. When we begin to stretch and crack open this area with the back-bending postures of the Second Series, we actually begin to "open the heart" (as I mentioned in the last chapter when we were doing Upward Bow Posture).

In chapter 2, where I first began the discussion of breathing and how people breathe, I talked a little bit about why people may breathe "backward" or shallowly. And I mentioned that for a variety of physiological or psychological reasons, it might be the result of a shutdown in the navel or *manipura chakra,* the area of the solar plexus. This, then, not only deprives the abdominal organs of full nourishment, but our "feeling" center of full capacity as well. We began to work on energizing and awakening this third *chakra* with our *ujjayi* breathing, the *bandhas*, and the Primary Series of postures.

In the same way with some of the Second Series postures, still using *ujjayi* breathing and the *bandhas*, we start to "open" (put some energy into) the fourth, or heart, *chakra*. You may remember this *chakra* is called in Sanskrit *anahata,* and is represented by the element air. In the most fundamental sense, opening this area structurally means simply getting more air into the thoracic cavity!

There is an inclination that I see frequently in class among students just beginning Second Series work, to go about halfway into a posture, then recoil. Most often it is not pain or tightness that stops us, but fear. Fear of injury, perhaps, but more often fear of not knowing just where you are going. Fear of giving up some protected site in favor of vulnerability. On a deeper and less tangible level, there are ancient fears stored deep in the cells. The back-bending postures are, in their simplest terms, intended to conquer fear and open the heart.

LOOKING AT THE STARS

There are four basic curves in the spine. The cervical curve, at the back of the neck, and the lumbar curve, in the lower back, are called posterior curves. That is, they curve away from the posterior or back part of the body. The sacral curve, the flat place below the lumbar curve, and the thoracic curve, the middle back, are called anterior curves and curve away from the anterior or front part of the body.

Over the years what seems to happen as a result of stress, poor or weak posture, injury, fatigue, overtraining, or specificity of training is that the cervical and lumbar curve tend to decrease and the thoracic curve tends to increase. Regular practice of Second Series counteracts this degenerative tendency of the cervical and lumbar curves to diminish and the thoracic curve to increase.

Development of the strength, health, balance, clarity, and longevity of the spinal column is one of the main objectives of the yoga practice. The spine is meant to move in all directions. Often we forget that the spine is able, anatomically, to bend backward, because it is not something we generally do in our everyday activities. Students will often ask me in class after I have asked them to look up or back over their eyebrows, "Isn't that bad for my neck?"

"Do you have any neck injuries" I inquire.

"No," they generally respond.

"Does it hurt?" I continue.

"Um, no, it just feels tight," they say.

"It probably *is* tight. Is it bad to look at the stars? Don't you think we were meant to look up?"

"Um, well, yes, I guess so."

If you don't have a neck injury, it isn't bad to look up or back. We were designed to go that way. It's just that nothing we do in everyday life encourages us to move that way. Everything seems to persuade us to lean forward, whether to garden, plant, pick, sweep, change diapers, work at a desk or computer, or play piano. It certainly isn't a direction of movement found in most forms of athletic training, except possibly dance, gymnastics, high jumping, or pole vaulting.

As so much of everything we do is based on forward bending, one consequence over the years as the cervical and lumbar curves get flatter and the thoracic curve gets greater is that the front side of the spinal column begins to compress and the back side to separate. Can you visualize an evenly stacked column of vertebrae, one on top of another, all with nice little pads in between them, keeping things well cushioned? Then visualize that same column always bending forward and leaning in one direction. Can't you see that eventually the front part of the pads would begin to wear away and that the front edges of the vertebral bone would get closer together, imminently touching and beginning to grate against one another, while the back edges spread further apart?

Backward bending reverses this. Bending over

backward, or just simple back therapy strengthening (like lying on your stomach, with arms and legs extended, and then raising the arms and legs in the air) opens up the anterior spaces between the vertebrae and strengthens the muscles that hold the posterior spaces in place. This gives anteriorly compressed discs space to regenerate and heal and can eliminate pain caused from nerves pinched by collapsing or grating vertebrae.

A Prerace Workout

These next few paragraphs are primarily aimed at competitive runners or other competitive athletes who use their hamstring muscles as one of the prime movers of their sport: cross-country skiers, soccer players, and other running-sport participants. However, this general advice could apply to the primary muscles used in any sport.

Often in an intermediate class, when I know a number of the students are coming up on a competitive running event in which many of them are participating (like the week before the New York City Marathon), I will focus on the simple back-bending postures instead of the Primary Series. I have found over the years that contracting the hamstrings, as we do in the back-bending work, is a more appropriate prerace workout for them than stretching. In fact, it's better to rest the prime mover muscles from strong stretching for at least a few *days* before competition. *However, this only applies to an athlete who has been doing regular Power Yoga practice.*

For some reason, the contractions of the back-bending postures—like Postures 1 through 4, for example—wake up the hamstrings and get them used to the contracting they will have to do in the run. But since yoga requires a different kind of contraction than that required during running—a static contraction as opposed to a dynamic contraction—it exercis-

es the muscles in a different way and doesn't deplete them. It is like having a dress rehearsal that energizes the players instead of exhausting them. Doing these postures also doesn't produce lactic acid the way the dynamic contractions of running do, but rather cleanses the tissue of lactic acid buildup.

Consequently, I will invariably tell runners not to crank on (stretch out) their hamstring muscles for several days before an event. I *do* recommend the warm-ups and the standing postures as part of the prerace routine. But the focus in the standing postures should be only on the contraction of the quadriceps, not on the stretching of the hamstrings.

If you have been consistent with your yoga training, you don't need to be *so* concerned about stretching before an event—or before or after anything, for that matter. Your regular practice takes care of your stretching needs. You don't need to waste time stretching before your runs or after your bike rides or ballgames. Use Sun Salutations as a warm-up, as I have mentioned before, and do a few standing postures after the game or run. But keep up *regular* practice.

A Representative Sampling

One must train to prepare for the Second Series, as you have been doing by following the sequence given in this book. Backward bending, even the simple back-strengthening work that begins this chapter, is advanced practice. It cannot be attempted until the Primary Series becomes routine and familiar. That is why this is called *Second* Series.

Some of these postures are contraindicated for certain conditions and certainly should not be attempted by the untrained general public as isolated poses! More specifically, they should not be practiced by beginners, overweight persons, pregnant women, or people with back injuries, chronic spinal misalignment, or fused, slipped, inflamed, or removed disks. The Second Series may also be inappropriate for persons with certain conditions accompanied by vertiginous or unsteady symptoms or effects.

All of these groups require the one-on-one supervision of a professional yoga therapist trained in this method *and* the supportive enthusiasm of their physicians. If you have any doubts about whether or not you can do these postures, please check with your family doctor.

I have called this chapter an "Introduction to the Second Series," because it does not include the complete Second Series of postures. There are approximately thirty-eight postures in Second Series (including the various combinations and permutations), and I simply did not have the space to include them all. Also, since I wanted you to be able to carry this book home from the store and finish reading it in one lifetime, I decided to simply include a representative sampling of the Second Series postures for the Power Yoga workout.

I have followed the sequence and included all postures that are essential as counter postures to preceding poses. Often what happens in the Second Series, as in the Primary Series, is that there will be a basic posture and then two or three more advanced variations. In most cases what I have done is to only include the basic posture (plus a few of my own favorites). Another reason for omitting some of the more advanced postures is that many of them are almost impossible to learn without a coach or teacher helping or "spotting" for you.

Spotting is a fairly common term in gymnastics—for example, where you depend on the coach to keep you from falling or injuring yourself while you are learning a new move. This can mean help with holding your weight, maintaining balance, or achieving a particular position. It is the same in yoga. When you are hot and have been practicing regularly, a teacher can help put you into a posture, hold you in that posture, or help you achieve something (Handstand, for example), that you might not be able to do on your own. If you ever come to our advanced classes in New York City, we will be able to help you with these few intricate postures of the Second Series.

CONTINUING THE PRACTICE

When I was first learning this practice, each day I would do what I had done the day before. Then when I was ready, I'd add another posture or two. When I finished with the Primary Series, I would just keep on going into Second Series, and then end with Closing Sequence. Thus, my practice just kept getting longer and it was a great way to build mindfulness and endurance.

However, many of you might not have the time to go through the entire Primary Series just to get to the Second Series. Thus, once you have attained some proficiency in the Primary Series, you can begin to work with the Second Series postures. Moving up to the Second Series can require anywhere from six months to two or three years of prior Primary Series practice, depending on how *regular* your practice is and what shape you are in when you start. The Second Series is generally practiced directly after warm-ups *and* the standing postures from the Primary Series. You want to be really hot and sweaty when you start these postures, and doing the standing postures as part of the warm-up helps get you ready.

Often, just to loosen up a bit more, I will go one-third to one-half of the way through the Primary Series and then skip to the Second Series. Remember, no matter how long your practice is or what portion of the postures you do, you always end with Closing Sequence. (At this point it should be Complete Closing Sequence—and if you aren't doing the inverted postures, then possibly you shouldn't be doing the postures from this chapter either. It depends on the reason why you aren't doing inverted poses). So any Second Series work comes after warm-ups and standing postures, and before Closing Sequence.

THE POSTURES

Note of caution: The postures in this chapter require awareness, preparation, and prior training. Do not attempt to practice poses in this chapter without having first thoroughly read, studied, and practiced the preceding chapters for at least three to twelve months and attained proficiency in those postures.

1

LOCUST POSTURES A AND B: *SALABHASANA A AND B*

Salabha means "locust" or "grasshopper."

TECHNIQUE

Note: This posture begins a backward-bending series that continues through Posture 5, Beautiful Thunderbolt. It is probably best to do all the postures, one

after another, without too much interruption in between, as each one helps to warm up and prepare the spine for the next one in sequence. Most of you will be able to do at least Postures 1 through 4. Posture 5 will be the most difficult of the batch and could be omitted until the first four get easier. If this is all you can do when you first begin work with this chapter, make sure to leave time and energy to do Crane Posture (No. 6) and Intense West Stretch (Full Forward Bending) Posture (No. 14), both critical counterposes for the first four or five postures.

Preparation: Begin from *sama-sthiti,* or attention position. Do Sun Salutation A through to Position 7,

Figure 8.1

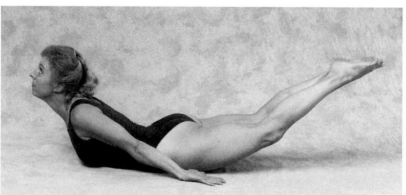

Face Down Dog. Then, instead of jumping through to a seated position, simply lie down on your tummy. Place arms back along sides with palms facing up, feet and shoulder blades pressing together, and middle of forehead resting on floor.

Inhale, raise head, shoulders, and legs in air.
Exhale, press back of hands down into floor. Gaze up (Figure 8.1).

THIS IS LOCUST POSTURE A—HOLD FOR FIVE BREATHS (FIGURE 8.1).

Inhale, hold posture but bend elbows, turn hands over so fingers point forward and palms are facedown. Hands should be at sides of waist so when you lift up, your arms look like grasshopper (or locust!) legs. Gaze is still up.
Exhale, hold.

THIS IS LOCUST POSTURE B—HOLD FOR FIVE BREATHS (This position is not pictured. Please follow instructions in text.)

Inhale, Face Up Dog.
Exhale, Face Down Dog
Inhale, lie down on tummy.

2

FROG POSTURE: *BHEKASANA*

Bheka means "frog." This posture stretches the thighs and the top of the feet in exactly the same way that Horizontal Facing One Leg Posture does in the Primary Series.

TECHNIQUE

Inhale, separate the legs slightly, bend the knees, reach back and grab the top of the feet with the hands (Figure 8.2). If possible, turn the hands around so that the wrist points back and the palms are on the upper part of the feet with fingers pointing front, as in close-up illustration (Figure 8.3).
Exhale, push down on the top of the feet, bending the elbows so that the front of the upper arms (bicep muscles) are engaged, bringing the toes and heels closer to the ground alongside the hips (Figure 8.4). Ultimately, the heels will touch the floor. Lift the head and shoulders. Gaze is up and back.

Note: Make absolutely sure the feet are correctly aligned before you begin pushing down on the feet.

Figure 8.2

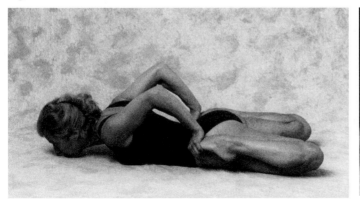

Figure 8.3

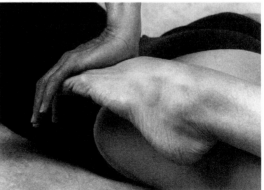

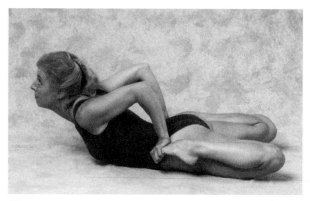

Figure 8.4

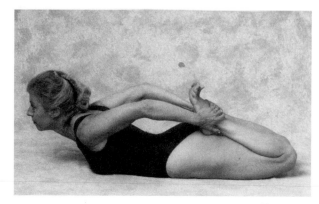

Figure 8.5

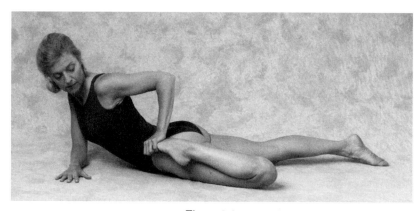

Figure 8.6

As I said in chapter 5, with regard to Horizontal Facing One Leg Posture, do not let the feet turn out to the sides. This throws the ankles and knees out of alignment. So if you find your heels turning in in this position, instead of pushing down on the feet, grab the heels and work to open them out.

Modification (somewhat easier):
Inhale, reach back and grab the feet.
Exhale, push the heels toward the buttocks. Be careful not to arch the back to inadvertently get "around" the quadriceps stretch. Instead, push the pubic bone into the floor (Figure 8.5). Breathe!

Modification (most easy):
Inhale, prop yourself up on your right forearm, and grab the left ankle with your left hand.

Exhale, push down on the left foot, trying to take the foot to the buttocks. Keep the left hip on the floor (Figure 8.6).

Note: Everyone is going to feel this stretch in the thighs to some degree! But pay attention to just exactly where you *are* feeling it. If you are a skater, skier, or cyclist, for example, most likely you will be feeling it most in the thighs. You should work to keep your heat up so you are able to get a good stretch without undue stress. If, however, you are a runner or skier, let's say, and you are feeling this most in your knees, readjust the leg position, roll out the calf muscle, and keep the foot parallel to the thigh. If this still bothers your knee, *back off!*

THIS IS FROG POSTURE—HOLD FOR FIVE BREATHS (FIGURE 8.4, 8.5, OR 8.6).

Inhale.
Exhale, release and come down.
Inhale, Face Up Dog.
Exhale, Face Down Dog.
Inhale, lie down on tummy.

3

BOW POSTURE: *DHANURASANA*

Dhanu means "bow." This is the reverse of *Urdhva Dhanurasana,* or Upward Bow, which was listed as an optional posture at the end of the Primary Series.

TECHNIQUE

Inhale, reach back and grab ankles (Figure 8.7).
Exhale, bring feet together, toes (and heels if possible) touching.
Inhale.
Exhale, lift the knees, thighs, and, eventually, even the pelvic bones off the floor. Use the arms to lift the legs up. Try to straighten the legs! Gaze is up

and back. Weight is on abdomen (Figure 8.8).

Note: Don't allow lower back to hyperextend. This can be prevented by holding *uddiyana bandha,* abdominal lock, with special emphasis on contraction of the obliques, as we have been attempting to remember throughout the practice.

THIS IS BOW POSTURE—HOLD FOR FIVE BREATHS (FIGURE 8.8).

Inhale.
Exhale, release, come down, let go of ankles, place hands alongside shoulders.
Inhale, Face Up Dog.
Exhale, Face Down Dog.
Inhale, lie down on tummy.

4

CAMEL POSTURE: *USTRASANA*

Ustra means "camel." This posture, along with the next posture, Beautiful Thunderbolt Posture, forms

Figure 8.7

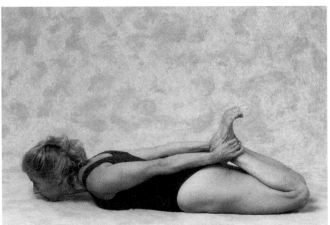

Figure 8.8

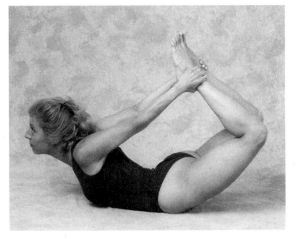

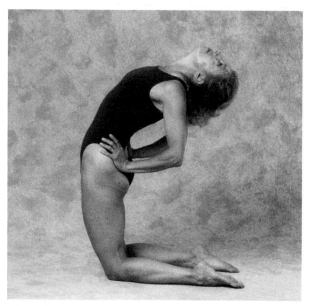

Figure 8.9

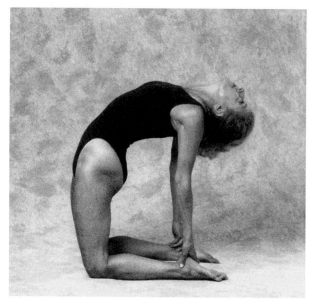

Figure 8.10

a duo of back-bending movements, with Camel Posture being the easiest and Beautiful Thunderbolt a little more difficult.

TECHNIQUE

Important note: The plan is that the preceding postures, such as Locust, Frog, and Bow, get you warmed up. If you manage okay in this posture, but the next one seems impossible, not to worry! It may not be a difficult posture for yogis, dancers, or gymnasts, but for just about anyone else—wrestlers, golfers, bodybuilders, runners, cyclists, well, you get the idea—it won't exactly be a cakewalk. But keep in mind that the Primary Series gets you ready for the Second Series. If you are feeling good about your long and diligent practice in the First Series, then at least give these a try using the modifications or help from a partner. Or if you prefer, you might skip this and the next posture and practice Hero Posture (chapter 5, Figure 5.18) and Reclining Hero (Figure 8.13 in this chapter) instead. Then continue with the next posture. Once Reclining Hero becomes easy,

you will be better able to start work with this and the posture that follows.

Inhale, kneel on floor, separating thighs and feet slightly, toes pointing straight back, with feet flat on floor.

Exhale, place palms on hips, press pelvis forward, lift the ribs, and begin to arch back (Figure 8.9).

Inhale.

Exhale, reach back and grab the right heel with the right hand and the left heel with the left hand. Thumbs go to the outside of the foot. Continue to press the pelvis forward. Be especially vigilant to hold root lock (squeezing the perineum) and abdominal lock (contracting abdominal muscles, especially oblique muscles), as this will protect the lower back from compression. This is extremely important. Almost all your focus should be on the *bandhas* here—especially the upper aspect of *uddiyana bandha* (abdominal lock). Gaze is back (at point between eyebrows) and extended out (Figure 8.10). With the spine and neck stretched back, and pressure on the abdominal area from the stretching of the front of the body, breathing may be difficult. Try to relax and breathe as deeply as possible. Every time you feel fear creeping up, *breathe and hold the locks!*

THIS IS CAMEL POSTURE—HOLD FOR FIVE BREATHS (FIGURE 8.10).

Inhale, return to starting position.

Note: If necessary, come to a counterposture called *Balasana,* or Pose of the Child, following Camel Posture. This will provide immediate relief of any stress in lower back. Come out of Camel Posture, bend forward, sit back on feet, and lower head to floor. Arms can be back along side or folded in front as a rest for the head. Hold for five to ten breaths.
Exhale, jump back.
Inhale, Face Up Dog.
Exhale, Face Down Dog.
Inhale, jump back to kneeling position.

5

BEAUTIFUL THUNDERBOLT POSTURE: *LAGHU VAJRASANA*

Laghu has a vast array of delightful meanings from "small and insignificant" through "light, quick, swift, nimble, not heavy or difficult" to "pleasing, agreeable, handsome, and beautiful." *Vajra* means "thunderbolt." Since this is such an awesome posture, I can't bring myself to call it Insignificant or Not Difficult Thunderbolt. So I call it Beautiful Thunderbolt.

TECHNIQUE

Inhale, kneel on floor with thighs and feet slightly apart. Keep hands on hips.
Exhale, arch back, pressing pelvis forward. Reach back and grab the calves, as close to the knees as possible, and lower the head to the floor (Figure 8.11). Most of the weight should be forward toward the knees, with very little to no weight on the head. (At first, because of tightness in the thighs, you will probably have a bit of weight on the head.) Gaze is back and extended out or at point between eyebrows (Figure 8.12).

Figure 8.11

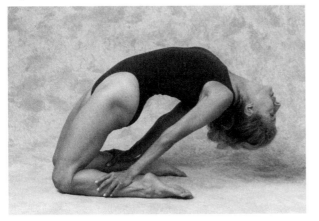

Figure 8.12

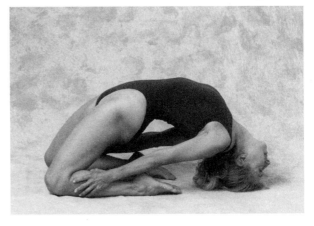

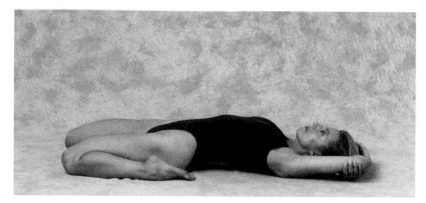

Figure 8.13

Important note of caution: This posture is almost impossible to exit from as you went into it, unless you do the pose nearly perfectly. All of the weight must be forward, with the thighs very close to vertical, or perpendicular, to the ground. Thus, the only other way to get out of this is to lie back down into Reclining Hero Posture, or *Supta Virasana* (Figure 8.13). Before you start, make sure you can do Reclining Hero *easily,* not straining.

Another option is to have a friend work with you as a spotter. Your friend then takes you down to the floor (Figure 8.14, as you see Thom doing for me), holds you there while you take five breaths, and then brings you back up again, letting go only when you are fully back in control. Depending on the flexibility and fear factors of the person you are working with, you may support him or her from behind the shoulder blades (with beginners) or at the back of the

Figure 8.14

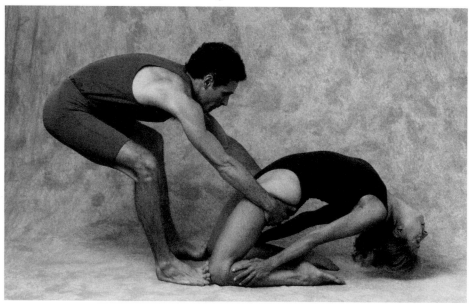

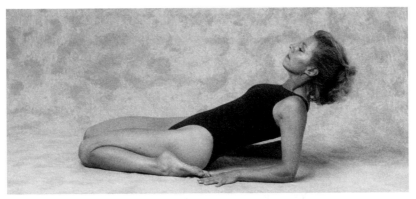

Figure 8.15

thighs (with more advanced students), as Thom does for me. Never support someone in this posture at the lower back. That is where 99.9 percent of people will feel compression in this posture, and holding them there just adds to the strain.

Modification:

If the thighs are either too tight or too weak to support the descent of the head to the floor, without bumping or crashing, sit back as far as possible (as in Hero Posture in chapter 5) and support yourself with your forearms (Figure 8.15). If possible, lie back down into Reclining Hero Posture (Figure 8.13). Press the knees and hips into the floor, stretching the thighs. Also, press the lower back into the floor. Hold the oblique contraction! The back should not be arched. If it is, you have to come back up to the position shown in Figure 8.15 and slowly work your way down. Once you are fairly comfortable in Reclining Hero, lift the chest, take the head back, raise the hips, and reach toward the calves with the arms, arching the spine and stretching or strengthening the thighs. Like the Bow and Camel, this posture contracts the spine backward and stretches the front of the body, which places a lot of pressure on the abdomen and diaphragm, making it difficult to breathe. Breathing will tend to be fast and shallow. Try to slow and deepen the breath, relaxing the mind and holding *mula bandha* and *uddiyana bandha*.

Note: This posture is interesting for a variety of reasons, but one aspect that fascinates me is that if your thighs are very tight (like mine are from ten years of skiing), then this will be an enormous stretch for the thighs. But once the thighs get opened up sufficiently, then the thighs are used, or contracted, to hold the body almost "hanging back" over the feet, and this enormously strengthens the thighs.

THIS IS BEAUTIFUL THUNDERBOLT POSTURE— HOLD FOR FIVE BREATHS (FIGURE 8.12, 8.13, 8.14, OR 8.15).

Inhale, come up, using the thighs or
   Exhale, lie back down between legs.
   Inhale, sit up.
Exhale, put hands down.
Inhale, take it up.
Exhale, and jump back.
Inhale, Face Up dog.
Exhale, Face Down Dog.
Inhale, jump to a squat.

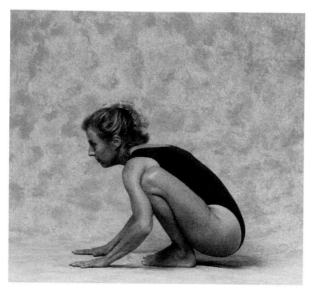

Figure 8.16

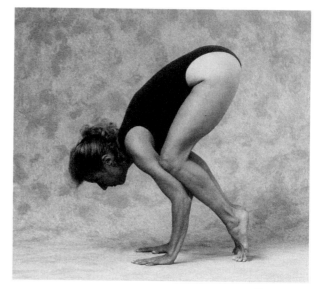

Figure 8.17

6

CRANE POSTURE: *BAKASANA*

Baka means "crane."

TECHNIQUE

Note: This is an *essential* counterpose to the postures that preceded it. That means you can't skip this, even if you can't "do" the posture. Work with the Modification.

Inhale, from a squat, with feet together (if possible) and/or parallel. Separate the knees and lean the torso forward between the thighs.

Exhale, continue to lean the trunk forward between the thighs, and maneuver the armpits to the inside of the knees. Place the palms on the floor (Figure 8.16).

Inhale, lean forward, lift up buttocks, come up on toes and press the knees into the back of the upper arm next to the armpits (Figure 8.17).

Exhale, continue to lean forward, lift the toes off the floor and balance (Figure 8.18). Work to straighten arms and raise feet (Figure 8.19). Head is up! Keep gaze up and out. This will help you to balance. Don't look back between your legs, as you will tend to tip over.

Modification:

After all the back-bending this posture feels terrific, since it serves as a counterpose for all those that have preceded it. Even if you are not able to position the knees on the back of the arms and balance, coming to a squat is the equivalent of a forward-bending pose. Try placing a little weight forward on the back of the arms, perhaps one leg at a time, hold, and breathe.

Slowly you will be able to lift one foot off the floor and then the other. If you are afraid of falling forward on your face, you might want to have someone stand in front of you with his or her hands under your shoulders to catch you if you start to tip forward (Figure 8.20). But your partner has to be alert. Spotting for someone in a yoga posture means being responsible for the other person's safety. If your spotter assures you that she will catch you, she must be ready

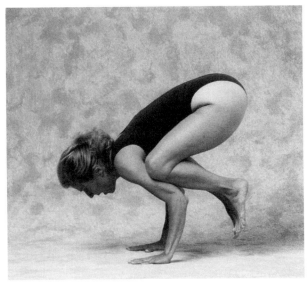

Figure 8.18

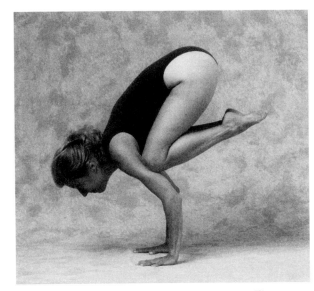

Figure 8.19

to catch you. You might try having your helper place her hands under and just lightly against your shoulders. Slowly tip forward so they can feel what holding your weight is like. Keep your gaze up and out.

Figure 8.20

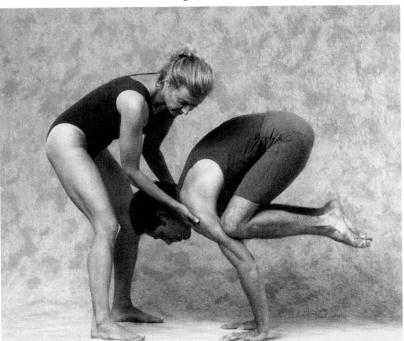

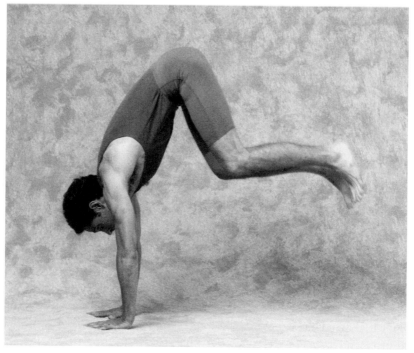

Figure 8.21

THIS IS CRANE POSTURE—HOLD FOR FIVE BREATHS (FIGURE 8.18, 8.19, OR 8.20).

Exhale, jump back out of Crane Posture if possible (Figure 8.21). If not, touch toes down and then jump back.
Inhale, Face Up Dog.
Exhale, Face Down Dog.
Inhale, jump through, sit down.

7

BHARADVAJASANA POSTURE

Bharadvaja was one of the heroes of the *Mahabharata* (literally, "great story"), one of the two great epics of India. It was written in Sanskrit around 200 B.C. Since this posture is a person's name, there is no translation.

TECHNIQUE

Inhale, fold the left leg back alongside the left thigh, so that the left foot is next to the left hip, as in Horizontal Facing One-Leg Posture. The left foot is parallel to the left thigh, with the toes pointing straight back. Take the right foot into half lotus position (place right foot on top of the left thigh, with the right heel near the navel) (Figure 8.22).
Exhale, reach around, and bind in half lotus position, taking the right foot with the right hand, if possible (Figure 8.23). Twist back to the right, reach across with the left arm, and place the left hand on the outer side of the right knee, with the fingers facing in. Tuck the left fingers underneath the knee and try to place palm flat on the floor. The wrist faces out, or away from the knee (Figure 8.24). If this is not possible with the hand, simply grab the right knee with the left hand. Look back over the right shoulder. Keep *both* buttock bones on the floor.

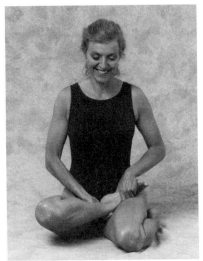
Figure 8.22

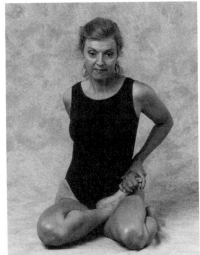
Figure 8.23

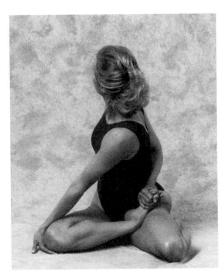
Figure 8.24

Note: This posture is a little tricky for persons with tight hips as it combines their two most difficult positions from the Primary Series, Bound Half Lotus and Horizontal Facing One-Leg. In most cases, when you first begin learning this, it is going to take two or three breaths, perhaps more, to get yourself assembled in the correct positions. However, once the hips get opened up and you can sit with one leg back and the other in Half Lotus a bit more easily, it should take only one full breath to come into the posture. If you cannot bind in the half lotus position, I suggest you simply face forward and work on Half Lotus as best you can.

For me, this posture is a great relief after the chain of back-bending poses. It soothes and laterally massages the vertebrae in the lower thoracic and lumbar zones of the back, as well as helping to develop suppleness in these same regions. It is also extremely beneficial to the kidneys. Due to the position of the legs, blood supply to the legs is reduced: therefore, circulation to the torso is increased. As the arm comes from behind to lock with the foot, there is pressure from the forearm on the kidneys—first one side, then the other—massaging and stimulating blood flow to these organs.

THIS IS BHARADVAJA-SANA POSTURE—HOLD FOR FIVE BREATHS (FIGURE 8.24).

Inhale.

Exhale, release, cross the legs (or release the upper body, but keep the legs as they are).

Inhale. If your legs are crossed, take it up (If you maintained leg position, put hands down, roll over, curl the back toe under, stand up on the left foot (Figure 8.25), and

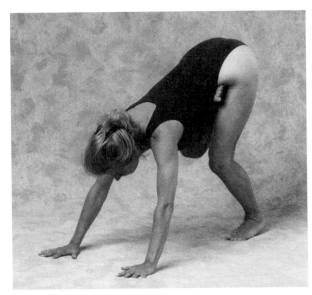
Figure 8.25

Exhale, jump back (disengaging half lotus position as
  you jump).
Inhale, Face Up Dog.
Exhale, Face Down Dog.
Inhale, jump through.
  Repeat instructions for the left side.

8

HALF LORD OF THE FISHES POSTURE:
ARDHA MATSYENDRASANA

Ardha means "half." *Matsya* means "fish." *Matsyendra* means "Lord of the Fishes." A simple fish, resting under a leaf in a pond, listened with rapt
attention and complete stillness as Lord Shiva, sitting
on the bank of the pond, explained the mysteries of
yoga to his consort, Parvati. Lord Shiva, who realized
that the fish had learned yoga while listening, be-
stowed divine form on the simple creature. Thus, the
fish became Matsyendra, the first teacher of yoga.

TECHNIQUE

Inhale, fold left leg under the right thigh, and bring
  the left heel alongside of right hip. Don't sit on the
  heel. Cross your right leg over the left knee. Put
  the bottom of the right foot on the floor next to
  the left thigh, so that the outer side of the right ankle touches the outer side of the left thigh near the
  left knee (Figure 8.26).
Exhale, twist to right.
Inhale, extend left arm from shoulder. Take back of
  upper arm (tricep) to outside of right thigh. Try to
  reach the left armpit to the outside of the right
  thigh. The left armpit should be flush against the
  bent right knee, with no space between the armpit
  and the knee. Clear chest past the thigh (Figure
  8.27).
Exhale, reach left hand to grasp right foot, taking the
  fingers under the outer side of the right foot. Keep
  arm straight (Figure 8.28). Internally rotate the
  inner side of the elbow inward so as not to
  hyperextend the elbow.
Inhale.
Exhale, twist farther to right, and reach the right arm

Figure 8.26

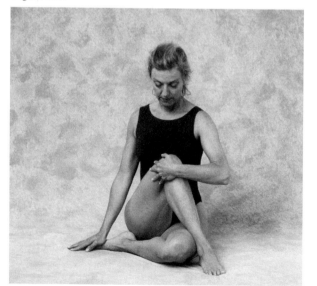

Figure 8.27

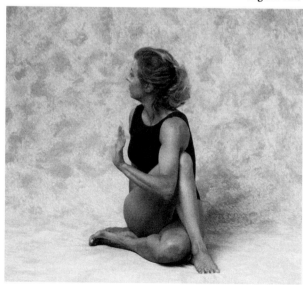

around behind your back at the waist. Try to touch left thigh with fingers of right hand. Stretch further and grip inner left thigh with right hand, if possible. Look back over right shoulder (Figure 8.29). Try to keep the left knee pressing down and both buttock bones on the floor.

Modification:

This is the same twist as we did in the Primary Series at the end of chapter 5, Marichyasana C Posture, so the twist should feel familiar. You are trying to clear both sides of the chest past the drawn-up thigh. Work the posture as best you can, focusing on the preliminary work as illustrated in Figure 8.27.

THIS IS HALF LORD OF THE FISHES POSTURE— HOLD FOR FIVE BREATHS (FIGURE 8.27 OR 8.29).

Inhale.
Exhale, release twist.
Inhale, place hands down, take it up.
Exhale, jump back.
Inhale, Face Up Dog.
Exhale, Face Down Dog.

Inhale, jump through.
Repeat instructions for the left side.

9

MODIFIED ONE FOOT BEHIND THE HEAD POSTURE: *EKA PADA SIRASANA*

Eka means "one." *Pada* can mean "leg" or "foot," as we have already learned in numerous preceding postures. *Sirsa* means "head." So *Eka Pada Sirsasana* means One Foot (Behind the) Head Posture.

Note: Very, very few of us, except maybe those who are either very flexible or have been doing yoga for a very long time, will be able to put their foot behind their head. *I* can barely put my foot behind my head without a lot of heat and help! But the modifications for this posture I give here are really terrific for the hips. We use them frequently in our classes at the New York Road Runners Club because they are ex-

Figure 8.28

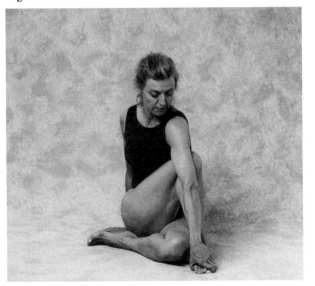

Figure 8.29

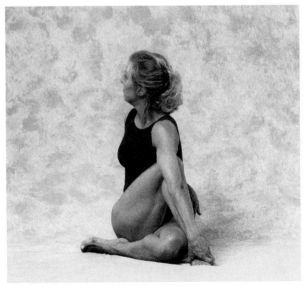

cellent for stretching out the tight hips of all the runners, skaters, skiers, etc., who come to those classes. So the following modifications are designed to continue the opening of the hamstrings and the hips, yet be realistically possible for most of us to practice.

TECHNIQUE

Modification:

Inhale, bring the right leg up into a cradle position. Put the right arm under the lower leg, and with the left hand grab the right foot.

Exhale, pull the foot in toward the middle of the chest. Take a few breaths (Figure 8.30). This might be enough of a stretch for many of you. In this case, take your five breaths in this position. Gaze out past end of nose.

More Advanced Modification:

Inhale, push the knee back and

Exhale, bring the bottom of the foot to the ear, as if you were talking into a telephone (Figure 8.31). Try to keep the chest lifted and the heart "open." Take five breaths in this position. Gaze

out past end of nose. Once you have practiced this for enough time that it becomes a little easier, you might want to go on to the third level of preparation for taking the foot behind the head.

Most Advanced Modification:

Inhale, bring the right leg up, and place the upper right arm in front of the back of the right thigh. Push back on the thigh with the arm and try to work the shoulder in front of the back of the thigh.

Exhale, then try to straighten the leg and reach behind the head with the left arm and try to grab the right foot with the left hand (Figure 8.32). Gaze is same as preceding modification.

THIS IS MODIFIED ONE FOOT BEHIND THE HEAD POSTURE—HOLD FOR FIVE BREATHS (FIGURE 8.30, 8.31, OR 8.32).

Inhale, extend the back, lift the chest as high as possible "into" the stretch.

Exhale, release the posture, placing the hands down with the right elbow in front of the back of the right thigh. If you did one of the two advanced

Figure 8.30

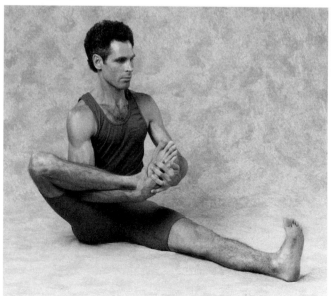

Figure 8.31

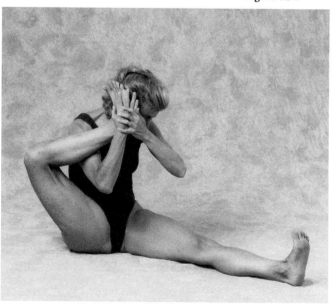

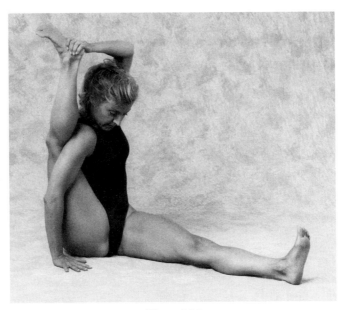

Figure 8.32

modifications, the back of the right thigh should still be up and over the back of the upper arm. Attempt to work the leg as high up on the arm/shoulder as possible.

Inhale, from this position, take it up into what is actually a posture called One Hand and Arm Posture, or *Eka Hasta Bhujasana* (Figure 8.33). Swing the right leg back over the top of the right arm, fold the left leg underneath you and bring it through (Figure 8.34).

Exhale, jump back.

Figure 8.33

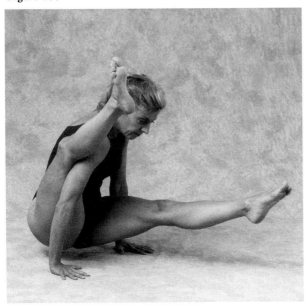

Figure 8.34

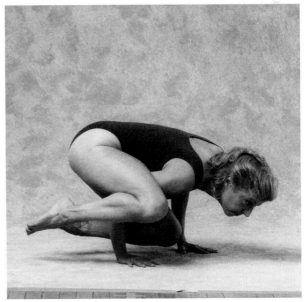

Note: This move might look extremely difficult, but actually once you get it, it's a lot of fun. The first time I did this without touching the floor with either foot, I felt like Rambo.

Inhale, Face Up Dog.
Exhale, Face Down Dog.
Inhale, jump through.
  Repeat instructions for left side.

10

FIREFLY POSTURE: *TITTIBHASANA*

In India, *tittibha* is a kind of bird and also an insect like a firefly. Your capability in this posture depends on regular practice of the two Tortoise Postures in the Primary Series, and all the preliminary work we have just done in the last posture. I love this pose. When I was first learning it, my legs would slip down and I always ended up toppling over backward. I didn't like it so much then. But once you can get the hips to cooperate, this posture is fabulous for strength and feels great.

TECHNIQUE

Inhale, jump to the outside of the arms, bring the legs up as high as possible on the back of the arms and then sit back (Figure 8.35).
Exhale, press forward, putting weight on hands, and lift up into the posture (Figure 8.36). Try to straighten legs and arms and lift the buttocks so that the legs are parallel to the floor. Gaze is up and out.

Note: Theoretically, here you jump into the posture on one breath from Face Down Dog of the preceding *vinyasa*. But since most of us need to struggle a bit to get the shoulders under the knees (Figure 8.37), as we did in Pressure on the Shoulders Posture back in the Primary Series, take as many breaths as you need here to prepare for the lift up into the *asana*. You should be familiar enough with the Primary Series that you will remember how to work yourself into preparation for this position.

THIS IS FIREFLY POSTURE—HOLD FOR FIVE BREATHS.

Inhale, lift up and tip forward.

Figure 8.35

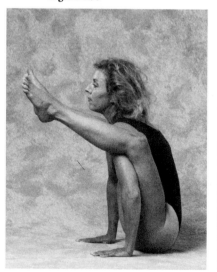

Figure 8.36

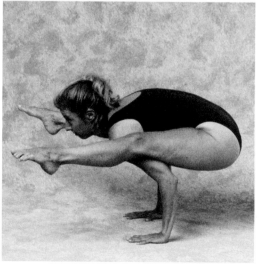

Figure 8.37

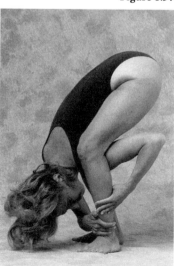

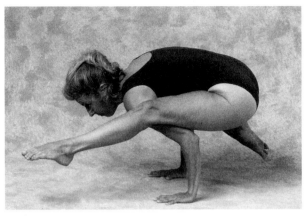

Figure 8.38

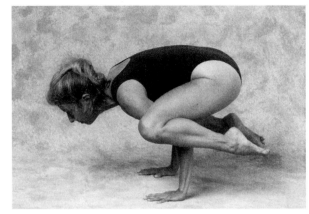

Figure 8.39

Exhale, take one leg back (Figure 8.38) and then the other (Figure 8.39) and jump back.

Inhale, Face Up Dog.

Exhale, Face Down Dog.

Inhale, jump through.

11

Peacock Feathers Posture: *Pincha Mayurasana*

As most words in Sanskrit, *pincha* has several meanings. In this usage, it means "feather," but it can also mean "chin." *Mayura* means "peacock." In this posture, as the legs and torso are lifted into the air, they resemble the majestic action of the peacock when it lifts and spreads its tail feathers.

Note: I love this posture. We always have a lot of fun with this in class, and people seem to enjoy learning it. I think it makes everyone feel strong and in control of life. At first many people see others doing it and think, Oh my God, I'll never be able to do *that.* But then a few weeks later they are doing it! Over the years I have seen this (and Handstand) consistently change people's image of themselves from

weak and fearful to strong and confident. It develops strength and courage and is an excellent posture for mental and physical powers.

Technique

Preparation: Begin by moving your mat to a clear and stable wall. From a kneeling position facing the wall, place the forearms on your mat, parallel to one another and about shoulders' width apart, with the fingertips a few inches away from the wall (Figure 8.40). Straighten the legs and hold this position (Figure 8.41). This will be similar to Face Down Dog Posture, except that the forearms will be on the ground. This position helps to open up tight shoulders (Figure 8.42), especially if you are able to employ the help of a training partner.

Inhale, walk the feet toward the elbows, moving the hips up over the head and

Exhale, kick the legs gently up into the air one at a time for balance (Figure 8.43). Don't crash into the wall. Go up and down a few times in control, trying to find the balance point without using the wall. (Use the wall for balance, if necessary.) You should be close enough to the wall so that your legs do not go way over your head, causing your

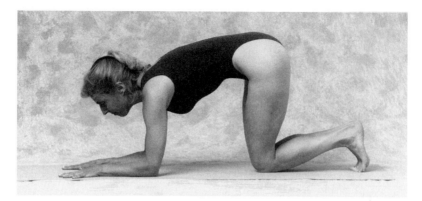

Figure 8.40

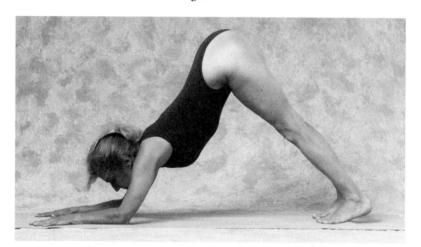

Figure 8.41

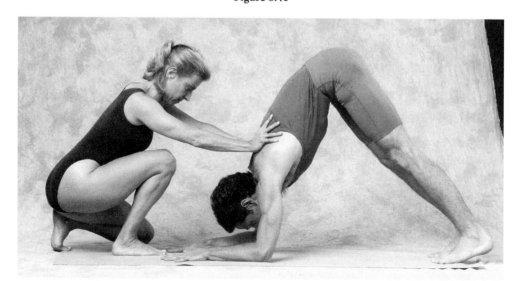

Figure 8.42

back to overarch, and far enough away from the wall so that you can find the balance point without hitting the wall and knocking yourself back down. Once you have correctly positioned yourself in relation to the wall, try taking the feet off the wall and finding balance (Figure 8.44). Gaze up as much as possible and straight ahead.

Note: Tight shoulders can be a real hindrance in this posture. Although you may have the strength to hold yourself in the posture, if the upper arms and shoulders cannot "open" enough to make a 180-degree angle, getting up into the pose and balancing will be difficult, and you will tend to "cave" or collapse in the shoulders, with the head unable to stay up off the floor. Balance is easiest when you are "stacked" correctly. "Perfect" form (which I am still working on) in this posture is a fairly straight torso with the feet, knees, hips, shoulders, and elbows all in line. Notice in the photo of me how my lower back has to compensate for my tight shoulders by slightly overarching. My work, and probably yours, too, is to lift up out of the shoulders and hold the *bandhas,* especially the abdominal lock, very strongly. The work illustrated in Figure 8.42 is extremely helpful for stretching out the shoulder joint.

THIS IS PEACOCK FEATHER POSTURE—HOLD FOR FIVE BREATHS (FIGURE 8.44).

Figure 8.43

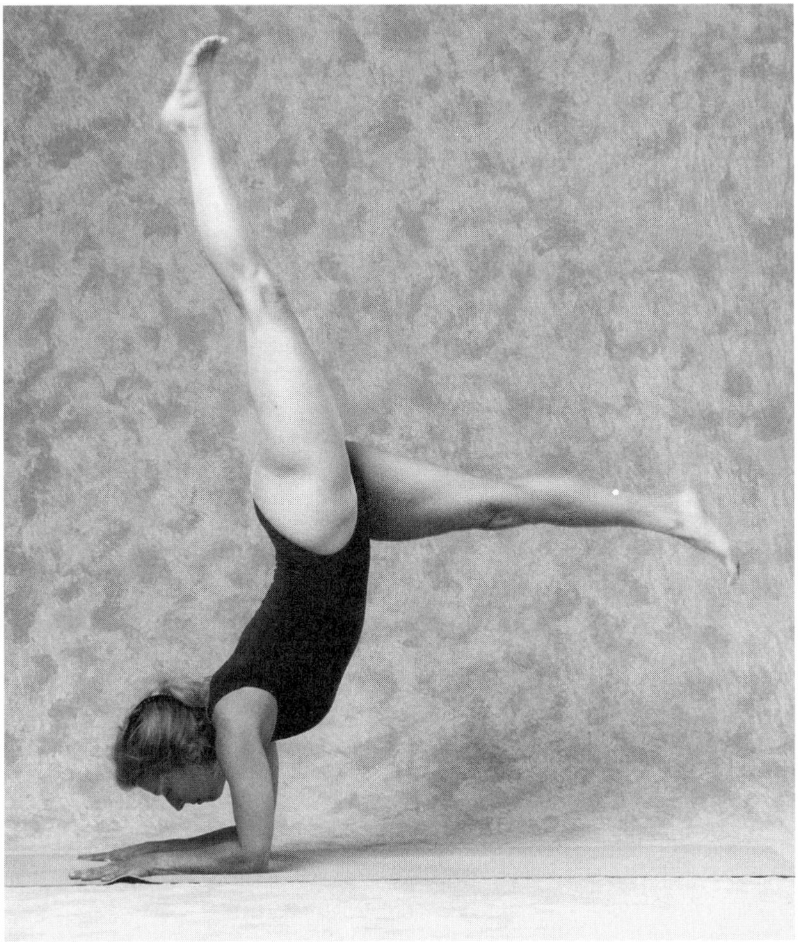

Figure 8.44

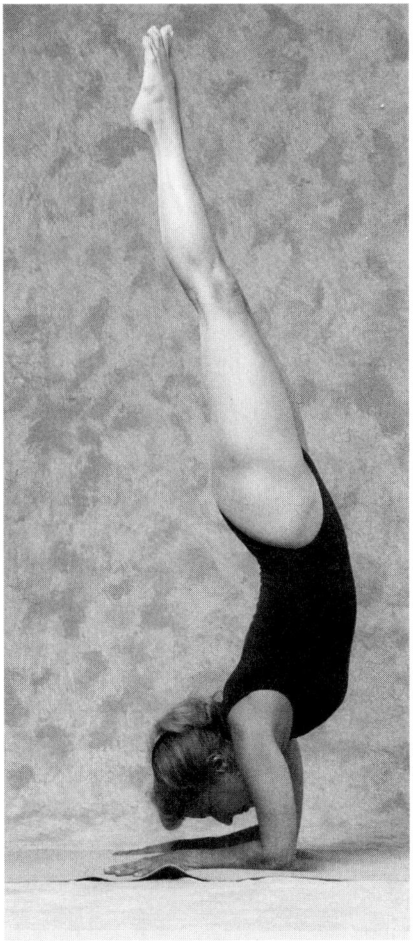

Inhale.

Exhale, release, bring legs to the ground one at a time, switch hands into *Chaturanga Dandasana,* or the push-up position.

Inhale, Face Up Dog.

Exhale, Face Down Dog.

Inhale, jump to standing, look up (as in Position 7 of Sun Salutation A).

Exhale, fold, nose to knees (as in Position 8 of Sun Salutation A). *Inhale,* return to *sama-sthiti,* attention position.

12

UPWARD-FACING TREE POSTURE (HANDSTAND): *URDHVA MUKA VRKSASANA*—OPTIONAL

Urdhva, as we know, means "upward." *Muka* means "face," as we also know by now. *Vrksa* means "tree." In yoga, the Upward-Facing Tree Posture is a handstand.

Important note: Perfectly practiced by superyogis, one comes into this posture from Upward-Facing Bow, the following posture, by simply kicking the legs up over the head from the backward-bending position, as a gymnast might do. Since this will be a little out of the realm for most of us, the posture is generally learned separately, and the best way to begin to practice is against a wall.

Find a wall that is free of pictures, nails, hooks, clocks, etc. Either place your nonskid mat up against the wall, or work on a wood or carpeted floor.

Here are three different methods for learning handstand:

METHOD 1 *(the easiest)*

Inhale, stand away from the wall, with the arms up in the air.

Exhale (with a little momentum), move the arms down to the floor, placing them shoulders' width apart, with the fingertips a few inches from the wall. Kick one leg up into the air, leaving the other leg down as ballast (as you did in Peacock Feather Posture) (Figure 8.45), and then come down again. Imagine, once your hands come to the floor, that you are pushing the floor away with your arms. This will help to engage the trapezius (top of the shoulder) muscles and keep your arms *straight.*

Practice this up-and-down movement, each time going a little higher with the lead leg and slowly taking the other leg up to meet it. Come down one leg at a time. Most important, this must be done in control! Do not hurl yourself up into the air, crashing against the wall. As you practice up and down, develop a graceful ascent and descent. Don't collide with the wall or crash back down to the floor. Feel the weight of your body on the hands, a little at a time. Finally, go all the way up, using the wall for balance. Hold as long as possible. Look at the floor between the hands. Come down one leg at a time. Don't crash.

Most of you will need to spend quite a bit of time simply getting comfortable with the idea of supporting yourself upside down on your hands and overcoming your fear. What is most helpful for this is the practice of Crane Posture, *Bakasana,* described earlier in this chapter.

METHOD 2 *(a little more difficult)*

In this version, you are starting with the hands on the floor instead of using the momentum that comes from a standing position. This requires a little more abdominal strength and a little more work and concentration.

Inhale, place your hands down on the floor, shoulders' width apart and a few inches from the wall.

Exhale, kick up into Handstand one leg at a time, in control (Figure 8.45). Balance against the wall.

Hold for as long as possible. Gaze at point of floor for balance (Figure 8.46). Come down one leg at a time, gracefully. Don't crash.

METHOD 3 *(the most difficult)*

Inhale, place your hands down on the floor, shoulders' width apart.

Exhale, bend the knees and jump up (Figure 8.47), taking the hips up over the head in a tuck position (Figure 8.48), and then pressing up into Handstand (Figure 8.49), using the wall for balance, if necessary. Hold for increasingly longer number of breaths. Gaze at point on floor between hands for balance. Come down with both legs together, bending knees to land lightly.

Figure 8.45

Figure 8.46

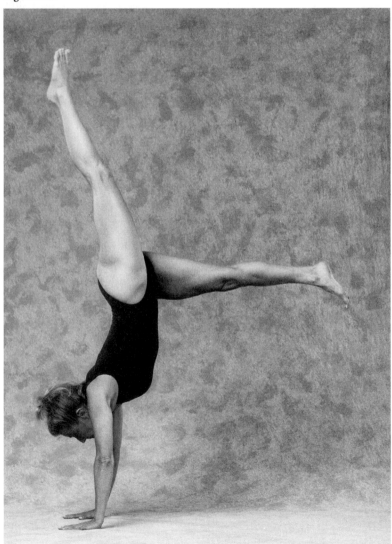

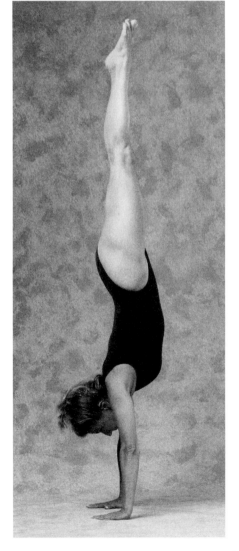

Work the Handstand (trapezius) muscles and attempt to push the floor away, using your strength to lift up out of the shoulders (Figure 8.50). Hold the *bandhas* strongly to keep the lower back lengthened.

THIS IS HANDSTAND POSTURE—HOLD AS LONG AS POSSIBLE (FIGURE 8.46 OR 8.49).

Return to mat, lie down.

Figure 8.47

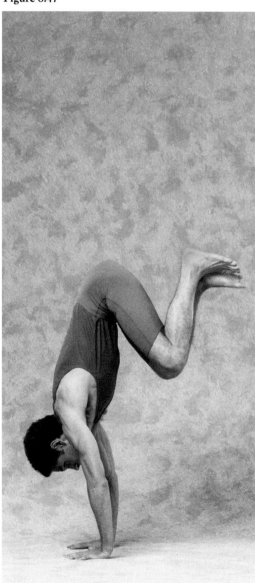

Figure 8.48

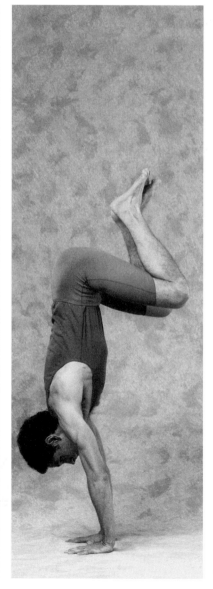

Figure 8.49

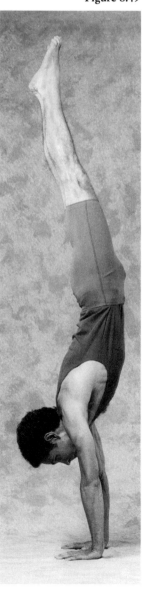

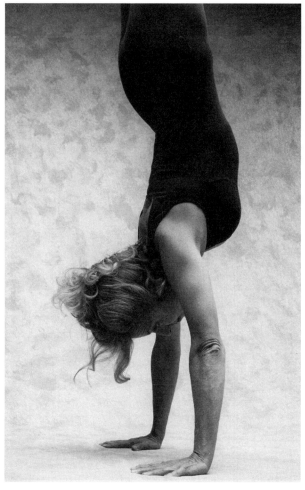

Figure 8.50

13

UPWARD-FACING BOW POSTURE: *URDHVA DHANURASANA*

Urdhva means "upward," as we have just seen in *Urdhva Muka Vrksasana,* Upward-Facing Tree Posture, or Handstand. *Dhanu* means "bow," as in the Bow Posture, *Dhanurasana,* in the last chapter. Many of you already began work on this posture at the end of Primary Series, where the complete instructions are given with various modifications. If you need to review these instructions or refer back to the detailed explanation of the posture, see chapter 6, Posture 20.

TECHNIQUE

Inhale. From lying down position, bring the feet up to the buttocks, and place palms of the hands alongside the ears.

Exhale, push with the arms and legs and press up into the pose. Feet are parallel! Then try to straighten arms and legs. Be sure to let your head relax, or hang back. Don't try to hold the head up. Gaze back down toward the floor (Figure 8.51).

Figure 8.51

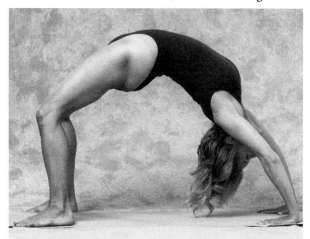

THIS IS UPWARD-FACING BOW POSTURE—TAKE FIVE BREATHS. (FIGURE 8.51).

Inhale.
Exhale, release, relax, and recover for a breath or two if necessary.

Repeat Upward-Facing Bow Posture two more times, for three repetitions altogether. Take five breaths for each repetition and try to lift higher each time.

Inhale.
Exhale, release, come down.
Sit up, extend legs straight out, and go directly into the next posture.

14

INTENSE WEST STRETCH (FULL FORWARD BENDING POSTURE): *PASCHIMOTTANASANA*

TECHNIQUE

Inhale, take the toes or sides of feet, or link hands around feet, straighten arms, look up.
Exhale, fold into Full Forward Bending Intense West Stretch Posture (Figure 8.52). Hold for ten breaths.

Note: Always follow Upward-Facing Bow Posture and Handstand, as well as the full selection of Second Series postures in this chapter, with Intense West

Stretch Posture, which you should remember is the first posture in chapter 5 (explained in full detail in chapter 5 and at the end of chapter 6). Intense West Stretch is a counterpose for all the intense "east" (front of the body) stretching we have just done. So forward bending balances the backward bending of Upward-Facing Bow, and in addition to simply feeling terrific after the backward bend, the posture returns the spine to neutral.

THIS IS THE END OF INTRODUCTION TO SECOND SERIES

The Second Series postures, like those in the Primary Series, are followed by the *Complete Closing Sequence.* Once you have become serious and progressed past the point of beginning-level practice, you should be doing the *Complete Closing Sequence* to end every practice. The *Modified* and *Amended Closings* are for beginners and persons with limited time and limited interest.

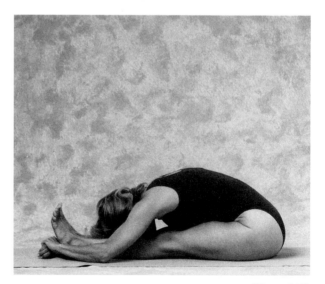

Figure 8.52

yoga therapy

*You have control over actions alone,
never over its fruits. Live not for
the fruits of action, nor attach
yourself to inaction. Established
in Yoga, O Arjuna, perform actions
having abandoned attachment and having
become balanced in success and failure,
for balance of mind is called Yoga.*

KRISHNA speaking to ARJUNA in *Bhagavad-Gita* (Chapter 2)

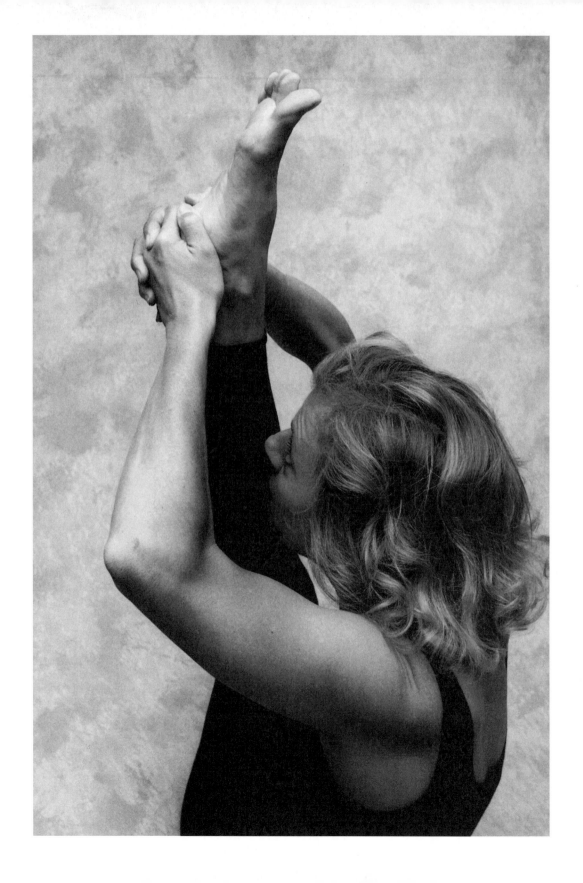

THE ORAL TRADITION

Astanga yoga, and consequently, the Power Yoga system, is based on an oral tradition. This means that knowledge of the form and the practice is directly passed along from teacher to student. The student then becomes a teacher and teaches her or his students, thus continuing the tradition. It is in this way that *astanga* has survived for 5,000 (and who knows how many more) years.

Apparently, the author of the *Yoga Korunta* foresaw that there might be a time when the link could be broken, when there would be no teacher to continue the lineage. In writing down the entire practice, he preserved the form for the future. Had it not been for the *Yoga Korunta,* the form of this original system of *hatha yoga* may well have been lost.

This book then represents, as far as I know, the first time since the writing of the *Yoga Korunta,* that the instructions for the Primary, and much of the Second, series of the practice have been formally written down in English in book form. At first, I felt a little uncomfortable trying to put on paper something that traditionally had only been taught orally. But then I remembered that the original manuscript of the *Yoga Korunta* was found only fifty years ago. What happened between the time it was written and the time it was uncovered? Was the *astanga* form lost? Was anyone doing it? If it weren't for that book, would I (or you) be doing *astanga yoga* or Power Yoga today? I don't know. So far, I haven't found anyone else who knows this form that didn't get it via Krishnamacharya, the man who saw and studied the original manuscript. And if it weren't for that book, many people who will discover, read, practice, and benefit from this system might otherwise go through life stiff, stressed, sick, injured, imbalanced, weak, polluted, asleep, and God knows what else!

However, for the form to be beneficial and to survive, it must come to life. If the *Yoga Korunta* had remained buried in the dark and dusty stacks of the National Library of India, would the form be alive today? No, it would probably be gone with the dinosaurs—extinct. It took one man to find it, study it, and recite it to his student, who then went on to learn it, practice it, bring it to life, and thus reestablish the oral tradition. The manuscript was possible as a result of the established oral tradition. The oral tradition was able to continue as a result of the manuscript. The two styles, the spoken word and the written word, came together to enable a discipline to flourish and evolve. When I realized this, I became much more comfortable with the awesome prospect of putting this form on paper. But putting it on paper is not enough. It must have spirit. It must be learned and practiced, by you and me and our children and their children's children.

FINDING A TEACHER

Astanga yoga is very much a hands-on discipline. A lot of the therapy comes from the guiding physical work of the teacher with the student. I, for example, learned the practice from a teacher who in turn learned from another teacher. We both were students of the oral tradition. But Krishnamacharya, although he had learned yoga and most of the postures originally from his teacher, did learn the *form* of this practice from a book. So whether you learn through written words or spoken words, the practice is still only words and it does not begin to speak to our hearts and souls until we ourselves begin practice!

As you work your way through this book, you may not have the added benefit of the hands-on guidance of a teacher, but you do have a form to follow. You can begin to practice, and you can instill the spirit of *astanga yoga* in yourself. As you go along, the day may come when you seek out a teacher. Qualified and sanctioned teachers of *astanga* are few and far between. It basically takes about ten years of training and practice to teach this well. This form is rapidly gaining in popularity, so more and more yoga studios and health clubs want to cash in on the growing interest. Many yoga centers are beginning to incorporate aspects of *astanga, vinyasa*, and Power Yoga into their classes to expand market appeal. In the coming years, increasing numbers of teachers will be jumping on the bandwagon. A few will be well trained and qualified, but most will not.

You tend to get the teacher you are ready for, so research your quest carefully. Don't be afraid to ask hard questions about qualifications, guiding organizational principles, and perhaps most important, whether the yoga school or organization is comprised of devotees who follow a particular religion, guru, or dogma. Not that there is anything wrong with being a devoted follower of a particular teacher, if that is what you are looking for. But if it isn't what you are looking for, you should know that before you sign up!

In the same way, I wouldn't recommend going to an eclectic yoga school to study *astanga* or the Power Yoga workout, unless you find a teacher there who is into *astanga* and seriously studying and teaching the form. Look for specifics. You should like the way your teacher looks and sounds as well as the way he or she conducts their life. Someone once asked Mahatma Gandhi what his religion was. He answered something to this effect: If you wish to know my religion, you must follow me around. You must watch the way I eat, the way I bathe, the way I walk, the way I speak, the way I treat my wife. My religion is a composite of the way I live my life.

▼

TRAINING FOR LIFE

At various times of the year, I often spend a bit of time at Columbia University doing swim workouts with the men's head coach up there, Jim Bolster, who is also a yoga student. After swimming practice Jim, my husband, Thom, and I would often do yoga practice by the pool. One day, after I had been coming quite regularly to practice for a few weeks, someone asked me what I was training for. "Life," was my response.

I will often say in class, "If your yoga practice isn't helping you to get your life together—physically, mentally, and spiritually—then you aren't practicing yoga." You may be stretching, you may be sweating, you may even be breathing a little, but something is missing. Certainly one important aspect of the practice of the postures is to train the mind and body for dealing with life. There *should* be carryover. You should notice that things you learn about yourself in practice pop up at the most unexpected moments—like on the freeway, on the phone, in bed, on the bus, on your bike, or at dinner. But this presumes that you will continue the custom of watching yourself throughout the day, as you do while practicing the postures. This means that your true "practice" starts the moment you end the Power Yoga workout for the day as I said at the end of chapter 7, or as I tell my students, "the moment you walk out of class." Once you begin to establish the routine of watching yourself, you will start to see that the other *angas,* or limbs, of this eight-limbed practice begin to reveal themselves in the most tangible ways. You may find that you are watching and controlling your breath at other times throughout the day, and thus practicing a natural form of *pranayama,* the fourth *anga.* You may notice that you are seeing your urges—the desire to run after this craving or that craving—as if they were somebody else's. This objective viewing of desires may help you to notice how your concentration gets sidetracked, how your peace of mind is disturbed by things that are not of the present moment. This is the practice of *pratyahara,* the fifth *anga,* or as I explained in the first chapter, a turning in, or refinement, of the senses. Slowly you realize that the mindfulness you practice when doing the form is beginning to seep imperceptibly into the cracks of your life. And that *this* practice is a great deal more than just postures.

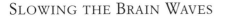

SLOWING THE BRAIN WAVES

The continuing practice of mindfulness develops concentration, or *dharana,* the sixth *anga,* which leads us into the seventh *anga, dhyana,* or meditation. It is important to remember that the techniques we practice to develop our mindfulness skills, such as watching the breath, are not meditation itself. Often people will come to class and tell me, "Oh, I have been meditating for years." After I ask them a bit about their methods, they might say, "Oh yes, I gaze at a candle and repeat a prayer over and over." Well, this is an excellent meditation technique, but it isn't meditation! It acts as the boat that carries the mind to the place where the state of meditation might begin, but repetition of a prayer, just like watching the breath, isn't itself meditation. When I worked as a biofeedback researcher in California in the early seventies, I was able to look in a fairly primitive way, but look nonetheless, at what happens to the brain when

we meditate. When we think or worry or relax or repeat a prayer or meditate, our brain cells are at work. Whatever the activity, many of the brain cells doing the same job will link up with neighboring cells and work at the same pace. This creates a "wave." When we are busy thinking or processing information, these waves tend to be small and fast, which means there are small groups of cells hammering out a variety of tasks. When we begin to practice a meditation technique, which usually involves focusing on one thing, and move toward relaxation, the waves get slower and bigger.

The *frequency* (or speed) of the wave is determined by the number of times per second that the brain cells in that wave "fire," or charge and discharge energy. As the mind becomes less active, the brain cells fire less frequently and the wave slows down.

The size of the wave is called the *amplitude.* In relaxation, more cells are freed up from other activities and tend to jump onto the wave to create greater amplitude, or strength. When we continue through relaxation into meditation, the frequency of the brain waves slows even more, and apparently the brain cells like what they see and jump on, and the wave gets bigger.

Thus, the so-called state of meditation isn't just some arbitrary, spaced-out state of mind. It is actually a measurable place where we can train ourselves to go. In fact, we all actually go to that place, in terms of frequency and amplitude, during sleep. The difference is that when we learn to meditate, we don't fall asleep. We achieve the same level of slowdown and power, but we remain "conscious" of what is happening.

So what is the point of doing all this watching and work to reach a place that at first might seem to be some artificially induced state of mind that is not in touch with what is really happening out there? Well, first of all, meditation is very much in touch with what is happening; more so in fact than any other state of mind you might experience. It is certainly a time when you are in the present moment, not distracted by worries of the future or regrets of the past. It is when you are most in touch with your inner self, so to speak. You have a direct line to your creative center. The "roof brain noise," as Robert deRopp calls it in his book, *The Master Game,* is quieted. You can "hear yourself think." If you read the journals and autobiographies of great minds, great achievers, great writers, great athletes, whatever, you will come across numerous accountings of what these people refer to as "peak experiences," or "altered states," or "contemplative moments," or "religious experiences," etc. All these moments, whether they were great moments in sports or great moments in literature or great personal moments, were times of meditation.

Meditation is soothing. It feels good. The mind rests, the body rests. It is a rejuvenative state. It is therapeutic. There are numerous studies and books on the biochemical state of meditation that show that the chemicals released into the body during meditation create relaxation and well-being. Chemicals that arouse, stimulate, and create feelings of anger, resentment, and bitterness are reduced. Stress is relieved. All stress-reduction programs are based on methods of meditation. Meditation is a time of healing. Positive images and thoughts can be planted and nurtured. For most people, once they get a glimpse of that "place" where meditation occurs, they want to go back. Not because it is an escape. Not because it is a high. Not because it is someplace else. But because it is so vividly "here" and so pleasantly soothing, healing, and balancing.

YOGA WORKS

For one to two weeks each summer since the middle eighties, Thom and I have been on the teaching faculty of a holistic learning center in Rhinebeck, New York, called Omega Institute. Omega offers courses in everything from massage to meditation, stress management to the Zen of baseball and boxing! One day a week they have what are called "sample" classes, where you can check out classes other than the one in which you are enrolled. One year after the samplers a few of our students came back and told other people in our yoga class what they had done.

"Well," said one, "I had my *chakras* balanced in an energy-balancing course."

"Oh, just like yoga!" said another.

"I took a class in mindfulness," said somebody else.

"Just like yoga!" chimed in two people simultaneously this time.

"I had some body work done, to balance my meridians and heal my liver."

"Just like yoga!" This time about four or five people said it together and started to laugh.

"I took a class in freeing up my inner child and learning to let my soul sing," contributed the last person, knowingly. Now everyone was laughing.

"Just like yoga," they all howled.

Astanga yoga was conceived as a pretty complete system. The practice leads us from balancing the body to balancing the mind. It is a path for life. Many of the alternative healing and treatment modalities becoming popular today have their roots in yoga. Power Yoga may not solve every problem in your life, but it's a start. It's certainly a good complement to other forms of exercise, therapy, and medicine.

Learn this and practice it, and encourage others to learn it and practice. The practice doesn't pollute. It doesn't use up natural resources. It doesn't diminish. It doesn't take more than it gives. It encourages awareness and develops consciousness. Through your practice you will set an example of personal ecology and self-reliance to others and be part of a planetary lineage older and wiser than any of us as individuals.

appendix

SPECIFICS FOR INJURIES

This is your life, and nobody is going to teach you, no book, no guru.
You have to learn from yourself, not from books. It is an endless thing, it is a fascinating thing,
and when you learn about yourself from yourself, out of that learning wisdom comes.
Then you can live a most extraordinary, happy, beautiful life. Right?

KRISHNAMURTI to young students in India,
from "Chop Wood, Carry Water," by the editors of *New Age Journal*

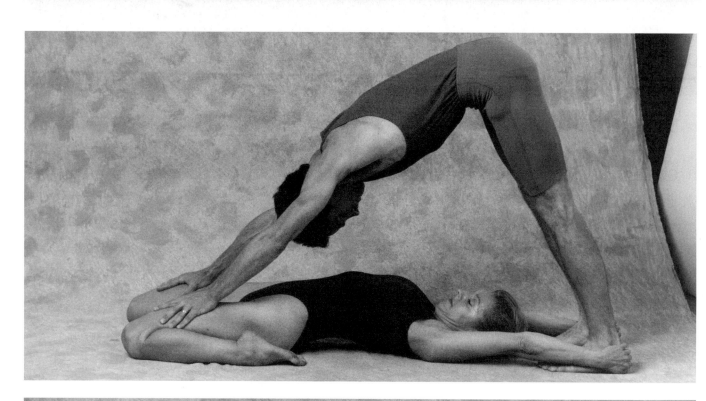

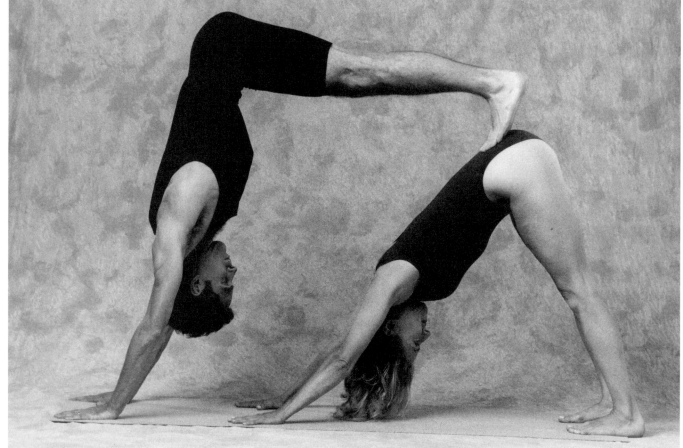

Specifics for Injuries

There are twelve specific injuries listed in this appendix, as well as general references to hip, shoulder, back, and neck "pain." These are:

1. Chondromalacia
2. Iliotibial band syndrome
3. Sciatica and piriformis syndrome
4. Shin splints
5. Hamstring muscle injury
6. Achilles tendinitis
7. Plantar fasciitis
8. Chronically sprained ankles
9. Stress fractures
10. Hip pain and greater trochanteric bursitis
11. Shoulder pain or rotator cuff injury
12. General tendinitis
13. Neck and back pain

Each injury is defined simply, yet accurately, so if you don't know what *chondromalacia* is, for example, you can look it up. There is also information on possible causes of each individual injury and what can be done (in terms of yoga practice or other modalities) to treat the condition.

If you have a specific problem, you might want to look it up and see what is recommended. Keep this as a reference source for yourself or friends. You will find detailed information about the relationship between a particular injury and the practice that is not included in any of the individual chapters. Of course, if you are doing regular practice, you probably won't need this at all. Over the years I have seen each of these injuries among hundreds of sports and fitness enthusiasts. Nearly everyone who has practiced regularly and stayed with the program has pretty much gotten rid of their injury and resumed training.

Out of the Blue

There are basically two types of injury that can happen to you as an athlete. One type is that which happens out of the blue. This can include fractures; contusions; torn muscles, tendons, and ligaments; dislocations; sprains; and bruises. This variety is generally called *acute,* and happens when you fall off a bike or break an arm while skiing. It usually needs immediate attention, in most cases by a physician, particularly if something is broken or bleeding or in need of diagnosis.

There isn't much yoga practice can do to prevent an accident, except possibly to make you more aware. It can make you more pliable and agile so that if you do take a tumble, you can actually lessen the risk of serious injury. It can also help you in coming back from a fall or accident in reestablishing range of motion and structural alignment, strengthening muscles, breaking up scar tissue, opening up tight, traumatized tissue, and generally rehabilitating the injured areas through strength and flexibility work.

CHRONIC IMBALANCE

The other type of injury is caused by structural abnormality or imbalance (from prior injury, specificity of training, poor posture, genetic idiosyncrasy, or lifestyle), and is the type I have referred to throughout this book. This is generally called a chronic injury. It comes on slowly, even though the pain may in some cases appear overnight. If the pain just started as a result, let's say, of a long run on the beach or a rough basketball game, I usually recommend stopping the activity that is causing the problem and doing more yoga. In our classes, whenever beginning students show up with an injury, provided nothing is swollen I generally ask them how many yoga classes they can take that week. If a person asking me about injury is a longtime student, the first thing I ask is how regularly he or she has been practicing.

Remember, there is a difference between "sore" and "swollen." If there is swelling, don't do anything—and that means no running *and* no yoga until the swelling is *gone.* Ice will help reduce inflammation. Once the swelling is gone, in most cases within a few days, you can begin yoga practice, easing into it slowly! Apply ice for fifteen to twenty minutes after your yoga practice.

Once the pain or soreness is gone, you can return slowly to your sport—tennis or soccer or whatever. This doesn't mean an afternoon of playing singles or soccer games, or a ten-mile run. It means gentle resumption of activity. A little volleying or a little running around the field with easy ball kicking, or a *short* jog. If the pain returns, stop. Slowly increase activity over the weeks. In most cases, the more yoga you do, the more quickly you can return to a sport. Always ice after activity, until the injury seems fully healed. If you happen to be at the beach or in the mountains, soaking your legs in the seawater or in those cold mountain streams has an excellent anti-inflammatory and therapeutic effect on the legs.

1

CHONDROMALACIA

Although often incorrectly used as a general term for any knee pain, *chondromalacia* is a tracking abnormality of the kneecap. Typically, when the knee extends and flexes (as in walking or running), the patella (kneecap) glides up and down in a cartilage-covered groove in the femur (upper leg bone). It is held in place by the quadriceps muscles and lateral (outside) and medial (inside) ligaments and tendons. There are certain structural or biomechanical imbalances (or old acute injuries) that can affect the normal tracking of the kneecap.

The most common chronic causes of chondromalacia are biomechanical processes such as tightness or weakness in the quadriceps muscles. Specifically, tightness in the outside thigh (vastus lateralis) muscle, the outside ligament of the knee (lateral retinaculum), and the iliotibial band (a thick strip of fascia, or muscle covering, that goes down the side of the thigh from the hip to the outside of the knee), coupled with weakness of the inside thigh muscle (vastus medialis), can all cause misalignment of the kneecap by moving it slightly to the side (and out of its groove) when the knee flexes. This misalignment causes the kneecap to rub on the underlying surface of cartilage, which softens it and causes pain. Ohhhhh!

What are the symptoms? Generally, there is a soreness around or under the kneecap, especially on the medial, or inside, of the knee. It is usually aggravated by hill running, stair climbing, or gardening (with squatting). The symptoms may go away while running and then come back at the end of the run, or the next day. But they won't just disappear. The knee may feel stiff after running or biking, or even after prolonged sitting, and may feel as though it has a tendency to "give out."

Fortunately, chondromalacia is one of the conditions that is most responsive to the effects of Power Yoga. Notice that nearly everything I mentioned as a fundamental contributing factor involved the word *tightness* or *weakness.* One of the first things a sports physician will tell you to do if you have gone to him or her for diagnosis and treatment is to strengthen the quadriceps, either through straight-leg weight lifting or static contraction of the quadriceps muscle. The reason Power Yoga works so quickly and well as an antidote for chondromalacia is because so much of the emphasis in the standing postures is on static contraction of the quadriceps, or *strengthening.*

However, strengthening alone is not enough, and only half the solution. If you simply do exercises to strengthen the quads, does that bring structural balance? No. It simply makes the quads tighter. The Introduction to the Second Series in chapter 8 begins the process of stretching the quadriceps as well. This brings balance between strength and flexibility and restores appropriate range of motion to the kneecaps, allowing them to return to their proper positioning.

result from overuse, speedwork on a bike or on foot, downhill running or racing, a hard race, or shoes worn on the outside. Even running or skating on the same side of the road will cause ITBS in the curbside knee. In classes and private work, I have also seen basketball players and tennis, racquetball, and squash players all with diagnosed ITBS.

As it comes on, most people tend to ignore it. But if you don't do anything about it, it will get worse. ITBS responds well to the practice of yoga. The standing postures require precise awareness of the balance and alignment in the feet. Consciously shifting and correcting subtle structural imbalances in the feet can begin to correct the problem almost immediately. All the standing postures will help and should feel good on the outside of the thigh. Marichyasana C, Posture 6 in chapter 5, will provide an excellent stretch for the outside of the thigh.

2

ILIOTIBIAL BAND SYNDROME

The iliotibial band is not a muscle. It is a thick strip of fascia, or muscle covering, that runs down the outside of the thigh from the hip to the side of the knee. It is an important knee stabilizer as the knee flexes during movement. It normally rubs back and forth across the outside of the knee, specifically where the femur (thigh bone) connects with the tibia (lower leg bone). Any stress in the zone where the iliotibial band moves over the bone can cause friction and resultant inflammation or irritation.

Generally, people with high arches, rigid feet, bowed legs, legs of different length, or pronating feet are most susceptible to *iliotibial band syndrome,* or ITBS. For skiers, skaters, runners, or cyclists, it can

3

SCIATICA AND PIRIFORMIS SYNDROME

The sciatic nerve starts on each side of the lower back at the lumbar vertebrae and continues down through the buttock and the back of the leg all the way to the foot. Any stress or strain anywhere along this nerve, whether it is caused by jarring from running, pressure from tight muscle tissue, flat feet, high arches, biomechanical imbalance, or misalignment of the spinal vertebrae, will cause *sciatica.* Any structural irregularity or imbalance in the legs can transmit the impact of repetitive sport to the lower back and irritate the sciatic nerve. Sciatica starts as a dull ache in the lower back, buttock, or back of the thigh. It gets worse if training continues.

The sciatic nerve passes out of the pelvis into the thigh under the cover of a deep buttock muscle called the piriformis. The piriformis is one of a group of hip rotator muscles. These muscles can get tight, especially from running, but also from skiing, basketball, golf, or any other sport where there is constant hip rotation. If the piriformis tightens up, it can press on the sciatic nerve and cause *piriformis syndrome.* This can also be a frequent cause of sciatic pain and is not easy to diagnose.

The Power Yoga practice is like a wonder drug for sciatica. Practically everything you need to do to prevent or treat sciatica involves strengthening and stretching. People usually begin to find relief from sciatic pain within a few weeks of starting regular practice. Some of the postures are positively dramatic in their effects. The standing postures are helpful in that they begin the process of opening the hip joints, elongating the spine, and stretching the back of the legs. The Bound Half Lotus Posture, both standing and seated, is also very therapeutic. All the seated forward bending postures are extremely helpful in that they stretch the buttocks and lower back. It is very important that the focus of the forward bend is on extension and elongation of the spine, as covered in chapter 4. *Incorrect forward bending or stretching can aggravate sciatica, especially if the cause of the sciatic pain stems from the spine, as in the rare case of a herniated disk, for example.*

There is also a particular sitting position in yoga that is extremely helpful in relieving constriction contributing to sciatica. It stretches the piriformis muscle and the other lateral hip rotator muscles, so if the cause of your sciatica is related to tight musculature from exercise, this will help.

From a seated position, fold the left leg under the right thigh so that the left foot is alongside the right hip. Don't sit on the foot. Then cross the right leg over the left and bring the right foot alongside the left hip. One knee will eventually be on top of the other. You may find that you are light-years away from this position. That's good. That means you will benefit. Practice this on both sides every day, as often and as long as possible. Once you can get one knee over the other, the sciatica should be gone!

Since the cause of sciatica can be something as simple as a tight muscle, or something as serious as a herniated disk, if indeed you do have serious pain that you suspect might be sciatica, it's important that you check with an orthopedist or sports medical specialist before beginning this practice.

4

SHIN SPLINTS

The first thing I look for when someone says they have shin splints is tight calves. Basically, the term *shin splints* refers to one of two conditions in the lower leg: anterior shin splints, also called anterior compartment syndrome (pain on the outside), and posterior shin splints (pain on the inside). Both of them, simply put, are generally caused by tight calf muscles. In one case, the calves simply overpower their opposing muscle partners in the front of the leg, and tear them from their connections to bone or membrane between bones. In the other case, the calves become so tight themselves that any stress or structural irregularity will cause them to pull or tear at their attachments.

In anterior shin splints, the pain is generally in the muscle tissue along the front outer (lateral) side of the lower leg and is usually due to small muscle tears in the area. The two main muscles (tibialis anterior and extensor digitorum longus) going down the front of the leg are not as strong (or as tight) as the muscles in the back of the legs (calves). Without Power Yoga to stretch the calves and strengthen the opposing muscles, this shortening and resultant tightness in the calves will eventually cause tiny tears or strains in the muscles at the front of the leg, and sometimes along the top outside edge of the tibia, or shinbone. (If the pain is in the tissue or muscle, it's probably shin splints. If the pain is in the bone, you had better investigate the possibility of a stress fracture.)

Pain in the soft tissue behind the bone on the inside (or medial) portion of the lower leg is referred to as posterior shin splints. The deepest muscle in the calf is called the tibialis posterior. It is actually right behind the tibia and fibula (lower leg) bones. It starts at the top end and in back of the shinbone, runs down the leg, turns into a tendon just above the ankle, where it winds around the ankle and inserts on the bottom of the foot. It has connections underneath the inside edge of the shinbone all the way down the leg. As it gets tight from running, skiing, or whatever, like the other calf muscles it is stressed at its attachment to the bone, and small tears or inflammation can occur.

What to do? Do your practice. Ice the pain area after practice and, if possible, one or two other times throughout the day. Stop running or playing your sport until the pain goes away. Do plantar flexion (Face Up Dog) and dorsiflexion (Face Down Dog) stretches every day. This will stretch *and* strengthen muscles on both sides of the bone. Depending on how bad your case is, the pain and inflammation could subside in a couple of days, at which time you could ease back into activity. Big Toe, Hand under Foot, Triangle, Inverted Triangle, and Intense Side Stretch Postures in the standing group all stretch the calf muscles. Face Down Dog Posture is probably the best single overall posture you can use, since it stretches the back of the lower legs and strengthens the front. All the seated forward-bending postures, like Intense West Stretch, will stretch the calves and contract the front of the thighs and shins.

Often, when people are new to classes and haven't yet learned the postures well enough to benefit dramatically from the practice, I will tell them about the *squat.* If you can't do the Power Yoga workout, the next best thing would be the squat. I used to do it for hours—at bus stops, in the subway, in the garden, after runs, cooking dinner, and any other time I could fit it in—to stretch out my calves and Achilles tendons (shortened from years of wearing high heels in the late sixties).

Two important things to note for the squat to work: (1) Your feet must be parallel and not turned out at the toes (once the toes turn out, you lose the effect), and (2) if you pronate, you *must* lift the arches up and shift the weight to the outside of your feet. Incorrect squatting, with feet pronating, will *not* help the problem. The ankles have to be lifted up, which strengthens the anterior tibialis muscle (front of the shin) and relieves the pressure on the posterior tibialis (back of the shin and part of the calf). *If squatting bothers your knees, don't do it.*

One more word: If you do *regular* practice, this is one injury you should never, ever be bothered with.

5

HAMSTRING MUSCLE INJURY

This is a nasty injury. I hate to tell you this, but most of you probably already know it. It can sideline you for a while and it takes a long time to heal. Sometimes in the case of a very small tear, this may be only a few months. But other times it takes two to three years! Why so long? I don't really know. Maybe because there is no way to really rest the hamstrings. We need to use them for walking. Injuries to the hamstring can range from microtears in the muscle fibers to severe tears! Which is *no* fun and happened to me as a cheerleader at Syracuse University back in 1963. I was doing a flying split (I shudder at the thought) in the old Archbald Stadium, landed on wet grass, and split a little further than the hamstrings could accommodate. R-r-r-rip. Oooooh, you will definitely feel it—a sudden, burning pain at the back of the thigh. Very painful.

In most recreational endurance athletes, like long-distance runners or cross-country skiers, the injury is usually a tiny tear, perhaps near the origin of the muscle at the buttock bone, or somewhere along the belly of the muscle. If soreness develops slowly, it often means that the hamstring muscles are simply getting tighter and tighter from running and need to be stretched regularly.

If the pain comes on suddenly, it is probably an acute strain and a classic example of a muscle tear, probably caused by speed work or hill training overloaded onto tight muscles. Severe tears are more frequently seen in sprinters or involve sprint conditions, such as on the football, soccer, or baseball field, where the athlete explodes into action, tears off for a short distance, then stops. In the case of a sprinter, both the hamstring and quadriceps muscles get tight from running. When the powerful quads contract and the hamstrings aren't flexible enough to accommodate this contraction, an injury can result.

Nearly all the standing postures and the Primary Series postures stretch the hamstrings. If you are having hamstring strains and injuries, you need regular, hot stretching. From Face Down Dog Posture to Intense West Stretch to Reclining Hand–to–Big Toe Posture, the practice works on the back of the legs. The first few weeks, you might be a bit sore from the stretching (not from microtearing!) Slowly you will loosen up and get used to the stretching process, and actually look forward to it.

When you first tear any muscle fiber, after the requisite few days of rest and ice, you need to begin to stretch the muscle—gently enough to avoid interrupting the healing process, but strongly enough to keep scar tissue from further shortening the muscle. The key is to make the process progressive. Each day you go a little deeper into the stretch, depending on what the muscle is telling you. As the tear heals, the stretching can become more intense. This is an excellent example of when it is pretty safe to say that nothing works quite as well as the Power Yoga workout for hamstring injuries, because of the heat. Without heat, stretching an injured hamstring is positively deadly.

Find a good massage therapist and see him or her regularly. Good old kneading, stroking, and deep tissue work will help to loosen the muscles and increase circulation. It doesn't replace yoga, however! (See Achilles Tendinitis below for more on massage.)

6

ACHILLES TENDINITIS

The Achilles tendon connects the calf muscles to the heel bone. *Achilles tendinitis* is a painful inflammation, with or without swelling, and is caused by microtearing in the tendon. This is such an easy injury to avoid, and so many people, who aren't aware that there is anything they can do to avoid it, get injured! Although most of the people I see with this injury are runners, it can affect all track-and-field athletes, soccer and lacrosse players, tennis players, dancers, and almost anyone who runs around in their sport. Even climbers, from hanging the heel below the toe and supporting body weight with the toe, can develop Achilles tendinitis. There are a number of little environmental encounters that can put strain on the Achilles tendon: Running uphill in rigid shoes or running downhill, where all the weight lands on the heel and the impact goes straight into the tendon, are two common ones. While running on the beach might sound sexy and serene, it can be hell on the Achilles tendon. As the foot lands, it sinks into the sand, putting untold stress on not only the Achilles but the plantar fascia tendon as well (see following section).

Without a doubt, the single most common contributing factor to Achilles tendinitis is tight muscles in the back of the leg, especially the calves, that have become shortened through training. These muscles are continuously pulling on, and creating a burden for, the tendon. There is no slack and no relief. Eventually, even though the Achilles is a big, strong tendon, it begins to tear.

The pain starts out with a slowly increasing "awareness" of the tendon, which leads to soreness and pain. It may go away as you run or play and the tendon warms up, but as you cool down, the pain will come back. Every time you reach out with the lead foot to take a step, the foot dorsiflexes (the toes come up). The Achilles tendon should be relaxed in this position, with enough slack granted it by the calf muscles, so that it can stretch to its fullest and allow full flexion on the other side of the foot. However, if the calf is tight, the Achilles has to extend against resistance. Strength and flexibility in opposing and partnering muscles have to be equal, or you're in trouble.

Nearly all the Primary Series postures work on stretching the back of the body. Do as much yoga as you can, as frequently as you can. If there is swelling present, or little bumps on the tendon, you most likely have a fairly severe and chronic case of Achilles tendinitis. Stop running or stop your sport. Ice until the swelling is gone (fifteen to twenty minutes two to three times per day). Then begin ankle rotations and easy Sun Salutations. This will begin the process of dorsiflexion and plantar flexion. Build up the yoga practice. Once the pain is gone and it doesn't hurt to the touch, start easy training—very easy. Rush to your nearest massage therapist and ask for deep tissue and transverse friction massage, as well as kneading and efflurage (stroking). Your therapist should always start with easy stroking to lessen the defensive tension against deeper work. Though you need the deeper work, it shouldn't be so deep that it causes bruising. However, it may not always be totally comfortable. Work on the back of the legs will relieve the tension immediately on the Achilles. As Ida Rolf, a master body worker and originator of the Rolfing technique, used to say, "Work where the pain isn't." If your tendon is still very inflamed, your therapist probably can't and won't work directly on the injured or torn tissue, but around it. After the pain stops, she or he will then begin the transverse friction massage to break up forming scar tissue and to encourage circulation. Massage helps. It isn't a substitute for yoga, but an excellent adjunctive therapy.

Oh, by the way, check your training shoes. If they lack good heel support or look like bedroom slippers, throw them out and buy new ones! Heel lifts inserted into your training shoes can help in the beginning, as they elevate the heel and reduce the distance the tendon has to go during extension. This will facilitate healing. However, eventually you should use the lifts less and less, relying more on the yoga to stretch out the tendon and muscles.

7

PLANTAR FASCIITIS

The plantar fascia tendon runs along the bottom of the foot from the base of each toe to the heelbone. If you have tendinitis in this tendon (sometimes called "heel spur syndrome"), you'll feel pain under the arch or in the heel area that spreads out to the central part of the tendon. The tendinitis or inflammation is caused by microtears in the tendon at its insertion into the calcaneus, or heelbone, or along the thick ropy part of the tendon under the arch. A heel "spur" can develop at the insertion of the tendon into the heelbone. This is usually sore as hell and is not helped by jumping and landing on the heels, as in hurdling, basketball, volleyball, and the like, or in any kind of running.

This injury is similar to Achilles tendinitis in that it is an overuse syndrome and can be caused or aggravated by all the same conditions, such as flat feet, high arched feet, or overpronation, which pulls on the plantar fascia tendon in the same way it pulls on the Achilles tendon.

The plantar fascia tendon is less directly affected by tightness in the back of the leg, because it is protected by the heelbone that is between the tendon itself and the shortening muscles at the back of the legs. However, hamstring and calf tightness can begin to limit the range of motion at the ankle, causing imbalance between pointing (plantar flexion) and flexing (dorsiflexion) of the foot. This can cause stress, tears, and inflammation in the plantar fascia tendon.

The injury usually comes on slowly, as Achilles

tendinitis does, and consequently takes time to heal. Heel pads, which cushion the heel and fat pad where the tendon inserts, can help. But nothing replaces rest and discontinuance of activity. Remember, rest, ice, and yoga will get you back into training faster than anything else, and perhaps as quickly as a few days. Transverse friction massage on the tendon—not necessarily on the "sore" spot, but around it—can reduce tension on the tendon and increase circulation, thus speeding recovery. Massage work on the ankle and legs can reduce tightness, increase range of motion, and indirectly relieve stress in the injured area.

Don't forget that you need good arch support for your feet. Shoes that look as if they were run over by a truck should be pitched out. Switch to another activity like water running or swimming until you can return to soccer or running or skating.

8

CHRONICALLY SPRAINED ANKLES

Usually, people who chronically sprain their ankles do so because their ankles are weak or tight (perhaps from prior injury), or because they have biomechanical imbalances in the feet such as have been described above—flat feet, high arched rigid feet, or hyperpronating feet. You can't always avoid a twist or a hole when running down a soccer or lacrosse field, or running cross-country, but you *can* develop strength and flexibility to increase your chances of withstanding duress.

The advice here is the same as for most of the other injuries: Stop training until there is no swelling or pain. Start icing immediately. Start simple ankle rotations after the swelling is gone. Do these for a few days, then start the Sun Salutations. Build the yoga practice gradually. Don't immobilize the foot for

longer than it takes for the swelling to go away. Healing through movement is the ideal way to rehabilitate a sprain or strain.

The Sun Salutations begin to stretch and strengthen the feet and ankles. The standing postures continue the strengthening of the ankles by developing awareness of structural imbalance in the feet and emphasizing correct "posture" of the feet. The seated postures then take the feet through an entire range of motion. Thus, doing the practice will strengthen the ankles and reduce rigidity.

9

STRESS FRACTURES

A stress fracture is the most common high-impact injury to occur in bone. It generally results from some type of jumping or pounding, whether in running, skateboarding, windsurfing, or whatever, and is actually a tiny crack in a bone. It can occur from doing too much too fast. Obviously, a runner is at higher risk of stress fracture than a Rollerblader. However, it is not an uncommon injury in football, basketball, and to a lesser extent, baseball. A stress fracture can happen in the sacroiliac joint (lower back), the lower leg bones, the metatarsal (foot) bones, a lumbar vertebra, or the pubic symphysis, the point where the two hipbones come together. The most common spots are the feet and lower leg bones.

Stress fractures are hard to diagnose, as they don't really show up on X rays for three to four weeks after the symptoms have started. Treatment is complete rest from running or jarring of any kind. To maintain aerobic fitness, swimming, biking, or aqua jogging (running in water) can help until the fracture is healed.

Yoga doesn't do much to relieve symptoms right away. However, with regular practice, the body structure can be slowly changed for the better—thus, changing the way in which landing or foot plant occurs when running or jumping on a skateboard, for example. This will alter the point of impact and give the fracture site a chance to repair itself, plus prevent future injury at the same site.

10

Hip Pain and
Greater Trochanteric Bursitis

When an athlete says he or she has "hip pain," it is important to realize that this can refer to a wide variety of injuries. Is the pain really in the hip, or in the buttocks or lower back? If the pain is in the side of the hip, it could be a muscle strain in one of the abductor muscles (which open the legs away from each other), especially the gluteus medius. If this is the case, the standing postures and seated twisting postures should alleviate the problem. An excellent stretch for the abductors in the thighs is Pressure on Shoulders Posture from chapter 6. This strengthens the adductors and stretches the abductors.

Lateral hip pain could also be caused by bursitis of the hip, technically called *trochanteric bursitis,* or inflammation of the bursa (or sac) over the greater trochanter (the knobby top end of the thigh bone). This is not so uncommon as you might think.

I developed an acute case of trochanteric bursitis in 1971, when I was playing tennis every day for a few weeks on concrete courts in Los Angeles. I wasn't doing regular yoga practice at the time, and the pain was so bad that at the peak of the inflammation, I woke up one morning, tried to stand up, and fell down. After extensive X rays of my spine and hips found nothing out of order, I was diagnosed with bursitis. I stopped playing tennis and went to Colorado for a month, and the symptoms went away.

It flared up once ten years later, after a summer of quite a lot of mountain and hill running in Colorado. I had just run a PR (personal record) for a half-marathon in Ottawa, and had returned to New York City. I was running the Central Park loop, and about halfway around, my hip started to hurt. Every time I ran in the next few weeks, it bothered me. This was before I knew about ice, but I did know about yoga. So I did more yoga, cut back on my mileage, ran in the opposite direction, and eventually the bursitis went away. All the postures that stretched the side of the hip, especially Extended Triangle and Inverted Triangle Postures, felt really terrific for me.

Ice will usually help get rid of inflammation. A number of structural imbalances such as leg length inconsistencies, irregularities in the running gait, or city running, where you have to go up and down off sidewalk curbs, can aggravate the bursa and cause bursitis. Thus, if the cause of the inflammation is biomechanical imbalance, the yoga practice will eventually correct the imbalance, and the cause of the bursitis will disappear.

11

Shoulder Pain
or Rotator Cuff Injury

Pain in the shoulder joint is similar to pain in the hip joint, and can be caused by a wide range of problems. The most common is probably tears and strains to any of the four muscles in the shoulder cuff that rotate the joint. This yoga practice is great for regaining range of motion in the shoulders and rehabilitating an injury. Postures like Face Down Dog, Extended Side Angle, Expanded Leg Stretch C, Parsvatanasana, and the Marichyasana series work miracles on the shoulders.

One of our oldest friends, Clifford Sweatte, is an

awesome yogi and triathlete now living in Oregon. He was one of the first people in the United States to study *astanga yoga,* and started in the early seventies in California and Hawaii. He tells this incredible story about one of his more formidable bike crashes, which dramatically illustrates the power of this practice: "Stitches in the head, hairline fracture of the left scapula, *wasted rotator cuff,* which could only, according to the doctors, be repaired by surgery. Sri K. P. Jois [Pattabhi Jois] showed up from India three weeks later and wanted to know why when I couldn't raise my left arm for Sun Salutations. Well, four weeks later, after two hours of practice per day, I was in Kona [Hawaii] swimming two miles across Kealakekua Bay and doing advanced series practice daily. Yes, big yoga therapy! The doctors couldn't believe it!"

12

GENERAL TENDINITIS

While writing this book on my laptop computer, I began to develop first, tendinitis, and then, the early symptoms of carpal tunnel syndrome. Both wrists were affected, but the right one was especially bad. The wrists would ache and the pain would frequently wake me up at night. When I wasn't writing, I would sit and hold my right wrist with my left hand or carry it around in a makeshift sling. The symptoms were the most severe over the summer of 1992, when I was doing long stretches of writing and editing, and would spend hours scrolling through the copy using only my right forefinger and the Cursor Up and Cursor Down buttons.

I stopped writing and began using my left hand to do all scrolling with the Cursor Up and Cursor Down buttons. I iced the wrists every day and did yoga. The pain went away after about three weeks and I haven't been bothered since, although I haven't reached the same density of hours of writing per day as I did at the peak of usage.

Rest, ice, and yoga. This is the general formula for almost all injury, and tendinitis is no exception. (While a strained ligament isn't correctly called "tendinitis," I have included it in this section with recommendations for tendinitis, because it generally responds to the same treatment patterns.) As you work with this yoga, pay attention to correct alignment, particularly in things like the push-up position of the Sun Salutations. If done incorrectly, this can aggravate a shoulder imbalance or inflammation, for instance. Even though the Sun Salutations may feel as if they are placing a great load on the wrists, this practice will eventually strengthen the wrists and make them more resistant to stress and strain. I had one akido practitioner in yoga classes for years. He would periodically turn up with wrist injuries from akido practice, and would then use the yoga practice for several weeks to rehabilitate the wrist for akido.

Injuries and soreness to the elbow and lower arm can frequently occur to sports participants who throw or hit baseballs, volleyballs, basketballs, or tennis, racket, and squash balls. Or they can happen to cross-country skiers, for example, from the stress of thrusting out with the ski poles. These injuries usually happen for pretty uncomplicated reasons—simply because greater stress is endured by the muscles, tendons, and ligaments than they can actually tolerate.

You can imagine the considerable strain on the extensor (throwing) muscles, the tendon insertions, and the ligaments involved in repeatedly throwing a baseball, for example—particularly if the muscles and connective tissue have become tight with the effects of training, which is almost always the case. So yoga helps.

13

NECK AND BACK PAIN

Many, many people begin yoga practice to try and get rid of back or neck pain. The pain may be anywhere from the back of the neck to the lower back or anywhere in between, and can be caused by anything from injury and stress to genetic degeneration of the spine. One night in class at the start of a new spring semester, I particularly remember looking around the gym at sixty beginners doing Face Down Dog Posture for the first time. That night happened to coincide with writing this chapter on injuries and I was thinking about back problems as I gazed out over a sea of tight, weak, crooked, imbalanced, misaligned, injured, stressed, overtrained, and generally screwed-up backs stretching out for what seemed like miles in front of me. So few people have perfect posture and correct spinal structure, I thought, that it is amazing that everyone isn't doing yoga, just for the therapeutic alignment of the body.

This topic is the subject of thousands of books and articles, and is absolutely too big a subject to cover here. In our classes, I generally recommend that all persons with any back, neck, or spinal injuries or pain have several private sessions and consultations with me before beginning group work. This is to doubly assure them and me that we understand the specifics of their problem and know how to modify specific postures to accommodate their individual needs.

I have talked throughout this book about the hows and whys of the practice. Consult your medical professional. Get all the information you can. Educate yourself. Then do the Power Yoga workout—forever! The documentation is ample. It works!

Axioms of Power Yoga

▼

1. You have to be hot to stretch.

2. Strength, not gravity, develops flexibility.

3. Sports do not get us in shape. In fact, sports get us out of shape.

4. All injury in sports is caused by structural and muscular imbalance.

5. Muscular imbalance and structural irregularities don't fix themselves.

6. Even iron will bend if you heat it up.

7. Stopping training doesn't correct an imbalance.

8. No matter how fit you are at what you do, when you start something new you have to ease into it.

9. Stretching doesn't equal warm-up.

BIBLIOGRAPHY

Arya, Pandit Usharbudh, D. Litt. *Philosophy of Hatha Yoga*. Honesdale, Pa.: Himalayan International Institute of Yoga, Science, and Philosophy of the U.S.A., 1985.

Bailey, Alice. *Initiation: Human and Solar*. New York: Lucis Publishing Co., 1922.

Bevan, Dr. James. *The Simon and Schuster Handbook of Anatomy & Physiology,* New York: Simon & Schuster, Inc., 1978.

Campbell, Joseph. *The Mythic Image*. Princeton, N.J.: Princeton University Press, 1974.

Chitrabhanu, Gurudev Shree. *The Psychology of Enlightenment: Meditations on the Seven Energy Centers*. New York: Dodd, Mead, & Company, 1979.

Chopra, Deepak. *Quantum Healing*. New York: Bantam Books, 1989.

Crowther, Finaly, Raj, and Wheeler. *India: A Travel Survival Kit*. Berkeley, Calif.: Lonely Planet Publications, 1990.

Feuerstein, George. *Encyclopedic Dictionary of Yoga*. New York: Paragon House, 1990.

Gray, Henry, F.R.S. *Gray's Anatomy*. New York: Bounty Books, 1977.

Houston, Vyaas, M.A. (ed.) *What Is Sanskrit? A Collection of Essays, Articles, and Quotes on Sanskrit*. Warwick, N.Y.: American Sanskrit Institute, n.d.

Iyengar, B.K.S. *Light on Yoga*. New York: Schocken Books, 1979.

Kapit, Wynn and Elson, Lawrence M. *The Anatomy Coloring Book*. New York: HarperCollins Publishers, 1977.

Krishna, Gopi. *The Awakening of the Kundalini*. New York: Kundalini Research Foundation, 1975.

Luk, Charles (Lu K'uan Yu). *Taoist Yoga: The Alchemy of Immortality*. York Beach, Me.: Samuel Weiser, 1970.

Maharishi Mahesh Yogi, *The Bhagavad-Gita* (translation and commentary). New York: Viking Penguin and Arkana Books, 1990.

Mishra, Rammurti, S., M.D. *Fundamentals of Yoga: A Handbook of Theory, Practice, and Application*. New York: Harmony Books, 1987.

Monier-Williams, Sir Monier. *Sanskrit-English Dictionary*. New Delhi: Munshiram Nancharlal Publishers Pvt. Ltd., 1988. (Originally published in 1899 by Clarenden Press, Oxford, England.)

Motoyama, Hiroshi. *Theories of the Chakra: Bridge to Higher Consciousness*. Wheaton, Ill.: Theosophical Publishing House / Quest Books, 1981.

Nikhilananda, Swami (chosen and with a biography by). *Vivekananda. The Yogas and Other Works*. New York: Ramakrishna-Vivekananda Center, 1953.

Ornish, Dean. *Program for Reversing Heart Disease*. New York: Random House, 1990.

Prabhavananda, Swami, and Christopher Isherwood. *Shankara's Crest Jewel of Discrimination (Viveka-Chudamani)* (translation). Hollywood, Calif.: Vedanta Press, 1978.

Reader's Digest Family Guide to Natural Medicine. Pleasantville, N.Y.: Reader's Digest, 1993.

Rieker, Hans-Ulrich. *The Yoga of Light: Hatha Yoga Pradipika, India's Classical Handbook* (commentary). London: Unwin Hyman Limited, 1989.

Satchidananda, Sri Swami. *The Yoga Sutras of Patanjali* (translation and commentary). Buckingham, Va.: Integral Yoga Publications, 1990.

Slater, Wallace. *Raja Yoga*. Wheaton, Ill.: Theosophical Publishing House / Quest Books, 1968.

Strauss, Richard, ed., *Sports Medicine*. Philadelphia: W. B. Saunders Company, 1984.

Taimni, I. K. *The Science of Yoga: The Yoga Sutras of Patanjali* (in Sanskrit, with transliteration in Roman, translation in English and commentary). Wheaton, Ill.: Theosophical Publishing House / Quest Books, 1961.

Wood, Ernest. *The Seven Rays*. Wheaton, Ill.: Theosophical Publishing House / Quest Books, 1925.

Zinn, Jon-Kabat. *Full Catastrophe Living*. New York: Dell Publishing, 1990.

index

INDEX